STANDING UP FOR SCIENCE

ABOUT THE AUTHOR

Salim S. Abdool Karim FRS is a South African clinical infectious diseases epidemiologist widely recognised for his scientific contributions to AIDS and Covid-19.

He serves as a Special Adviser on pandemics to the Director-General of the World Health Organization (WHO).

He is the Director of the Centre for the AIDS Programme of Research in South Africa (CAPRISA) and CAPRISA Professor of Global Health at Columbia University. He is an Adjunct Professor of Immunology and Infectious Diseases at Harvard University, Adjunct Professor of Medicine at Cornell University and Pro Vice-Chancellor at the University of KwaZulu-Natal.

He is Vice-President of the International Science Council and serves as a member of the WHO Science Council and the Advisory Board of Physicians for Human Rights. He previously served as President of the South African Medical Research Council and as Chair of the South African Ministerial Advisory Committee on Covid-19. He is a board member of the *New England Journal of Medicine*, *The Lancet Global Health* and *The Lancet HIV*. He is a member of the US National Academy of Medicine and The World Academy of Sciences. He is a Fellow of the Royal Society.

He is a visionary leader, scientist, human rights advocate and institution-builder whose scientific contributions have impacted on the global response to the HIV and Covid-19 pandemics.

STANDING UP FOR SCIENCE

A Voice of Reason

South Africa's Chief Covid-19 Science Adviser at
the Frontlines of the Pandemic

SALIM S. ABDOOL KARIM

MACMILLAN

First published in 2023 by Pan Macmillan South Africa
Private Bag X19, Northlands
Johannesburg
2116
South Africa

www.panmacmillan.co.za

TPB ISBN 978-1-77010-823-3
HB ISBN 978-1-77010-890-5
E-ISBN 978-1-77010-824-0

Editing by Alison Lowry
Proofreading by Sally Hines
Indexing by Judith Shier
Design and typesetting by Triple M Design, Johannesburg
Cover design by publicide
Cover photograph by Rajesh Jantilal

'We're Building the Ship as We Sail It' from
The Best of It © 2010 by Kay Ryan.
Used by permission of Grove/Atlantic, Inc.

*At the time of publication, all the website and article links
provided in the book were live.*

Dedicated to health care workers, scientists and essential workers for their personal sacrifice and unwavering, selfless commitment during the Covid-19 pandemic.

Contents

Foreword

When I was putting together the WHO Science Council in 2021, I asked Professor Salim Abdool Karim – better known to all as Slim – to serve as a member of the Council, recognising his important contributions in several scientific advisory positions in the WHO over the past two decades. The following year, 2022, I asked him to serve as my Special Adviser on pandemics, drawing on his leadership during Covid-19 and his years of experience in dealing with epidemics and pandemics.

Slim's contributions to health research – both in his own country of South Africa and on the African continent – are held in high regard. Slim and his wife Quarraisha have worked steadfastly and with deep commitment over several decades to curb the impact of HIV, advancing HIV research, developing new technologies and approaches for HIV prevention and treatment, advocating for local and global action, and bringing hope for a better future.

Throughout his career, Slim has faced both political and scientific challenges with equanimity. When the Covid-19 pandemic erupted and created upheaval in people's lives, Slim was able to use his well-honed scientific knowledge to distil complex scientific concepts as well as help educate, inspire and reassure.

As I know from personal experience, he is also unafraid of using science to speak truth to power. His strong sense of social justice is tempered by a commitment to remain true to the science. As this book illustrates, Slim does not shy away from highlighting the injustices that often attend those inequalities, including those inequities that emerged so starkly, particularly in the early phases of the global distribution of the Covid-19 vaccine.

At the close of the first meeting of the WHO Science Council in April 2021, I quoted Louis Pasteur, who said: 'Science knows no country, because knowledge belongs to humanity, and is the torch which illuminates the world.' In this way, science can rise above partisan politics and geopolitical interests and remind us that we are all citizens of one planet, linked by our humanity. This is a lesson that Slim knows well from a lifetime of experience. His work is a reminder of the enduring value of science in the service of global health.

Tedros Adhanom Ghebreyesus
Director-General, World Health Organization
May 2023

Acknowledgements

My decision to pen my thoughts was made on the principle I hold dear – 'mutual interdependence' – the belief that each of us should act to benefit the collective, not just ourselves. This principle is the foundation for justice, peace, health and prosperity in the world. I have sought to follow this guiding principle with the help of three fundamental concepts that have guided my life's work and scientific contributions – passion, excellence and perseverance.

Writing this book was a journey that started with a discussion I had with the indomitable Smita Maharaj in 2020. I am deeply indebted to her for omnisciently facilitating this book and prodigiously providing encouragement to get it published.

Besides Smita, four people have been key to making this book possible. I deeply value their contributions and their personal commitment to this book project.

Sharon Dell, who began this project over two-and-a-half years ago with me. She is a gifted writer and captured my innermost thoughts and reflections through our numerous discussions. Her drafts had the uncanny ability to convey the complexities of scientific concepts almost effortlessly, belying the intricacy and enormity of the task.

Alison Lowry, who did a great job, working with the Pan Macmillan team to edit the manuscript, enhancing its flow and coherence.

Aisha Abdool Karim, who worked alongside me with her masterly editing, creating continuity and lucidity in the drafts of each chapter.

Safura Abdool Karim, whose superb writing skills I took advantage of to get text drafted and edited for the final section of the book.

Anyone who has authored a book will know that inspiration is a prerequisite to complete and publish a book. My inspiring life partner and scientific collaborator, Quarraisha, was unstinting in her support and encouragement.

My thanks to Pan Macmillan and, in particular, Andrea Nattrass for her continual encouragement and for publishing my manuscript. She is the firm but generous taskmaster who ensured that I met deadlines for submissions.

Thanks to Nikita Devnarain for her help with the appendices and references. And my appreciation to those in the Presidency, the Ministry of Health, Department of Health and the many other government officials I worked with for giving me the opportunity to make a scientific contribution to South Africa's pandemic response.

It was an honour and a pleasure to serve with each and every member of the South African Ministerial Advisory Committee on Covid-19. Thank you for the opportunity to work with you, to learn from you and to provide advice with you on the Covid-19 response, of which I am proud. We produced 119 advisories in its first year, thanks to the hard work and dedication of the MAC secretariat, Jane Ridden, Janine Jugathpal and Amanda Brewer. Many thanks also to my friends and colleagues across the world for all their help and support.

My gratitude to the media – to the numerous journalists in South Africa and internationally who interviewed me and did such a sterling job of translating complex science for the general public. They created the opportunities to educate people with stories that shaped the public understanding of the epidemic and ushered in a new era on science communication. To each of them, I owe a debt of gratitude for their relentless and tireless efforts. Arguably, the media transformed public accessibility to science when it mattered most.

And, finally, I want to convey my appreciation to the countless people who have come up to me in the streets, restaurants, shopping malls and elsewhere to express their gratitude for my accessible scientific explanations in the media. Their feedback highlights the importance of public engagement with science.

This is an unvarnished account of my personal reflections during the first three years of the pandemic. It has been a labour of love.

Acronyms and abbreviations

ARV	antiretroviral
bnAb	broadly neutralising antibody
BSL-3	Biosafety Level Three
CAPRISA	Centre for the AIDS Programme of Research in South Africa
CCC	Coronavirus Command Council
CDC	Centers for Disease Control and Prevention
CERSA	Centre for Epidemiological Research in South Africa
CFR	case fatality rate
CoP	Correlate of Protection
CPAP	continuous positive airway pressure
CPHIA	Conference on Public Health in Africa
CROI	Conference on Retroviruses and Opportunistic Infections
DG	director-general
DUT	Durban University of Technology
EFF	Economic Freedom Fighters
ER	emergency room
EUA	Emergency Use Authorisation
FDA	Food and Drug Administration
HFNC	high-flow nasal cannula
HHMI	Howard Hughes Medical Institute
HOD	head of department
HPV	human papillomavirus
ICU	intensive care unit
IPC	Infection Prevention and Control
KRISP	KwaZulu-Natal Research Innovation and Sequencing Platform

LSHTM	London School of Hygiene & Tropical Medicine
MAC	Ministerial Advisory Committee
MERS	Middle East Respiratory Syndrome
MPP	Medicines Patent Pool
MRC	Medical Research Council
mRNA	messenger RNA
NAGI	National Advisory Group on Immunisation
NATJOINTS	National Joint Operational and Intelligence Structure
NCCC	National Coronavirus Command Council
NEHAWU	National Education, Health and Allied Workers' Union
NEMLC	National Essential Medicines List Committee
NGS-SA	Network for Genomics Surveillance in South Africa
NHLS	National Health Laboratory Service
NIAID	National Institute of Allergy and Infectious Diseases
NICD	National Institute for Communicable Diseases
NIH	National Institutes of Health
NRF	National Research Foundation
Panda	Pandemic data and analytics
PCR	polymerase chain reaction
PEPFAR	President's Emergency Plan for Aids Relief
PPE	personal protective equipment
PrEP	pre-exposure prophylaxis
R_0	reproduction rate
RBD	receptor-binding domain
RNA	ribonucleic acid
SAHPRA	South African Health Products Regulatory Authority
SARS	South African Revenue Service
SARS	Sudden Acute Respiratory Syndrome
TWG	technical working group
UNAIDS	Joint United Nations Programme on HIV/AIDS
UNISA	University of South Africa
VRC	Vaccine Research Center
WHO	World Health Organization

A new pandemic arrives: The first 100 days

CHAPTER 1

Alert!

It was the middle of a blistering hot summer when I got an alert that would change my life. My family and I had retreated to the soaring mountain vistas of the Drakensberg to find some relief from the oppressive heat on the coast in Durban. Halfway through a mountain hike one day, I heard the soft ping of a notification on my smart watch. I glanced down to see the words: 'ProMED alert! Undiagnosed pneumonia – China'. I gave it a cursory read before quickly rejoining my family along the path. This was the first public announcement of a disease that would later be named Covid-19.

It was 30 December 2019 and the entire Abdool Karim family was taking a long-awaited holiday. On the way to the mountains, we stopped for a few days at the Anglo-Zulu battlefield site at Rorke's Drift for guided tours with historians who fired up our imaginations by bringing the battles to life with their vivid accounts of events. We had then meandered through the Midlands enjoying a sampling of local cheeses before reaching our final stop: the Cleopatra Mountain Farmhouse, a hotel named after the mountain at its entrance that resembles a beautiful face.

It was in this part of the Drakensberg escarpment that I found myself on one of the many hiking trails when I got the ProMED alert. Another case of SARS [Severe Acute Respiratory Syndrome – that was first reported in China in 2002], I thought, not realising that this was in fact a new disease entirely. Instead, I filed away a mental note to follow up on the notice once I had returned to work in the new year and didn't give it a second thought. My determination to complete the hike came in part because of what lay at the end. This was not just to get some exercise in but was my way of building up an appetite for that evening's seven-course dinner. This boutique hotel is famed for its cuisine and each evening is a three-hour treat to a chef's menu bulging with exotic dishes, with ingredients fresh from the surrounds.

The Abdool Karims all share an appreciation for good food – whether it's a seven-course dinner or a simple home-cooked meal. The mission, put simply, is to strive for excellence. That doesn't apply only to my work but to all facets of my life. It is a drive that I share with my wife, Quarraisha, who is an infectious diseases epidemiologist like me. We have been married and have worked side by side for over three decades, including the founding of the Centre for the AIDS Programme of Research in South Africa (CAPRISA) together in 2002.

We have three children. Our eldest daughter, Safura, is a lawyer who has a master's degree in public health law from Georgetown Law School in Washington and a PhD in law from the University of KwaZulu-Natal, after completing a clerkship at the Constitutional Court and enrolling as an advocate at the Johannesburg Bar. Her sister, Aisha, has a master's degree in journalism from Columbia University in New York and has since concentrated on health, writing for, among others, *Daily Maverick*, *Bhekisisa*, *Spotlight*, *AVAC* and the AmaBhungane Centre for Investigative Journalism. Our youngest, Wasim, has a degree in computer science and statistics from the University of Cape Town and an honours degree in computational biology from Stellenbosch University, focusing on developing websites, especially for health information dashboards. Joining us on this road trip was a more recent addition to our family: Safura's husband Ivo, who took up a position as a computer programmer at a global software company after completing his studies in computer science.

It was typical for us to spend holidays together, with a strict no-work rule in place. For most of the year, we try to balance family time with the ever-growing mountains of work. But for those few days in December, the only acceptable use of computers is to watch movies on Netflix. Cell phone use is also restricted, with the limited signal in the mountains helping reduce the chances of a work call coming through. It was for this reason that the alert on my phone – along with any ponderings about a possible new virus – would have to wait until the new year.

A week later, I was back at work. Even as I tried to catch up on the work I had missed during the break, I was aware of increasing media reports around the still-unknown virus causing pneumonia in China. I'm something of a news junkie, so my inbox is always brimming with alerts from the daily publications to which I subscribe – *The New York Times*, *The Economist*, *Nature Briefing*, Associated Press's *AP Morning Wire*, *LegalBrief*, *M&G Mornings*, *News24*, *Daily Maverick*, *TimesLive* and the daily Meltwater search of articles across the globe. Aside from these digital updates, I start every morning by waking to the news bulletin on East Coast Radio and reading a hard copy of *The Mercury* newspaper during breakfast. In the evenings, I tune in to eTV, eNCA or Newzroom Afrika for the evening news. It's a habit I developed as part of my commitment to staying abreast of global events. Still, even as I followed the coverage of this unfolding outbreak in my daily news sources, I was not expecting anything near what unfolded – after all, how often does one expect a pandemic?

It was while at my office at CAPRISA that I learned the ProMED alert came from machine translations of Chinese media reports. These reports were based on leaked notices from the Wuhan Municipal Health Commission to hospitals in that city, alerting them to cases of atypical pneumonia associated with the Huanan Seafood Market.

ProMED is an early-warning programme of the International Society for Infectious Diseases.[1] It reports and monitors emerging infectious diseases around the world. I had subscribed to the programme when I served as an editor of the society's scientific journal several years ago. In a world where new disease outbreaks are increasing as humans encroach ever more into animal habitats, the alerts have helped me to timeously keep up with new infectious disease developments and threats. And this instance was no different. It was probably the first global communication about the virus, and it set off a chain of events.

Staff at the World Health Organization (WHO) headquarters in Geneva picked up the warning and instructed the WHO China Country Office to request verification of the outbreak from China's government. The Wuhan Municipal Health Commission then issued its first public statement on the outbreak, saying it had identified 27 cases. A day later, the Wuhan authorities shut down the market and a team from China's Center for Disease Control and Prevention (CDC) collected environmental samples for analysis. One thing to remember is that with Covid-19, everything moved at speed. There was a staggering amount of information generated rapidly within the first two weeks of that ProMED announcement.

Perhaps the most shocking development came on 11 January 2020. Professor Tulio de Oliveira bounded into my office clutching his mobile phone. De Oliveira, who is a friend and mentee, is a leading bioinformaticist and Director of the KwaZulu-Natal Research Innovation and Sequencing Platform (KRISP) as well as a Research Associate at CAPRISA. KRISP is just one floor below CAPRISA at the Doris Duke Medical Research Institute building at the Nelson R. Mandela Medical School in Durban, making it easy for him to pop into my office on short notice. Always energetic, De Oliveira seemed to be even more ebullient than usual that day. His eyes alight, he announced that the genetic sequence of a novel coronavirus causing the pneumonia outbreaks in Wuhan was on Twitter.

Genetic sequencing is no small task. It involves pulling apart the genetic material of the virus and identifying its unique pattern. Everything has its own coding, so knowing the virus's genetic code helps reveal what we're dealing with. KRISP uses Genome Detective software, an automated system for high-speed virus identification from sequencing data, and it offers advanced genetic sequencing systems to support genomics research in Africa. It would later create the South African Network for Genomics Surveillance that discovered the Beta and Omicron variants.

That year, my son Wasim was using his summer vacation to work part-time doing computer programming at KRISP. When I asked Wasim over dinner one evening about the specifics of the work they were doing, it emerged that Wasim and the De Oliveira team were actually at the forefront of global efforts to develop genomic methods to identify the new virus. Their focus was on adapting the genome detective software to enable it to use data at high speeds to separate the new coronavirus found in Wuhan from other coronaviruses, according to genetic sequences. 'That's how we will know it's new,' he told me. 'We've got to be able to separate it and show whether the gene sequence is sufficiently different from all the other known coronaviruses.'

So, when De Oliveira came in a few days later with his announcement, I was taken aback for two reasons. Firstly, I had to grapple with the fact that we had confirmation that this was indeed a new virus. We now knew it was not SARS, although it was very similar to SARS. It was a close cousin to SARS – but a new virus nonetheless. For a virologist and epidemiologist like me, the discovery of a new virus that can infect and was infecting humans is a highly significant event as it captures the nexus between both disciplines. As a medical virologist, I was fascinated to learn more about this new virus – to know how it spread, what it looked like. But as an epidemiologist, I wanted to take a closer look at what it would mean for prevention, public health and people's lives. Any illnesses caused by the new virus would come with enormous implications in terms of the global and local public health response. That's because no one had ever experienced the new virus before and there was no existing protection against the disease. In the absence of any immunity to the new virus, the entire world's population was literally a 'sitting duck'.

Secondly, I had to understand the news that the sequence – all 30 000 base pairs of it – had been mapped by Chinese scientists *and* was available on Twitter in a post that links to Virological.org. Sequencing can take years to achieve, and coronaviruses are among the longest RNA viruses in the world. In 2003, it took scientists about six months to publish the full sequence of the SARS coronavirus and even the speed of that process was considered groundbreaking. Now we had the genome, the full genetic material of the new virus, in just over a week. And it was on Twitter. Has the world gone mad? I wondered. Given my enduring suspicion of social media in all its forms, Twitter is not a space I gravitate towards or would naturally turn to for information. I had never used Twitter and so did not really understand how this Nobel Prize-winning information could be in such a short message. It dawned on me much later that this was the start of the revolution I would soon witness in the way medical research would now be conveyed and shared.

While it seemed like an overnight discovery, I later learned that scientists in China had sequenced the genome of the virus as early as 5 January 2020, almost a week prior to it being shared publicly. The first known case of what we now know to be Covid-19 may have gone as far back as 16 November 2019 to a patient with atypical pneumonia in Foshan City, China, but the first known patient was picked up by doctors on 8 December. However, it was places like Twitter and open-access forums that allowed the information to circulate as widely and quickly as it did later that month.

While there is also some contestation as to whether the first genetic sequence of this coronavirus was that by Yong-Zhen Zhang of Fudan University in Shanghai on Virological.org, or by the China CDC on the GISAID database, the available evidence suggests that Zhang's sequence was the first sequence that came to the attention of the scientific world. Sydney-based virologist and evolutionary biologist Edward Holmes FRS was the one who first tweeted about the sequence, making it international public property on 10 January 2020. He posted the sequence from Zhang on Virological.org, an open-access discussion forum for the analysis and interpretation of virus molecular evolution and epidemiology, on behalf of a Chinese-Australian consortium led by scientists at Fudan University. The sequence was also deposited on GenBank, the publicly available database of the National Institutes of Health (NIH), which contains nucleotide sequences for hundreds of thousands of organisms. Holmes subsequently tweeted the link to the sequence from his own Twitter account. Around the same time, the consortium posted these findings on the biological pre-print server, bioRxiv (pronounced 'bio-archive'). The findings were later accepted for publication by the journal *Nature* on 3 February 2020.[2]

The fast pace at which things were moving was a strong signal that evidence for the existence of a new virus – one with unknown impact – was substantial, and there was concern about its potential to spread. At this point, though, I was mostly ignoring the new virus – principally because there had not yet been any person-to-person transmission. That changed on 20 January 2020 when Dr Zhong Nanshan, a respiratory expert, told the media that two people in Guangdong province in southern China caught the virus from family members and that some medical workers had also tested positive for the virus. I realised that I could ignore it no longer. I needed to remain continuously aware of developments in this new disease. The next day, 21 January, the United States reported its first case – a Washington State resident who had returned from Wuhan. At that stage, it was reported that six people had died and 291 had been infected in China. Country after country followed with reports of their first cases.

It was becoming clear that the virus now posed a worldwide threat. One month after the first public reports of the disease, on 30 January, the WHO declared Covid-19 a public health emergency of international concern. The WHO had come under pressure to make this decision as cases were rising rapidly. This designation activates the International Health Regulations, whereby all member states are obligated to report epidemiological information on Covid-19 to the WHO. This enables global surveillance so that reliable data on the scale and nature of the pandemic can be continuously monitored – without this, we would be trying to fight the pandemic without knowing the full extent of where the virus is spreading.

Using the genetic code now available, De Oliveira and his team, including Wasim, had successfully developed an algorithm to identify whether the genetic sequence of the virus belonged to any of the existing known coronaviruses or the new coronavirus (which was now being referred to as 'novel coronavirus'). They deposited their findings on bioRxiv on 31 January with the details of their coronavirus typing tool, which could identify the novel coronavirus's nucleotide sequence within minutes.

All of these developments meant that by 11 February the genetic make-up of the virus was sufficiently established to enable the International Committee on Taxonomy of Viruses to give it a name: Severe Acute Respiratory Syndrome Coronavirus 2 or SARS-CoV-2. The name reflected its close genetic link to SARS, but also highlighted its difference from SARS. On the same day, the WHO announced the name of the new disease caused by SARS-CoV-2, Coronavirus disease 2019, abbreviated to Covid-19.

On 17 February, De Oliveira's manuscript was accepted for publication in the prestigious *Bioinformatics* journal with the title 'Genome Detective Coronavirus Typing Tool for rapid identification and characterization of novel coronavirus genomes'.[3] Not only is it a typing tool to accurately classify all the SARS-related coronaviruses, but it also facilitates the accurate tracking of new viral mutations – these were expected as the outbreak continued to spread globally. This is essential for the development of new diagnostics, drugs and, of course, vaccines.

In a sense, De Oliveira and his team were ready for the arrival of the novel coronavirus. They had developed substantial gene sequencing capabilities over the past years in order to monitor genetic changes in HIV that would confer resistance to antiretroviral (ARV) treatment. They had the bioinformatics capabilities and had used these successfully in outbreaks of the Zika virus in 2015–16, and Yellow Fever in 2016. By the time SARS-CoV-2 made its appearance, they had experienced the benefits of sharing information outside of formal structures and procedures and were able to work at breakneck speed. Wasim, who had the right skills and was in the right place at the right time, was fortunate enough to contribute, as an undergraduate student, to a groundbreaking scientific effort that was published in a highly cited paper.

I, on the other hand, was a lot slower out of the starting blocks. I am often referred to as a 'leading scientist', but, in respect of Covid-19, I was effectively upstaged in February 2020 regarding publishing scientific articles on the pandemic, not only by Wasim, but by all three of my children. Before now, we had all worked in very different spaces and had little overlap in our work – with Quarraisha being the one exception.

But that was starting to change. Each of them working in their respective fields had been quick to understand the significance of Covid-19 and its potential to disrupt the world.

Safura, who was a senior researcher at the Wits Centre for Health Economics and Decision Science, very quickly embarked on her own research in the area of Covid-19, going on to publish an article in the *South African Medical Journal* about the implications of criminalising Covid-19 transmission. This was followed by subsequent Covid-19-related papers in the *Journal of Law, Medicine and Ethics*. Later, she published an important article on the looming challenges that would contribute to vaccine inequity in the prestigious medical journal *The Lancet*. Not only was this unusual because it was a lawyer publishing in a medical journal, but it was also a publication related to intellectual property and vaccine inequity long before Covid-19 vaccines were available or shown to be effective. She was well ahead of the game.

By February, after Wasim featured as a co-author on the coronavirus Genome Detective paper, articles on Covid-19 written by Aisha started to appear regularly. If you go back to some of her earliest pieces, you will be struck by how well she was able to articulate what needed to be done in the midst of uncertainty. Her television appearance educating people on 'washing hands' still rings in my ear. Aisha's many media appearances helped to me to see how rapidly the scientific world was expanding that knowledge base and how the media played a big role in tapping into that expanding resource to disseminate critically important information to the public.

For my part, I watched in awe as all three of my children were making important scientific contributions. I cheered them on. I had resolved to keep a watching brief, but not do anything too dramatic just yet – a resolve that would prove difficult to maintain much longer, as the pandemic loomed.

CHAPTER 2

The reality of the pandemic dawns

*As epidemiologists, our responsibility is to think ahead and
stay several steps in front of a problem.*

In early February 2020, things started to escalate, and staying on the
sidelines was becoming a harder option. Both eNCA and Newzroom
Afrika, national television news channels in South Africa, approached me
to comment on the potential impact of the coronavirus in South Africa.
There was concern about how the virus, once it arrived, might affect
the millions of people in South Africa whose immune responses were
compromised through HIV and TB infection. Those interviews were the
first of a steady trickle that I fitted into my normal work routine. Published
scientific research was scarce at the time, and the need for information was
growing at all levels. Being one of the voices sharing that information
began to slowly consume my time – as more of my day went to reading,
assimilating, analysing and publicly sharing available information about
the pandemic.

This marked the start of a push-pull tussle on my time and focus
between Covid-19 and HIV. But, during this early period, my HIV
research was the clear winner. It was a critical time for HIV researchers
and there were a number of important HIV and TB research projects
under way. The discovery of broadly neutralising antibodies (bnAbs) had
opened new pathways to us and formed the basis for exciting clinical trials
at CAPRISA – I could not ignore this key research.

With these important new HIV-prevention prospects on the horizon,
it was hard to devote more of my time to the novel coronavirus. In part,

this reluctance was due to the thinking that I, among others, was still expecting that the virus might be contained before it even reached us. It was difficult to know how much effort to devote to the issue of a nascent global pandemic in early 2020 that was yet to announce its presence within our national borders. But as the days passed, it became clearer that we were dealing with something quite significant – and fate was pushing me towards what was becoming a more pressing need.

The wake-up call came on 24 February 2020 in an article that provided the first data on how deadly this disease was.[1] The paper, published in the *Journal of the American Medical Association*, was co-authored by my friend and colleague Professor Zunyou Wu, chief epidemiologist and head of AIDS at China's CDC. The study revealed that the virus had a case fatality rate (CFR, the number of fatalities divided by the number of infections) of 2.3%. I emailed him to discuss the findings and was reassured by his reply that his analysis was scientifically sound – although I'd expected nothing less. Goodness! I thought. If one in 40 people who get infected die, this is a serious problem. Could we really be looking at a disease that may kill more than a million South Africans?

A month prior to Wu's publication, there were two seminal papers on the novel coronavirus, both shared on the same day in *The Lancet*. But neither had enough patients to raise alarm bells in the way that Wu's data had. The first-ever scientific publication on Covid-19, an account of 41 patients from Jin Yin-tan Hospital in Wuhan, had appeared in *The Lancet* on 24 January 2020.[2] That issue of *The Lancet* included a publication by my colleague Professor George Gao FRS, who is the head of China CDC.[3] I thanked him for it later when I wrote to congratulate him on his election as a Fellow of the Royal Society. His article in *The Lancet* provided very important insights on the novel coronavirus (as it was referred to before being named SARS-CoV-2) and raised the alarm, but, like the other papers that followed, the number of patients described was still small. Both articles in *The Lancet* brought home the foreboding that we were about to see a serious new disease, and Wu's paper left little doubt about how serious it was going to be.

The Wu article held some early clues as to the dangers of Covid-19 and provided a much more granular look at the deadly toll this disease could take, particularly on the elderly. It also showed the ways that Covid-19 differed from other respiratory diseases, including influenza. Just to give you some point of reference, the CFR for seasonal influenza is 0.1%, which translates to one death for every thousand people infected. Wu's data, which chronicled China's early experience with the virus, found that the CFR for 70–80-year-old people was 8% (one in 12 infected people died), going up to 14.8% (one in seven infected people died) in those over 80 years old. Worryingly, Wu also reported that in critical cases, where patients were admitted to the intensive care unit (ICU), nearly half were dying. This study's findings have been borne out over time. The average global Covid-19 CFR during the first six months when the original strain was predominant was also between 2% and 3% worldwide, noting that this does not factor in the large number of asymptomatic infections. This epidemiological study emanating from China in the early days of the pandemic gave me cause for concern. Influenza does not kill like that, I thought. This is a different order of magnitude.

The epidemiological data from China clearly indicated that there was no room for a casual approach. I needed to act. As epidemiologists, our responsibility is to think ahead and stay several steps in front of a problem. Such foresight can mean the difference between life and death, not just of individuals, but entire populations. At CAPRISA, Quarraisha and I sat down that same Monday afternoon in February after reading the Wu article to contemplate what these data would mean if applied to our country. Meeting at short notice is easy for both of us as our offices are next to each other and we share a secretary. It was a sombre discussion. The reality of a potentially devastating impact of the pandemic in South Africa dawned on me. Always one step ahead of me, Quarraisha had already arrived at this conclusion days earlier. We knew that we needed to start preparing right away for what lay ahead. Our actions were predicated on an understanding that the virus, once in South Africa, was likely to spread like wildfire – as it was starting to do in Europe, especially Italy, and in the US.

Now the clock was ticking. We knew it was only a matter of time before we had our first case in South Africa, given the influx of foreign travellers into the country. Wishful thinking that the virus would not reach us was now well and truly behind us. This virus was coming – and we had to be prepared. The priority was to establish surveillance for the virus and contribute early evidence on its transmission in our setting in order to guide prevention strategies. It wasn't just about identifying cases but being ready to test tens of thousands of South Africans a day if we wanted to get a handle on the virus.

From my regular communications with Professor Lynn Morris, a world-class immunologist, who was at the time the head of the National Institute for Communicable Diseases (NICD) and a Research Associate at CAPRISA, I knew that testing was available at the NICD and capacity was being established at the National Health Laboratory Service (NHLS). Quarraisha and I agreed that we should be using the time before the virus arrived to develop testing capacity at the CAPRISA laboratory to support the NICD's efforts. Since the CAPRISA laboratory has substantial capacity to undertake polymerase chain reaction (PCR) testing for HIV and TB, we could make a helpful contribution if we converted one section of our laboratory to conduct testing for SARS-CoV-2.

Ms Natasha Samsunder, head of the CAPRISA laboratory, was charged with this complex task. She arranged for one section of the laboratory to be partitioned off to do only SARS-CoV-2 PCR testing. This section included our Biosafety Level Three (BSL-3) laboratory, which has all the precautions required to work with the infected swabs without placing the laboratory technicians at risk. BSL-3 laboratories are highly specialised sealed facilities with positive pressure airflow through HEPA filters. These high-containment laboratories can only be accessed in full protective gear through airlock chambers. Samsunder is a 'can do' person and no obstacle was too difficult for her; the newly partitioned SARS-CoV-2 laboratory was ready by the end of that week. Working with De Oliveira, we reached out to colleagues at the Beijing Genomics Institute in China and ordered batches of Covid-19 test kits and reagents for use in the CAPRISA laboratory. This was not straightforward as there were no flights out of Beijing. Despite this, we managed to get our kits when the Jack Ma Foundation sent planes loaded with supplies to Africa.

Quarraisha took the lead in developing a formal study protocol for the SARS-CoV-2 testing programme, which would include surveillance. To start with, we planned to regularly test all CAPRISA staff and patients with respiratory illness, and to conduct house-to-house community testing in Vulindlela, the rural community outside Pietermaritzburg where CAPRISA has an HIV research clinic. This proactive approach meant that we were not just going to sit in our offices and wait for the virus to descend on us. Instead, we were going to actively look for the virus in sick patients in the community in order to get a head start in responding to it.

Now we needed some funding to implement this. Sourcing the funding required to cover this testing initiative was not quite as straightforward as I had hoped. I made several unsuccessful attempts to get hold of the CEO of South Africa's National Research Foundation (NRF), which is the research funding agency of the Department of Science and Innovation, as it had already funded CAPRISA to host the DSI-NRF Centre of Excellence in HIV Prevention. Messages were left but never answered, despite assurances that he would call back. I was disappointed by the lack of responsiveness and more so in what it suggested about the lack of foresight and responsive leadership from the country's leading research agency, and I later told them so in a meeting at which senior NRF representatives were present. Given that the role of the NRF is to support and facilitate research, I argued that I had expected the NRF, under the circumstances, to be more proactive in its response to what was then an imminent public health threat.

Realising the futility of pursuing the NRF any further, I contacted Ms Glaudina Loots, the director for Health Innovation at the government's Department of Science and Innovation (DSI). I received a more encouraging response from Loots, who told me that the department had just allocated funding to the South African Medical Research Council (MRC) earmarked for Covid-19 research. She suggested that CAPRISA submit a funding proposal as soon as possible. I needed no further encouragement. We put together and successfully lodged an application for a grant. With the DSI funds secured from the MRC, we were able to go ahead and conduct laboratory testing ahead of the virus's arrival in the country.

By the beginning of March, the protocol developed by Quarraisha's team was finalised and had received ethics approval. The collection of swabs for SARS-CoV-2 began. The protocol had been written and implemented in the field at breakneck speed by any standard. Ordinarily, this would take several months, yet here we were, only a week later, beginning to run the first tests. Up to this day, I do not know how she did this – but it was not surprising as Quarraisha is not only a top-notch epidemiologist but also a wizard in getting the impossible done. It is therefore no small wonder that she has received more than twice as many science awards and prizes than me in the course of our careers as scientists. And this was a busy time for Quarraisha. Shortly thereafter she was appointed to the executive group of the International Steering Committee for the COVID-19 Solidarity Trial. Launched by the WHO and its partners to help find an effective treatment for Covid-19, it was one of the largest international randomised trials for Covid-19 treatments, involving thousands of patients in 30 countries.

On 5 March 2020, the first confirmed case of Covid-19 in South Africa was announced. It was a patient in the small village of Hilton, about 100km north-west of Durban. The first patient was a South African traveller who had recently returned from northern Italy. Both he and his wife were confirmed to be PCR positive by the NICD. Suddenly, South Africa had joined the ranks of countries affected by the virus and there was an uptick in interest from the media in hearing about Covid-19 in South Africa.

Just before this case had been identified, BBC journalist Andrew Harding, anxious to stay on top of a developing story, had contacted CAPRISA's communications manager, Smita Maharaj, asking to interview me about the virus in South Africa. Maharaj is amazing in her emotional intelligence when it comes to the media. She manages my media schedule, ensuring that all my limited media interaction time is used optimally. I told Maharaj that I thought the request was premature, given that we were yet to experience our first case, but she correctly persuaded me to grant the request. As it happened, Harding ended up interviewing me on 6 March, a day after the first case was reported in South Africa, and the story appeared, along with a short video, a few days later under the headline 'Coronavirus: South Africa braces for the worst'.

Harding's story emphasised that living conditions for large sectors of our poorer population rendered mitigation interventions difficult and made them acutely vulnerable to infection. My concern, which I shared with him, was for the estimated 2.5 million people in South Africa who were living with HIV but were not on ARV medication. In the interview, I also explained the benefits of having had a few extra weeks to prepare for the arrival of the virus in Africa and our decades of experience in fighting the world's worst combined epidemics of TB and HIV. 'If we take steps and ensure we react appropriately and take the necessary precautions, I think we'll be able to contain this infection,' I said. In hindsight, I am taken aback at my optimism at the time, which was based on the past successful containment of SARS in China.

That wasn't the only thing I was optimistic about in those early days. Having seen the strides made in HIV, I was perhaps misplaced in assuming that there would be less stigma surrounding this new virus. I was wrong. Shortly after the first case had been announced and the reality of this virus in our midst hit home, there was a great deal of anxiety around contracting the virus – and CAPRISA got its own reminder of this.

We had been ramping up the Covid-19 testing done at our laboratory, but the laboratory procedures were new and we were still gaining experience on how to perform the test reliably. In one of the tests in the CAPRISA laboratory, we unknowingly developed a contamination in the water bath we use to keep the test tubes at the correct temperature. Unfortunately, the contamination resulted in 10 false positives among CAPRISA staff. Before we could redo the tests to confirm the results, word was out. It set off alarm bells among administrators at the University of KwaZulu-Natal, who ordered us to shut down immediately. Provincial Health officials also expressed their disquiet at the 'outbreak' at CAPRISA. CAPRISA staff were castigated for being harbingers of infection – by health care professionals and leaders who should know better. In an effort to calm everyone down, I eventually had to write a formal letter to explain that there were no infections in CAPRISA as the tests were all false positive results. But I shouldn't have had to.

This episode was a useful illustration of the way in which people are quick to apportion blame for infection, and the way in which stigma can swiftly coalesce around a new disease. I had been through this in the early days of HIV, when children with HIV were not being allowed to attend school and positive individuals suffered both stigma and discrimination. The reactions to the short-lived SARS-CoV-2 'outbreak' in my research team was *déjà vu*. We all needed to move past this. Yet more countries were reporting their first cases and the virus was rapidly becoming widespread.

On 11 March 2020, it became official. The WHO announced that Covid-19 had the characteristics of a pandemic – a new disease spreading in multiple countries around the world at the same time.[4] By that time, the virus had infected around 118 000 people in 114 countries and had caused 4 291 deaths across six continents. Making the announcement, a sombre WHO Director-General Dr Tedros Adhanom Ghebreyesus (affectionately called Dr Tedros), explained that 'pandemic' was not a word to use 'lightly or carelessly'. It had the potential to cause 'unreasonable fear, or unjustified acceptance that the fight is over, leading to unnecessary suffering and death', he said.

As the WHO head implied, the word 'pandemic' has particular connotations, which might be better understood in the context of the devastation caused by disease pandemics throughout human history. One of the most serious global pandemics in human history dates back to the fourteenth century. An outbreak of the bubonic plague or Black Death caused by a bacterium carried by fleas living on the rats that travelled on merchant ships killed an estimated 75–200 million people in Eurasia, North Africa and Europe and caused enormous social upheaval.

A key feature of pandemics is their contemporaneous geographical spread and their ability to affect a large number of people. As outlined by Dr Tedros, a pandemic by definition affects multiple countries at the same time and is not contained within a season. While diseases such as Ebola in West Africa, Zika virus in Brazil, SARS in China, and Middle East Respiratory Syndrome (MERS) in Saudi Arabia have been regarded as significant threats to human health and human populations, these have been largely contained within a geographical area or over time and are therefore not classified as pandemics.

Serious pandemics in the past have been caused by influenza-type viruses. Since the outbreak of the 1918 Spanish flu pandemic, which was estimated to have killed around 50 million people, there have been three other influenza pandemics: the 1957 Asian flu (H_2N_2), the 1968 Hong Kong flu (H_3N_2) and the 2009 Pandemic flu (H_1N_1), which caused an estimated 1.5 million, 1 million, and 300 000 human deaths, respectively. Rather than a coronavirus, the next likely global pandemic, like the Spanish flu, was also expected to come in the form of influenza – and the Global Influenza Programme was launched in 1947 by the WHO to deal with just such a threat.

Covid-19 was by no means my first time having to confront a pandemic. In the early 1990s, I was the chair of the government committee that developed South Africa's preparedness plans for pandemic influenza. But for the better part of my life, I have been on the frontlines of another pandemic – AIDS – a responsibility that I was trying to juggle as Covid-19 came to the fore. Because HIV has been with us for some time, people tend to forget that we are still living through a prevalent and deadly pandemic, even though the WHO currently uses the term 'global epidemic' to refer to HIV/AIDS. However AIDS is defined, the numbers are staggering.

According to the Joint United Nations Programme on HIV/AIDS (UNAIDS), an estimated 32.7 million people had died from AIDS-related illnesses by the end of 2019 since the epidemic first started in the early 1980s. In the year 2019, there were 1.7 million new cases. That roughly translates into 4 600 new infections per day. Nearly 38 million people around the world are currently living with HIV – one-fifth of them live in

South Africa. These figures are cause for ongoing alarm, but the concern should not and does not end there: among those new infections in sub-Saharan Africa, one in four affects girls and young women. Through our CAPRISA studies, we've learned it's not just about identifying problems or understanding a pandemic but also trying to find solutions. CAPRISA prioritises the most vulnerable and our research has helped test and develop technologies that empower young women to protect themselves from HIV.

While all of these past experiences with the epidemics of HIV, influenza, haemorrhagic fever and many other viruses helped to some extent, nothing could really prepare us for this new coronavirus. How we responded as a country would be critical to its impact. Days after the WHO's declaration, my mind was racing with ideas as I mulled over what we should do and how South Africa could respond. But the contemplation was short-lived. The President was going to make an announcement on Covid-19, that evening, 15 March 2020. As I, along with the rest of the country, anxiously waited for what would be the first of many late-night addresses, I wondered what measures the President was going to take.

CHAPTER 3

The pandemic response – science advice needed

As a scientist aware of the coronavirus threat and committed to helping the country, the next steps were not clear. I had never heard of a 'lockdown' to curb the spread of disease – it sounded like something from a movie.

In pandemics, decisions need to be made in the interest of public health and these are determined by the government or governmental agencies. The government's response to a public health crisis should be informed by evidence as far as possible. Yet, this isn't always the case. For example, the initial HIV response in South Africa led to life-saving treatment being withheld from people living with HIV. AIDS denialism stemmed from those in positions of power and came with its own dose of harmful misinformation about ways that you could prevent infection through home remedies, including the use of garlic, lemons and beetroot. That was a difficult time for me, as I was the head of AIDS research at the MRC and was among those in the frontlines of challenging the government's AIDS denial. Thankfully, that time has passed and the country's fight against HIV has turned to the side of science. But we all need to remain ever vigilant and hold governments accountable for their decisions, even in the midst of a rapidly growing pandemic, whether it's AIDS, Covid-19 or something else.

With the bitter lessons of HIV still ringing loud, South Africa's Covid-19 response was dialectically opposite. Far from being one characterised by denial or phoney vegetable-based prevention, the government's response to this looming threat was much more considered and proactive. The President declared a state of disaster on 15 March, as the country's case load was starting to escalate and cases were doubling every second day. The state of disaster included 'The Big 10', a euphemistic name for the Coronavirus Emergency Plan that included travel bans from high-risk countries, closure of schools and universities and restrictions on gatherings, among others. These measures were intended to slow viral spread and buy us time to better prepare our health system for a possible pandemic onslaught.

The President was sombre in his message. 'Never before in the history of our democracy has our country been confronted with such a severe situation.' He announced the creation of the Coronavirus Command Council (CCC) and recommended three public health measures: avoidance of close contact with any symptomatic people, cough etiquette using elbows, and washing of hands. And in a flash, he ended the ritual friendship greeting of handshakes when he said, 'In essence, we are calling for a change of behaviour among all South Africans. We must minimise physical contact with other people and encourage the elbow greeting rather than shaking hands.'

I did not know what to make of this announcement. Most of the measures seemed well reasoned but some felt like overkill at a time when South Africa only had 61 cases. One thing was *certain* though – the future looked deeply *uncertain*.

However, not everyone was on the same page. At this early stage of the pandemic, and later too, people argued that these drastic containment measures could not be justified as they curtailed individual freedoms and damaged the economy. Former US President Donald Trump was one of those people. UK Prime Minister Boris Johnson was another. Brazilian President Jair Bolsonaro was a third. Even in South Africa some people argued that the state of disaster was too extreme a response. The reasoning was that Covid-19 was a mild disease and most people would not be at risk for complications or serious health problems.

As the pandemic progressed, however, the reality sank in. With each successive wave of infections witnessed around the world, specious arguments questioning the seriousness of Covid-19 began to abate. The exception was, and remains, among 'flat earth' type groups, including one in South Africa led by actuaries, who still argue to this day that Covid-19 is no worse than the 'flu'. One of the Covid-19 denialist groups has been particularly vocal – blatantly refusing to acknowledge the strong evidence we have on the virology or epidemiology of SARS-CoV-2, choosing instead to repeatedly spout outright lies in their desperate attempts to downplay the infection and deny the efficacy of public health measures or vaccines. But the numbers speak for themselves and the toll that Covid-19 took is truly sobering. The global reported death toll stood at over 2 million after one year of the virus spreading throughout the world, and another year later, by January 2022, it rose to 6 million. Two years after the first case in South Africa, there were nearly 100 000 reported Covid-19 deaths in the country – more than 10 times higher than the number of deaths expected each year from 'flu'. If we take account of excess deaths – the difference between the number of actual deaths and the number of historically expected deaths – the toll would be almost triple this number. While the medical conditions responsible for the excess deaths are not known, most are likely to be due to Covid-19 as excess deaths have varied in proportion to the number of cases. But we don't need to treble the number of deaths to establish that this is a serious disease; 100 000 deaths is serious enough. No person or government can in good conscience allow such loss of life without doing what it can to ameliorate viral spread, particularly when public health measures have been used effectively in other countries to achieve this.

Among the naysayers, there were also those who were keen to point out supposed contradictions in the way in which the government was dealing with Covid-19 compared with diseases such as TB and influenza. These were, at root, ideological arguments rather than scientific. The fact is that all diseases are different and require different responses. A state of disaster or a lockdown would never be considered for either TB or influenza. In the case of influenza, it does not overwhelm hospitals and deaths are too few to justify such drastic measures. In the case of TB, its status as a chronic disease that has existed in human communities for centuries meant that a lockdown would have some, though limited, impact and only in the short term. Covid-19, on the other hand, was a rapidly spreading disease that could be stopped in its tracks by eliminating person-to-person contact while the opportunity still existed before the virus became widespread. The way in which this could be achieved, however, was still somewhat uncharted territory.

In the early months of 2020, the only thing we knew for sure was that we had our work cut out for us.

On 19 March 2020, as the state of disaster was being implemented, I received a call from the Office of the President. On the line was Professor Olive Shisana. I had known Shisana from well before she became Director-General in the Department of Health in the 1990s and subsequently the CEO of the Human Sciences Research Council. In her capacity as an adviser to the President, she asked me to prepare some written information on prevention and infection control of Covid-19. Shisana typically demanded rapid turnaround times, and this was no exception. I helped as best as I could, given the time constraints. And so, it began – I was now providing the government with scientific information to help guide the Covid-19 response!

The next day brought with it another request. Late in the afternoon on Friday, 20 March, an email from Shisana arrived in my inbox. This message came with an attachment – the official *Handbook on Prevention and Treatment of Covid-19*, which had been compiled by clinicians from the First Affiliated Hospital, Zhejiang University School of Medicine, in the interests of sharing the experience of health care workers in China with the rest of the world. Shisana had distributed the document to a dozen or so people, including myself. She asked for assistance in identifying the key lessons from the Chinese approach, so that these could be adapted for the local context. We also received a copy of the Chinese plan for managing Covid-19, a comprehensive strategy document that covered issues ranging from protection of health care workers to quarantine arrangements, housing of the homeless and ensuring access to clean water during a 'lockdown'. She needed it ready by 5am on Sunday morning. I got to work.

During my training and in all my years as an epidemiologist, I had never heard of a 'lockdown' as a measure to curb the spread of disease. I was aware of curfews and limitations on movement as strategies to contain dangerous contagious diseases like drug-resistant tuberculosis, but I had never heard the word 'lockdown' used in this context. To me it sounded like a military or law enforcement term. My mind drifted to the 2019 movie *21 Bridges* where Chadwick Boseman (of *Black Panther* fame) plays the New York policeman who is trying to capture the gunmen responsible for the deaths of several colleagues and calls for a lockdown of the city at all its bridges. I searched the internet for information that might enlighten me. I found only three articles that had some relevance: the first was an article in the online *Guardian* newspaper referring to a lockdown in Mexico to contain swine flu; the second was a paper in the *International Journal of Epidemiology* concerning a lockdown in Sierra Leone to contain Ebola; and the third was this handbook dealing with Covid-19 prepared by the Chinese authorities, which was publicly available on the internet. In short, there was little, if anything, to go on in trying to understand a lockdown. Evidence for decision-making was limited.

On reading the Chinese strategy document, I was impressed with the level of detail and high level of organisation it reflected. I was intrigued in particular with the red flag system they used in China. For people confined to their homes for long periods, they designed a flag system so that people in need of medical help, food or anything else could be easily identified by the red flags placed outside their homes and apartments. The Chinese government deployed mobile teams to monitor the flags and to provide whatever assistance was required. The document also described in meticulous and systematic detail the correct process to be followed in the case of food delivery by restaurants and takeaway outlets. At no stage in China was the sale of hot meals by food outlets restricted as it was in South Africa; in fact, those outlets performed a valuable service in terms of keeping people supplied with cooked meals in lockdown.

But how helpful had such a drastic approach actually been in China? One answer to this question had been provided by the report of the WHO mission to China that had just been released in early March 2020.[1] 'China's bold approach to contain the rapid spread of this new respiratory pathogen has changed the course of a rapidly escalating and deadly epidemic,' the report said. 'This decline in COVID-19 cases across China is real.' The more complicated question was whether China's approach would work in other countries, given that few countries had strong government control over social behaviour. Could this be done in South Africa? I wondered. This was a harder answer to know, as it had not been done here before. The closest I could think of was the hospital quarantine applied to extremely drug-resistant tuberculosis in the last few years. This had not worked well as patients in the Eastern Cape and KwaZulu-Natal hospitals had simply walked out the door. If that approach hadn't worked then, what would? How would this plan need to be adapted? What was reasonable or possible to get people to follow? The questions buzzed incessantly in my mind. I played out multiple different scenarios over and over in my head. The key conclusion I reached was that whatever path South Africa chose, it would be difficult, with no guarantees that it would work. I could see that there was no *one* perfect solution. Most of the alternatives I could imagine ended with the measures slowing the spread of the virus but not containing it. If we could not contain the virus, then it would continue spreading. My hope was that we could slow the spread down, even if we could not contain it.

In the end, my advice came down to finding a balance of measures. The draft strategy document for the government that I worked on, alongside other experts, incorporated advice from the WHO and advocated for a 'careful strategy that minimises spread of the disease and reduces the burden on strained health care systems'. The document's tone conveyed some of the stress and uncertainty that defined that period and, given the high uncertainty, a conservative approach was among the least of the many distressing options available.

This approach would use some of the measures that had worked in China, including the stay-at-home lockdown. The recommendation to go this route stemmed heavily from legitimate concerns for the large pool of HIV-infected people, especially those who were not on treatment, as this group was immunocompromised and may experience high death rates. There was particular concern for the large number of impoverished communities, especially those in informal settlements, as the virus was expected to spread rapidly in overcrowded settings. Behind our advice was the acknowledgement that there would be regional implications too: South Africa's actions would likely be emulated in many other countries in Africa in dealing with the pandemic. The need to take action was growing, as each evening we witnessed the trauma of this disease being portrayed on our television screens. Countries around the world, like Italy, which had suffered a heavy blow during their first wave and paid a huge price in terms of loss of life and pressure on health care services, were now regretting not having locked down sooner.

On the evening of Monday, 23 March 2020, a 21-day stay-at-home stringent lockdown was announced by the President.

Only hours before I had been appointed Chair of the Ministerial Advisory Committee on Covid-19 (MAC), a new committee and a new role for me. Given the timing of the announcement and the rapid move to a lockdown, it was perhaps no surprise that people assumed I had been the driver behind the concept. 'Karim called it and the President locked down,' one newspaper columnist declared, ascribing far more authority to me than I had.

In truth, I had little to do with the government's lockdown decision, which actually preceded the creation of the MAC. The MAC was not even aware that the announcement was imminent. For myself, I was one of many who had provided the President's adviser what little advice I could on possible steps to take for Covid-19, acknowledging the uncertainty and the lack of evidence. But I was not involved in any way in the decision to impose a stay-at-home lockdown and I did not know it was about to be announced.

When the announcement came, we had reached a point where there was no option for the government but to take action. The doubling time for infections was rapidly increasing. We knew from observing the experiences of other countries such as the United Kingdom, which was running two to three weeks ahead of us, that if action was not taken, the epidemic would take off rapidly. Even though I didn't have any say in the decision to impose a lockdown, I supported the measure fully when it was officially declared that evening. Still, this was the first indicator of what was to come; a misunderstanding of the role of the MAC and an over-estimation of its influence on political decisions.

The decision to create a MAC was an indicator of the Department of Health's desire to make sure they were armed with as much knowledge as possible when dealing with this deadly disease. I had been prepared for the role to some degree because I was already providing advice on Covid-19 to several others, including my friend and former colleague at the Nelson Mandela Medical School, Dr Barry Kistnasamy, who is the head of occupational health in the National Department of Health. I had reconnected with Kistnasamy on the unfortunate occasion of the death (unrelated to Covid-19) of his sister Joy Kistnasamy in Durban on 11 March. While I was assisting him with the funeral arrangements, he asked if I might make myself available to provide scientific advice to the occupational health unit of the department in its response to Covid-19. Naturally, I agreed, and I put forward the names of other people whom I thought might also be able to help. So, to some extent, I was being asked for scientific advice and therefore knew what this would involve. Or at least, I felt so at the time.

My invitation to serve on the MAC was more understated than many people realise. A week prior to my appointment, on 16 March, my personal assistant, Ms Norma Hatcher, popped her head into my office to let me know that the Health minister's office had called asking for my contact details: they wanted to invite me to a meeting the following day. I assured Norma that I was available and had no problem with her giving the minister's office my details as I knew the Minister of Health, Dr

Zweli Mkhize, well. He had been a year ahead of me at medical school and we had both been anti-apartheid activists in the Medical Students Representative Council. He left the country to join the African National Congress (ANC) in exile shortly after graduating from medical school. His wife, Dr May Mashego-Mkhize, was his medical school classmate and a fellow activist who went into exile with him. In 2002, I had recruited Mashego-Mkhize to join CAPRISA to run our rural research clinic, which was close to her home on the outskirts of Pietermaritzburg. In the years that she ran the clinic, it became a highly sought-after source of medical care in the community.

As it happened, the invitation to the mysterious meeting scheduled for 17 March never arrived, although I was made aware afterwards that the meeting had in fact taken place. I assumed that somebody had forgotten to send me the invitation. A follow-up virtual meeting was scheduled. This time the invitation arrived, and when I joined the minister's conference call that morning, I found myself among about 50 to 60 other participants, most of whom were clinicians, virologists and epidemiologists. I knew almost everyone at the meeting from their involvement in HIV or TB care or research. After being welcomed by the minister, we were given a short presentation on the latest global and national situation on Covid-19. The Acting Director-General for Health at the time, Dr Anban Pillay, then announced the formation of a ministerial advisory committee. It would comprise three groups, he said: clinicians; pathologists and laboratory experts; and public health experts. Later, a research group was also created. A notice would be sent to all participants after the meeting asking them to indicate their preferred group membership. Once the group membership was settled, there would be a process to elect a chair for each of the sub-groups, said Pillay.

Towards the end of the meeting, he announced that 'Professor Salim Abdool Karim would be the overall chair of the MAC'. It was unexpected. I was surprised. The thought of turning it down never occurred to me at the time. In any event, if I had been asked beforehand, I would have agreed without hesitation. As scientists, we were all aware of the serious challenge the new coronavirus presented to the country, and I think I can confidently say that we were all committed to playing any role we could to help the country meet the challenge. It had been very clear during the meeting that the government was taking the Covid-19 threat very seriously. The scientific community was being asked to step up and assist and, under those kinds of circumstances, one does so.

But exactly what kind of help was required? What was the committee's mandate? How could we make best use of the scientific expertise available on the committee? I contacted Pillay later in the day to get clarity on some of these questions. I was given carte blanche to organise the committee as best I could. I started to put things in place for what I anticipated might involve a whole new experience. Along with concerns about the enormity of the problem came trepidation at the daunting task being set before us.

I was thinking about my advisory role in the way I had previously provided scientific advice to others, namely, that this would be a quiet backroom activity where I would write up some literature reviews and summarise their implications. No way. I was about to learn that this would be a task like no other.

CHAPTER 4

Building while sailing

We're Building the Ship as We Sail It

… It's awkward
to have to do one's
planning in extremis
in the early years –
so hard to hide later:
sleekening the hull,
making things
more gracious.

(Poem by Kay Ryan, a former US poet laureate)

In its essence, the poem that heads this chapter speaks to the angst involved in growing up ('the early years') and forging one's own identity from raw materials. Among a host of other insights, it reveals how the survivalist response to fear or crisis often produces a particular shape or form – 'a foundational raft', if you will, that is difficult to disguise once the crisis has passed and the vessel is required to adapt to a more sophisticated function.

The metaphor of an incompletely built ship needing to sail turbulent seas fitted the reality of the MAC well and even our national Covid-19 response, forged 'in extremis' in early 2020. As a new and unknown disease started to spread, there was little time for meticulous design, or a focus on form and aesthetics. We simply had to climb on board, work as hard as possible to make our craft seaworthy and chart a sensible way forward. There was little time for grand designs, carefully mulled plans, or to ensure that we all shared the same expectations of our vessel. We were charting a course in the treacherous seas of limited evidence and high scientific uncertainty. Despite the dangers, we had an imperative to act, and this meant 'building the ship while sailing it'. I borrowed and quoted this term frequently at MAC meetings to capture the unique and often frustrating circumstances in which we found ourselves. Everything we were doing for the first few months was based on very little evidence related to the novel coronavirus.

Fortunately, as chair of the MAC, I had been allocated some excellent 'shipmates', selected by the Minister of Health. These members comprised some of the country's senior clinicians, virologists, epidemiologists, mathematical modellers, public health practitioners and other experts.

The MAC was a repository of the country's highly accomplished medical scientific expertise – a brains trust – and they were a capable group. It was a positive reflection on the country that the government was able to call upon such vast expertise in a time of crisis. It spoke to the research investment South Africa has made in its medical academics and researchers. You cannot produce scientists and academics overnight – they spend years honing their expertise and reputations – so this is something we should treasure. I was often struck during that time at how fortunate we were in South Africa to have such an abundance of accomplished scientists that the minister could easily have his pick of talented individuals at short notice.

I knew almost all of the MAC members – some as close colleagues. Several had, like me, cut their teeth as infectious disease specialists and researchers during the HIV pandemic that ravaged South Africa during the 1990s and still represents one of its biggest disease burdens. Despite its ravages, HIV had also built a strong national capacity in medical science and had spawned a generation of scientists who understood the ins and outs of a viral epidemic. Granted, HIV was a different kind of epidemic when compared with Covid-19, but there were many common elements. Much of our advice in the early phases of the epidemic was drawn from our collective experience of dealing with HIV as well as influenza. This was a huge advantage for a country poised to deal with Covid-19.

The MAC members proved to be, in the vast majority, a hard-working bunch who willingly pulled their weight and accepted with dedication, enthusiasm and grace the extra – and unpaid – responsibility of serving on the MAC. I valued their collective wisdom and deeply appreciated working with them. I would often marvel at some of their insights in our discussions and I learned a lot from them. There were also a fair share of challenges, as would be expected in any group dynamic, principally when egos came to the fore. But there was nothing I could not handle.

I was concerned, however, that the MAC was very 'medical' as there were few social or behavioural scientists on board. I later raised this concern with the minister and he addressed it, initially with the creation of a separate social and behavioural MAC and, secondly, by adjusting the membership of the MAC on Covid-19 after the first six months to include behavioural science and ethics.

The purpose of the MAC meetings was first and foremost the development of advisories for the government. Initially, I received the questions requiring MAC advice verbally from the Minister of Health or the Acting DG and I would provide verbal responses within a day or two. But it became obvious to me quite quickly that we needed a system to document the questions and the advice so that there was a formal response that did not need word-of-mouth for dissemination to everyone who needed to know the advice. Also, a written reply would afford us the opportunity to update the advice as needed.

In the beginning, the queries came fast and furious from the Department of Health. We were kept very busy dealing with the multitude of queries – from providing a definition of exposure to qualify for quarantine to providing estimates on how people would likely be hospitalised in the first wave. But as the pace slowed and queries came at a more realistic rate, there came a point at which we also offered unsolicited advice. But our *raison d'être* was to provide advice. The MAC was not a talk shop. Advisories were our end product.

Among my initial administrative tasks was getting to grips with who was or was not a real member of the MAC. An invaluable resource when it came to not only this but all our duties was the MAC secretariat constituted by the Department of Health and made up of three exceptionally talented and hard-working individuals: Mrs Jane Ridden, Mrs Janine Jugathpal and Ms Amanda Brewer. All qualified pharmacists, they worked as a secretariat for various existing ministerial advisories committees, including the NEMLC (National Essential Medicines List Committee) on antimicrobial resistance, and they had ample experience with governance and policy work at the level required by the Covid-19 MAC. Their responsibilities included arranging meetings, engaging with stakeholders and drafting advisories and presenting them to the Incident Management Team of the Department of Health responsible for implementation. In particular, their expertise and efficiency showed in their ability to produce accurate minutes of all meetings of the MAC and its sub-groups – almost as soon as a meeting was over. The meticulous work of the secretariat came in handy when trying to ascertain who did, in fact, belong to the MAC.

Attendance at the first two MAC meetings had been based on invitations issued by the Department of Health and I had patchy information on who was on those lists and what the criteria for selection had been. Later, the secretariat discovered that there had been some variation in the two invitation lists, with the second meeting having more participants than the first. There was precious little time for consultation, so I simply combined the list of attendees at both meetings and declared that anyone who had attended one or both of those meetings was an official member of the MAC. Those who were invited but hadn't attended were left off the list. That gave us a total of 51 members. Because it was a departmental committee, the membership needed to be a Department of Health decision. So, I ran this rather unsophisticated selection procedure past the Acting DG and it was duly endorsed.

To give a human face to the MAC, the secretariat started to collect photographs and primary affiliations of all members for display on the Department of Health website. I knew most of them, but one name was not known to me and stood out – 'Lindiwe Ringane Ka Seme', whose title was 'external advisory on Health and Presidency'. She attended one of the two first meetings, which was how she had secured her place on the MAC. I anticipated that I would get to meet her and learn more about her medical expertise during the upcoming MAC meetings. The MAC secretariat kept accurate information on meeting attendance and a later analysis showed that Ka Seme's attendance was almost non-existent. After consulting with the Acting DG, I dropped her from the MAC membership, which meant we stopped sending her information, minutes and notices of meetings. I didn't think much more about the matter until early October 2020, when I received a call from a newspaper journalist asking me about Ka Seme's contribution to the MAC. By that time, I could barely remember her name let alone comment on her performance. Apparently, Ka Seme had no medical qualification, contrary to her claims. I felt that this was not worthy of any more of my time and effort and felt vindicated in dropping her from the MAC to focus on more important issues. But the experience of having to deal with this matter made me much more wary about taking things in the MAC for granted – I realised that I needed to be much more vigilant on even the most elementary matters in the MAC.

After confirming the membership of the MAC, the next step was to allocate all members to four sub-committees. These included a patholo-gists and laboratory sub-committee, chaired by Professor Koleka Mlisana, a microbiologist from the NHLS; a clinicians' sub-group, chaired by Professor Marc Mendelson, an infectious diseases specialist from the University of Cape Town; a public health sub-committee chaired by Professor Shabir Madhi, a paediatrician from Wits University; and a research sub-committee, chaired by Professor Glenda Gray, a paediatri-cian who was the president of the MRC. As soon as these allocations took place and chairs were elected, we hit the ground running. I tried to attend as many of the meetings as I could. This included working groups and sub-committees and, later, technical working groups. There would be several meetings of the MAC and its sub-groups during the course of the week, and sometimes there were two or three in one day. This meant I had to literally drop everything else. For a period of about four months – meetings started to tail off in August 2020 when infection rates started to drop – my secretary Norma simply cleared my usual schedule to ensure that I would be available for MAC meetings as and when they were scheduled.

The minister sometimes attended the MAC meetings, the acting DG more often, but questions from both came thick and fast for the first few months. The MAC was functioning at a high level almost immediately from set-up. It quickly became all-consuming, demanding vast amounts of time and almost all my attention. About three months after the MAC had been created, I asked the secretariat to provide me with an analysis of MAC members' attendance so that I could include it in my update presentation to the MAC. It emerged from that process that the vast majority of members had exemplary attendance, with most exceeding 80%. Only five members had attendance that fell below 50%. They included some very busy members of the NICD and NHLS and one or two clinicians, with substantial clinical duties at their hospitals. I think this was testimony to the calibre of MAC members and their commitment to assisting the national Covid-19 response.

Given the unprecedented circumstances, and the speed and pressure under which we were working, I sounded a warning bell to the minister and MAC members that we should expect to make mistakes – after all 'to err is human'. But we could learn quickly from those mistakes and make the necessary amends. To some extent that's the nature of the scientific process. Our success would be measured by how we minimised our mistakes, by learning from the mistakes we made, guided by an improved understanding of the issues involved, close observation and careful analysis of outcomes.

Because it so aptly captured the 'work-in-progress' nature of our activities, I borrowed Kay Ryan's 'building while sailing' metaphor (although at the time I had no idea it was hers – it had become part of my brain's lexicon) for my first Covid-19-related publication: a short article for the *New England Journal of Medicine* published in May 2020.[1] The piece arose out of a conversation I had with Dr Yogan Pillay, Deputy DG in the

Department of Health, not long after I was appointed to the MAC. We were trying to pinpoint and stack our priorities in the national Covid-19 response. Out of a need to ensure that nothing slipped through the cracks, I jotted down a checklist comprising eight overlapping stages, which provided a broad canvas for the South African response for a slide-set I was making (more on this in Chapter 7). I used this eight-stage plan to outline a way forward so that we could prepare for the anticipated next set of tasks in the national Covid-19 response.

The framework proved over time to have covered all the bases for the first wave, but it did not factor in the as-yet-unknown variants that would drive successive waves. In my early discussions with Pillay, a day or two after being appointed to the MAC, it occurred to me that a public health goal was already in place – even if it had not been articulated in any formal way. That plan at the beginning was, quite simply, to 'flatten the curve'. This refrain reverberated around the world as countries started to grapple with their epidemic curves. Flattening the curve is a public health strategy that involves slowing the spread of a virus so that the number of people needing health care is delayed and those seeking health care services are spread over a longer period. It is aimed at protecting vulnerable members of the population in particular, giving the health system critical time to prepare, and carving out more time for the development of a possible vaccine and other treatment options. Although it is on the same continuum, and involves the same mitigation strategies, it is a less ambitious strategy than containment or elimination; the latter was the goal adopted by some countries like New Zealand, Taiwan and Australia. Island nations naturally tend to do much better with elimination and containment strategies because it is easier to close off borders and their population density tends to be lower.

For us, however, there was general consensus that 'flattening the curve' was the best option to follow, as elimination was not a realistic goal for South Africa. The consensus was that this approach would be a more practical one for the country to take and not because, as one newspaper columnist tried to suggest in a political viewpoint article, the government had embraced a defeatist approach in order to absolve itself of ultimate responsibility for the outcome, whatever it might be.[2]

There were several factors to be considered. A major problem was South Africa's leaky land borders. There was also the issue of living conditions: large swathes of the South African population live in impoverished and overcrowded conditions that are not conducive to elimination or containment. Another consideration was the high economic costs to implement the kind of restrictions needed for viral elimination. Not only would economic activity be negatively affected, but social security costs would also soar. Additionally, more resources and infrastructure would be required to scale up contact tracing and testing – requiring levels of testing that were not feasible when South Africa could not secure an adequate supply of test kits in the context of huge global demand. All of these factors, together with what we knew thus far about the high transmissibility of the virus, led us to believe it was unlikely that we could contain the virus.

It is not unusual to be criticised. The process of arriving at an appropriate approach, when providing advice, is complex and factors in many variables, including an understanding of the virus, medical care needs, efficacy of individual prevention interventions and prospects of adherence to prevention measures, among others. It would be challenging to grapple with these multiple dimensions of evidence and uncertainty, expecting that everyone would have all this information or, if they did, would arrive at the same conclusion. In fact, criticism, even when misinformed, is important to guide reflection and helps to revisit advice provided and decisions made. With the Covid-19 pandemic, a major challenge was criticism that was not intended to be constructive or helpful but was rather driven by the need to feel important or by 'know-it-alls'. As scientists, we deal with this, even from fellow scientists, all the time and so this was to be expected.

Flattening the curve relies heavily on measures aimed at minimising the spread of the virus through testing, quarantine and contact tracing, handwashing and social distancing. Most of these measures had been in place since the first case of the virus was reported on 5 March. At that stage, face masks were not yet an official part of the prevention toolkit. Given what we had seen of the rapid spread of the virus in the UK, we knew that we needed to intensify our mitigation strategy beyond hand hygiene and social distancing, particularly because both of these measures were difficult and even impossible for some sectors of South Africa's poorer population to implement. We needed to reduce human mobility and interaction to reduce human-to-human contact so that any infected individuals would not be able to infect others beyond their immediate confines. We knew we could not rely on voluntary behaviour change as this takes a long time to achieve.

Flattening the curve is a recognised public health strategy, but I had no direct experience of such a rapidly spreading epidemic. Up to that point, I had never come across a disease that was able to overwhelm health care facilities in developed countries in the way that SARS-CoV-2 was doing in Europe and the US. Every year, South Africa sees a spike in hospitalisations for influenza, but nothing on the scale that we were witnessing for SARS-CoV-2 in other countries. I had some understanding of the impact of Ebola, which had overwhelmed health care systems in West Africa, largely because it was the health care workers that fell to the disease, but in Covid-19 we anticipated a much greater challenge in terms of patient numbers. On this basis, flattening the curve was not only our best option, but it was also a necessary step in anticipation of a rapidly growing pandemic that puts enormous pressure on hospitals. And as pressure on hospitals increases, the deaths rise.

MAC members were supportive of this approach when Pillay presented it to the MAC. So, we proceeded on that basis, asking the next question: how far do we need to flatten the curve? It then became obvious that our primary national goal had no quantitative dimensions. We had no idea what our curve would look like without intervention; without a benchmark, it was impossible to attach any precise goals to our plan. I suggested we focus on two key issues: pushing back the peak – if the peak came in April, health care systems would likely not be ready – and lowering the peak.

When I look back with hindsight, we achieved both of these goals during South Africa's first surge in a way that served us well: we delayed the peak by about six to eight weeks, pushing it from April/May to July, and we also managed to dampen the peak to the extent that field hospitals in Cape Town, Johannesburg and Pietermaritzburg that were set up in preparation for the surge were never actually filled to capacity. In Cape Town, roughly 450 out of the 800 beds made available were used during the first wave. That our field hospitals did not reach maximum capacity was not a problem for me; I would rather we had spare capacity than have someone die because there wasn't a hospital bed available.

I have been repeatedly asked if we really did succeed through our mitigation techniques, particularly the stay-at-home lockdown, in flattening the curve in that first wave or whether it would have happened anyway. The answer is: we simply do not and cannot know definitively. To make a conclusive determination that could withstand the rigours of scientific enquiry would have required us to have a control group with no stay-at-home lockdown. That was simply not possible. What I do know is that we were compelled to act, and that the curve did flatten following our actions.

But I tried to provide some comparisons, even though they were not perfect. One approach to estimate the effect of an intervention is to use an external control group from another country, though this has its own limitations. Comparisons between the trajectory of the South African epidemic and the epidemic in the UK in the early stages were particularly revealing and, in my view, vindicated the actions we took. Logarithmic graphs showed both countries were initially on the same trajectory, but South Africa's curve flattened off in late March, while the UK's curve continued to rise. The inflection point at which the rate of growth of the epidemic in South Africa in the first wave starts to level off, and when public health measures are starting to have an effect, coincides with the implementation of the hard lockdown on 26 March 2020, which means that at least part of the process likely started with the onset of the state of disaster 10 days earlier, allowing for an incubation period. In the case of the UK, where lockdown measures were implemented much later in the trajectory of their epidemic, the curve continues to rise sharply before flattening out, and at a much higher level.

The evidence at our disposal suggests that South Africa did indeed succeed in what it set out to do – namely, flatten the curve. During 35 days of stringent stay-at-home lockdown, the doubling time slowed from 2 days to 15 days by 30 April. The peak, which was pushed back by six to eight weeks, reached 13 944 cases per day on 24 July 2020, before dropping back down to just over 2 000 per day in early September. In the absence of any definitive evidence at the time or any advice from the MAC (which didn't exist then), the government's proactive approach, erring on the side of caution, of declaring a state of disaster on 16 March 2020, followed 10 days later by a stay-at-home lockdown, had in all likelihood flattened the curve.

In those early days of the pandemic there were simply too many hypotheticals and unknowns, which meant the MAC had to accept that we were working with high levels of uncertainty. We were still grappling with many basic questions about Covid-19. How the virus spread was one: was there faecal-oral transmission; mother-to-child transmission; could pets transmit the disease? Should we be offering assisted isolation to individuals or insisting on whole-household quarantine? And so the questions grew. The more we learned about this virus, the more we realised how little we knew. It would never be smooth sailing. The waters were murky and choppy, and our crew was still learning how to navigate using a makeshift boat; nevertheless we were satisfied that we did the best we could under the circumstances. And as the storm clouds of uncertainty gathered, I was negotiating our half-built vessel, the MAC, through the challenges of providing scientific advice.

Scientific advice comes from a good understanding of multiple aspects of the disease and its challenges. In trying to understand the disease up to this point, I had been looking at the statistics and the biology of the virus in order to provide evidence-based advice. Surely I needed to know as much as I could about the number of tests, infections, hospital admissions and deaths to understand this disease, I thought. Yet, even with all the information I had available to me, I could never have been armed with enough facts to feel prepared for the shock I got when I learned about the challenges in dealing with Covid-19 in hospitals – this was what opened my eyes to what we were really dealing with.

CHAPTER 5

More than an infection

Covid-19 at that time was not just an infection. It was stigmatising.
Further, St Augustine's Hospital highlighted the problem that infected
or exposed doctors and nurses had to go into quarantine just when they
were needed most in hospitals under pressure from Covid-19 cases.

On 21 March, about a week before South Africa entered its initial stay-at-home stringent lockdown, there were a total of 240 confirmed Covid-19 cases (identified from 7 425 tests) reported in the country. I had not yet seen any of these 240 patients, nor did I know anyone who had been infected at that stage. But that would soon change, and the reality that Covid-19 went beyond just clinical illness became clear.

While I was in the midst of pondering the complexities of what we should do as the coronavirus was spreading in our country and providing some information to Olive Shisana, I got my first insights into what the reality of Covid-19 might entail beyond the clinical illness – a glimpse into what this virus meant for people's lives and what it could do to the country's health care system if unprepared. I woke up that morning to a phone call from my son, Wasim, in Cape Town. He wasn't feeling well and some of his symptoms – fever, cough and sore throat – matched those of Covid-19. At that point, I was well aware of the common presenting symptoms and the potential of this virus to progress quickly to respiratory distress.

My immediate response was, as usual, to calmly make a plan. While still on the phone with him, I began outlining the steps that Wasim should follow: avoid public transport, get on your bicycle, ride slowly to the hospital, explain your symptoms and get yourself tested. While he set out to the hospital, I called ahead to let them know that a suspected Covid-19 patient was coming in. Despite this forewarning, Wasim's arrival seemed to prompt pandemonium. Judging from Wasim's account, his admission to the health care facility had created fear and concern, and so it wasn't entirely smooth. The staff were unprepared for exactly how to handle his case and were seemingly scared to deal with him. The necessary protocols might have been in place, but the staff reacted as if a leper had arrived at their doorstep.

However, when the emergency room doctor, Dr Jocelyn Hellig, took charge of treating him, she calmed things down and handled the situation well. His care greatly improved once Wasim was moved to an isolation ward where the ward staff were familiar with barrier nursing, a well-established method of managing highly infectious patients and providing them with care while also exercising caution to keep everyone safe. He was that hospital's first suspected Covid-19 patient, and the experience was a warning of what was to come if hospitals were not properly prepared to deal with potential cases.

Wasim's negative PCR test result arrived late the next day while I was reading Safura's prophetic article on *The Hill* website on the future affordability of Covid-19 vaccines and the US government's decision not to impose any price controls on Covid-19 vaccines, thereby giving the pharmaceutical industry free rein on the vaccine market. Her article read: '... without price controls it may not matter whether a coronavirus vaccine is developed because it will be out of reach to millions across the world who cannot afford it. This is why, despite concerns about losses of potential profits and overzealous government regulation, the vaccine price is critical. Being a South African, I have witnessed the impact laws allowing price controls and parallel imports can have on people's health ... Intellectual property protection on medicines and vaccines can make life-saving interventions completely inaccessible.'[1] *The Hill* is an influential source of information on Capitol Hill, the seat of government decision-making in the US, and Safura's article would ring in my ears many months later, in

September 2020, when I attended my first meeting with a pharmaceutical company to learn of their supply and pricing plans should their vaccine prove to be effective.

On Sunday evening, just days before the President announced South Africa's lockdown, Quarraisha and I were watching our daughter Aisha's television interview on Covid-19, where she was describing droplet spread. At the same time, we chatted about Wasim's experience. We realised that it would be much better if all of our children came back home. That way, we could at least be assured of their safety and could manage any Covid-19-related infection should it arise. And so, Wasim flew back to Durban once he had been discharged from hospital on Monday, and a day or so later, both Aisha and Safura, along with Ivo, left Gauteng by car and returned to the family fold. This turned out to be an unexpected big bonus – we had our family together again.

Wasim's experience reminded me of the time I dealt with the initial AIDS cases. People are scared of the unknown and their mental images of Covid-19 at that time were quite scary. Covid-19 at that time was not just an infection, it was stigmatising. In a health care setting, some staff were concerned, especially those who were older or had comorbidities, about their own safety. I was beginning to understand that care of Covid-19 patients would be challenging, but I was not prepared for what followed a few days later at St Augustine's Hospital.

My second experience of how Covid-19 played out in a hospital also started with a phone call – except this time it was from the National Health Department's Acting DG. Late in the evening on Friday, 3 April, about a week into the stay-at-home lockdown, he rang to inform me that there was a crisis brewing at St Augustine's, a large private hospital in Durban. At that stage, there had been 13 reported cases with three deaths in the hospital's outbreak. He asked me to investigate this spate of infections and report back to him and the minister. It was arranged with Dr Richard Friedland, the CEO of Netcare, that I would meet Craig Murphy of Netcare early the next morning at the hospital.

The first hurdle came with actually getting into the building. The hospital was like Fort Knox – security was not allowing anyone to enter, no exceptions, not even for the chair of the MAC. The irony of the moment was not lost on me: while most people were giving the area a wide berth, I was doing my best to get in for a closer look. Epidemiology can be similar to firefighting in that sense. My mind flashed to the imagery of those going towards the fire while everyone else is trying to get away from the flames. As I was trying to talk my way in and deal with security, Murphy arrived to let me in.

Murphy introduced me to his team working on the hospital's outbreak. The team was led by Sister Liza Sitharam, the regional Netcare Infection Prevention and Control (IPC) manager, and included hospital practitioners Sister Nicole Govender and Sister Maryann Maistry. The four of us sat down in the boardroom and spent over an hour going through the whole history of the outbreak with a fine-tooth comb. No detail could be spared if I was going to get to the bottom of what happened in the hospital. After our lengthy conversation, Sitharam took me on a walk-through, where we retraced the movement of the virus from its first entry into the hospital.

We arrived at the conclusion that the outbreak likely started on 9 March, when a patient who had just returned from the UK called the hospital to let them know that he was coming in for a Covid-19 test. The hospital had already established a screening tent outside the emergency room (ER) for Covid-19 screening. From there, any suspected cases were directed through a separate entrance into the ER procedure room for a swab. This patient zero, who was later found to be PCR positive, had followed all the procedures that were in place. The next case, patient one, was a woman from a Durban nursing home for the elderly who was in the ER for a transient ischaemic attack. Neither patient ever made contact with one another during their stay at the hospital but both were being attended to by the same doctor and nurse and were in different sections of the ER at the same time. In fact, after examining and swabbing patient zero, this health care duo then took care of patient one in the ER. She was then admitted to the cardiac ICU where she developed Covid-19 symptoms a few days later. In the meantime, three other patients, including two men in a distant section of the cardiac ICU, acquired the infection. Patient one was then transferred to a ward where the person in the bed next to hers became infected. At least five more patients, including some who were in distant sections of the same ward, subsequently became infected. When she was discharged and returned to the nursing home, the infection spread to several others in the nursing home for the elderly – with a high case fatality rate.

As I walked through the ER, the corridors, cardiac ICU and wards, I could almost see how the virus was spreading sometimes by direct contact and sometimes through staff members or contaminated equipment sharing. It was almost a virtual reality playback for me. At the end of the almost two-hour walk-through, we had traced the virus's path and I had all I needed for now. I stopped by the hospital's Covid-19 ward to see the patients – the first Covid-19 patients that I attended. Two were on oxygen but were otherwise well, though I heard crackles on inhalation with my stethoscope and found clinical signs of pneumonia in both patients. The third patient in the ward had been maintaining her oxygen saturation within an acceptable range without oxygen supplementation. Things turned out to be very different when I got to the ICU. It was full. The ward was abuzz with staff scuttling around dealing with their very ill patients. I discussed the presentations of the patients with the ICU doctors, who confirmed that prone positioning, which is lying the patients on their stomachs and not their backs, was helping.

On leaving the ICU, I thought I had done as much as I could. It was time to call in a team who could get a more detailed investigation under way. It was urgent that we get hold of the swabs from patient zero onwards to determine if it was the same virus in each of the other patients to work out the chains of transmission. I called Dr Richard Lessells, who is a first-rate UK-trained infectious diseases physician based at KRISP, and his boss, De Oliveira. The pair arrived about 40 minutes later and I handed the outbreak investigation over to them. They drew in Professor Yunus Moosa, the head of the Infectious Diseases Department at the Nelson Mandela Medical School. This was a top-notch threesome doing the outbreak investigation and they did an exceptional job.

A few weeks later, the report was ready.[2] Their investigation confirmed that the virus had spread from the traveller who came to the ER for a Covid-19 test to the elderly woman in the ER, as I had originally postulated during my walk-through, but their detailed analysis showed that 80 staff and a total of 39 patients were infected in at least five wards between 9 March and 30 April just in this one outbreak. There had been 12 deaths in these cases. And the outbreak hadn't ended there, and it led to an additional 21 cases in people outside the hospital. This included the four residents at the Durban nursing home for the elderly, along with 17 patients and staff at St Augustine's outpatient dialysis unit.

By the time of the report, approximately 4% of all staff being tested for SARS-CoV-2 were coming back positive. The infection then moved rapidly through the hospital since the first suspected case on 9 March. This was facilitated by the frequent shuffling of patients and health care workers between different wards. The evidence suggested that the virus was mainly spreading through direct contact between people and in a few cases possibly by touching contaminated surfaces. A few of the cases did not have proximity to an infected individual in hospital and were mostly likely infected through airborne transmission. The investigating team managed to get some of the positive swabs from patients and staff for genetic analysis. Through this, they were able to show that everyone had the same or very similar virus constituting a single cluster, supporting the contention that it was a single-source outbreak. The report is an exemplary example of how 'shoe leather' epidemiology – tracing the movements of each patient involved – can illuminate fundamental understandings of the virus. To this day, it is one of the most scientifically rigorous Covid-19 outbreak investigations that I have seen in South Africa.

The report also provided a list of opportunities that were missed to stop this outbreak. One of these opportunities was to create a process whereby patients would be separated out to reduce the risk of the virus spreading in hospitals. Before handing the investigation over to Lessells, I had taken the St Augustine's staff through the importance of identifying at-risk areas and then designating green, red and orange zones in the hospital. Green was for all those who screened negative at the entrance, while red was for those considered to be SARS-CoV-2 infected – referred to as patients under investigation. Orange would be a mixed zone. The hospital was quick to implement the process. Within a few days there was coloured tape on the floor demarcating the three zones. For me, this outbreak highlighted the ease and rapidity with which SARS-CoV-2 can spread through a hospital, requiring improved IPC measures. I came to see first-hand how nosocomial (originating in a hospital) transmission could be important for the virus spreading in South Africa.

The investigation report noted: 'There is no reason to believe that a similar outbreak cannot and will not happen in other hospitals and institutions in South Africa, in both the private and public sector.'[3] Unfortunately, this proved to be correct. Two of Durban's public hospitals – RK Khan Hospital in Chatsworth and Addington Hospital in central Durban – later reported having over 50 health care professionals, including nurses and doctors, infected with Covid-19.

This experience highlighted the often-hidden problem in nosocomial SARS-CoV-2 transmission – impact on staff. Nursing and cleaning staff were at risk of acquiring infection and, when they did, they exposed several of their colleagues either over lunch in the staff canteen or through carpooling. This meant that staff were confined to quarantine either from infection or from contact exposure just at the time that they were needed most in hospitals to deal with the multitude of Covid-19 cases. The enormity of this problem dawned as South Africa went into the first wave and a sizeable number of staff were in quarantine. It was during this wave that I learned my third lesson about Covid-19 patients.

Once again, my phone was the connecting point to the lesson. In early April I got a call from a prominent Durban businessman, who had picked up Covid-19 in the UK but was only diagnosed on his return to South Africa. He was looking for my advice because after quarantining for two weeks, he was still testing PCR positive. Another week passed and he still didn't have a negative result. He was growing concerned about exposing his family and didn't know what to do. Not exactly sure what was happening and if maybe it was a false positive, I arranged for him to come to CAPRISA, where we took a swab and a blood sample for antibodies. Our PCR test simply confirmed that now, a month after his initial diagnosis, he was indeed still PCR positive. This was both a mystery and surprise to me as it wasn't a phenomenon I had been expecting.

Shortly thereafter, while reading a report from South Korea, the light bulb went on in my brain. The report described over 100 patients who were still PCR positive three months after being diagnosed with Covid-19. The catch was that the virus in the tested swabs could not be grown in the laboratory. This can only mean that the person isn't actually infectious or capable of spreading the virus, but the sensitive nature of the test was picking up traces of the virus's RNA but not actual viable viruses in their body.

Unfortunately, this wasn't a test that we could run in the CAPRISA laboratory to see if the same was true of the businessman. We didn't have the ability to culture the virus at that time, meaning we wouldn't know if it was possible to grow it in a lab or not. So, I called Professor Penny Moore, one of our country's leading B-cell immunologists and a CAPRISA associate, to ask if she could measure the viral antibodies for this patient. She agreed without hesitation. It turned out that his antibody levels were quite low. But all was not lost. This provided us with a clue that his body was still actively trying to clear the virus out of his system, even if that hadn't been fully accomplished yet.

Since his immune system was producing antibodies against SARS-CoV-2, it was most likely that the antibodies were attaching to the virus and so the viruses that the PCR was picking up were most likely not alive. It meant that even though the PCR continued to come back positive, he was not likely to put anyone at risk of getting infected. We didn't know how long the possibly dead virus fragments would remain in his system, but it seemed safe for him to exit isolation and go back to his family. It was only several weeks later that he finally tested negative. This was one of the first curveballs I encountered with the virus – seeing how widely its presentation could differ from person to person. Monitoring that case for so long helped me to understand that Covid-19 is not simply a two-week acute illness. Instead, I realised that a person could potentially be sick for months – and that in these cases, the viruses being shed are not viable. In this case, that person didn't need to be in quarantine for months at a time.

Fear of the unknown shouldn't fly in the face of logic. That is what each of these three cases taught me. Covid-19 came with many unknowns and people were scared and worried enough about being infected with the virus without having to deal with additional obstacles – whether that be health care professionals being too afraid to interact with patients, hospitals not being ready to reduce the risk of the virus spreading, or keeping people separated from their loved ones when they didn't pose a threat.

Behind the bluster of facts and evidence, each Covid-19 case was also a person. They weren't just a number but someone who had family or loved ones or others who depended on them. Each infection came with consequences and a knock-on effect that was unimaginable to me. It was something I would become all too familiar with very soon.

CHAPTER 6

Not just a disease – an upheaval

Not only is Covid-19 a deadly serious disease,
but it had profound social consequences.
Nobody can come anywhere near you. You die alone.

It was easy to look at this virus through statistics and scientific analyses. Yet, there were more personal elements to a pandemic that no journal article or data point would ever be able to convey. I had been reading voraciously to understand as much about Covid-19 as possible. But this virus held many secrets and surprises that were not evident or obvious in any journal article or any statistical data. Nothing prepared me for the experience of the virus's deadly force hitting so close to home when two close friends got Covid-19.

Professor Peter Piot is one of the world's foremost experts on viral epidemics. Referred to as a 'rock-star virologist' by the *Financial Times*,[1] Piot co-discovered the Ebola virus and had served as the founding director of UNAIDS. Shortly after retiring as head of the London School of Hygiene & Tropical Medicine (LSHTM) in 2020, he was appointed coronavirus adviser to the European Commission president, Ursula von der Leyen. While Piot had spent his life fighting viruses, it was SARS-CoV-2 that finally caught up with him, infecting him in mid-March 2020. The way in which Piot's experience with Covid-19 unfolded revealed yet more secrets hidden by the virus. Piot, aged 71, had no other comorbidities, yet he found he simply couldn't shake the illness. He was hospitalised for a week and although he eventually recovered and tested negative for Covid-19, some of his symptoms lingered. Shortly after he'd been discharged from hospital and returned home, Quarraisha and I called him. We spoke at length to his partner, Dr Heidi Larson, who is a world-renowned expert on vaccine hesitancy. She described how Piot struggled for weeks to regain his strength and energy.

What Piot's illness suggested, and was subsequently confirmed more than a year later through the study of other similar and more recent cases, was that Covid-19 can precipitate a debilitating condition among certain patients known as 'Long Covid'. In these patients, symptoms such as malaise, fatigue and lack of concentration can persist for many months after the usual recovery period and affect quality of life. In Piot's case, it was seven weeks before he began to feel 'more or less in shape'. Through Piot's experience, I got to understand much more clearly that this virus was not simply an acute respiratory illness – it caused both acute and chronic illnesses that affected not just the lungs but almost every system within the human body, with heart disease being particularly prominent. Even more, I got to understand the suffering, the torment and the daily challenge of living with the long-term consequences of this viral infection.

Several months later, on 28 October 2020, Quarraisha and I shared a platform with Piot on a Gairdner Global Perspectives panel discussing the Sustainable Development Goals and global health through the lens of Covid-19. During this presentation, Piot explained how he suffered 'months of exhaustion, interstitial pneumonia and cardiac problems' in the wake of his infection. It was for this reason that he argued against a mitigation strategy based on herd immunity. As he noted in the Gairdner discussion, not only can Covid-19 place a burden on the individual who contracts it, it also has major public health ramifications, placing a burden on national health systems. This was, quite simply, not just another form of influenza. If even those who experienced a mild infection might still go on to suffer Long Covid, then it was better to avoid getting the disease altogether.

Piot's experience and his telling of it was another lesson for me in my journey towards the realisation that Covid-19 was not the kind of disease anyone should be wishing for, however facetiously. Right up to mid-February, my attitude towards the virus had been, I'm sad to say, more flippant. Like many people around the world, for me coming to terms with the seriousness of Covid-19 and perceiving it as more than 'just a kind of flu' was a shamefully slow process. I even remember jokingly saying to Quarraisha and some of my other colleagues early in the year, before Covid-19 had officially arrived in South Africa, that it might be good to 'get it over and done with'. At least if I contracted it early, there would be ventilators available in the event that I needed oxygen. That was more or less what I said. But the gravity of the situation was becoming unavoidable.

Unbeknown to us at the time, in March 2020 Piot had met with my close friend and colleague Dr Gita Ramjee, while they were both in London. I had known Gita for over 26 years and had recruited her into the MRC in 1996. She had been involved in almost every major HIV-prevention trial on microbicides and her determination, tenacity and commitment to improving the health of women was unwavering. On the last day of March 2020, Ramjee, then chief scientist at the Aurum Institute, died from complications arising from Covid-19. She was 63 years old. On the day of her death, the Health Department reported that confirmed Covid-19 cases in South Africa stood at 1 395 and the official number of deaths was five. Her death, which would have been among the following day's tally, might have been the sixth.

She was the first person I knew personally to die of Covid-19 – and her death came with some harsh truths.[2] Before that moment, I had not fully appreciated the potential deadliness of the disease. Ramjee's death made the grim reality of this disease personal. Her passing was a tragic wake-up call. Not only had she paid the ultimate sacrifice with her life, but she had suffered her final days in hospital in isolation and had died without the comfort of loved ones. It was not the kind of end I would wish for anyone, let alone a dear friend.

The last time I had spoken to her was in February. She was due to fly to Boston in the US to attend the annual Conference on Retroviruses and Opportunistic Infections – better known by its many regular attendees as

CROI – which was to be held over three days in early March. Given the number of coronavirus-related infections being reported in New York at the time, I was supportive of her decision to fly via London – where her sons and grandson were based – rather than New York, which was the usual route to Boston from South Africa.

As it happened, once she arrived in London, she was informed that her connecting flight to Boston had been cancelled owing to Covid-19 travel restrictions and that the main CROI meeting had been moved online. She was happy to stay on in London visiting her family for a few days. During this time, she also visited some of her colleagues at the LSHTM, where she held an honorary professorship. On 17 March, shortly after her return to South Africa, she delivered an online lecture to the LSHTM on HIV challenges among women and children. Soon after, she fell ill and was diagnosed with Covid-19.

I was told she was in Umhlanga Hospital, just outside the city, and I wasted no time in phoning the hospital to confirm that she was still there. A hospital staff member told me she was in ICU and my intention was to visit her as soon as possible. However, when I announced that I would be coming around shortly, I was told in no uncertain terms that visitors were not allowed. 'But I am a doctor – Professor Abdool Karim,' I said. My words meant little and even though the hospital staff knew who I was, I still received clear instructions to stay away. No one from outside the hospital, whatever their title, status or expertise, was permitted to enter the building. I was rendered ineffectual.

The restrictions, even more painfully, also applied to Ramjee's husband, Pravin, a Durban-based pharmacist. While he had been able to spend a short time with Gita before her admission to ICU, once her condition worsened, he had to take his leave and enter quarantine himself as he had been exposed. And so, Ramjee died alone in the ICU. A couple of days later, her body was cremated without a single family member or friend being there to witness it or say a few words.

Soon after I learned that Ramjee had died, I called Pravin on his cell phone. Unable to reach him, I drove round to the family home. A domestic worker answered the door but refused to let me in because, she told me, Pravin was still in quarantine. She handed me a piece of paper with a number on it and told me to use it to call him. I stood outside and from somewhere inside the house, where he was holed up, forced to deal with his grief in isolation, Pravin answered. Over the phone but within metres of each other, I tried to offer some solace. Pravin was understandably distraught about his wife's death and traumatised by the way she had died without being surrounded by loved ones. To add to his trauma, Pravin's pharmacy had suffered a notable drop in customers owing to the stigma attached to Covid-19 during those early days. Nobody wanted to frequent the place for fear of picking up the deadly virus. I could hear the anguish in his voice.

During that call, we also discussed aspects of the funeral arrangements. Dr Fazel Randera, a fellow anti-apartheid activist, an ANC stalwart and a former commissioner of South Africa's Truth and Reconciliation Commission, had been in touch with me to say that the ANC, which is the political party in power in South Africa, wanted to host a memorial service for Ramjee, and he asked me to liaise with the family. At the end of our telephone conversation, Pravin asked for a specific favour. Protocol at that time demanded that anyone with Covid-19 or suspected of having it needed to have a Covid-19 exit test after the infection period to confirm that they were infection free. Pravin asked me to organise this for himself. He also wanted his domestic worker to be tested. I arranged it. The swabs were duly taken and analysed in the laboratory at CAPRISA, where we had set up a testing facility. The results from both Pravin and his helper came back negative – they could safely de-quarantine.

Ramjee's death and my involvement in it, however tangential, was a turning point: it helped me to understand the disease for what it was and to appreciate more fully its dire repercussions. After that, there was no more talk from me of throwing myself in the line of infection and 'getting it over with'. Her death had brought a prompt end to such foolishness.

Now, it was becoming increasingly clear that not only was this a deadly serious disease, but it had profound social consequences. If you get this disease, it is like you are like a leper, I thought. Nobody can come anywhere near you. You die alone and people cannot even come to your funeral.

This was not just a disease; this was an upheaval.

CHAPTER 7

Making a plan

Public health action sometimes has to be taken even when evidence is incomplete, as exemplified by John Snow's removal of the handle of the Broad Street pump during the 1846 cholera pandemic.

Reeling from the upheaval being caused by Covid-19 as it impacted on someone close to me, I was now even more determined to do better in preventing infections. No one should have to go through what I had just seen. I redoubled my efforts to do my best to keep South Africans safe in the midst of this pandemic. The hot-button issue of the moment was whether people should be wearing masks to help reduce their risk of getting or spreading the virus.

There was a lot of debate around adopting a measure that had little evidence behind it. Mask-wearing – like many other measures at that time – had not yet been studied in this context. The other concern reigning at that time was that if there was a rush on medical-grade masks by the public, then those most in need, the health care workers, would run out of supply. In that situation, were there any other alternatives that could be offered? South Africa also had an extra layer to its argument in trying to find an option that would be easily accessible and affordable to everyone in the country. But soon masks would be lifted out of a purely scientific debate and cast into the political arena.

In South Africa, Health Minister Zweli Mkhize publicly endorsed the wearing of cloth masks on 1 April 2020 when he said they represented 'one of the best ways of preventing the spread of infection' and recommended them for people with symptoms of Covid-19 or where social distancing was difficult.[1] By then, the MAC had not yet provided any advice or guidance on masks and masks hadn't been endorsed yet by the WHO.

A day later, the US CDC recommended the use of non-medical masks for all members of the public – a reversal of their original advice, which was that healthy people did not need to wear them. At this stage, it was becoming clearer to scientists around the world that many of those responsible for transmitting the virus in the US were in fact asymptomatic and that masks could possibly serve as a partial barrier to transmission in public.

When he announced the CDC's recommendation at his press briefing the next day, on 3 April, President Trump took pains to emphasise that the recommendation was purely voluntary. He did not himself wear a mask during most of the event, thereby undermining the CDC's recommendation. It got worse. In that press conference, he announced that he personally would not be complying with the recommendation. He gave no real reason except that he was exercising his right not to wear a mask. In that moment, the face mask moved from being one part of a prevention toolkit against Covid-19 to being a political symbol in what was then an increasingly partisan political landscape in the US.

The MAC had been mulling over the issue of masks since its inception but had yet to reach a consensus on the complex question. For a group tasked with presenting evidence-based advice, the somewhat sketchy science behind masks was throwing us for a loop. At this stage, there was no support for general non-medical mask-wearing from the WHO, but we still felt it was necessary to investigate the matter thoroughly. If we were going to deviate from the WHO guidance, then we should have good grounds to do so.

In much of East Asia, particularly since the outbreak of SARS in 2002, masks are seen as a routine means to protect oneself but also, importantly, to prevent the transmission of influenza and other diseases to others. They are also often used to protect oneself from air pollution. On my part, a nagging question was why Southeast Asian countries were not being impacted on by Covid-19 like the rest of the world. Was it their routine use of masks when a person has a respiratory illness? I wondered. I thought that it could not be a coincidence that cities like Hong Kong and Singapore as well as countries such as Japan and Taiwan, which had managed to contain the virus during their first waves, had also donned masks early. In South Africa, however, mask-wearing as a means to avoid spreading any kind of disease was almost unheard of.

I personally felt that there are times when we have to act in the interest of public health, even in the face of incomplete evidence. The first example of this course of action comes from one of the founding fathers of public health, Dr John Snow. Eight years into the cholera pandemic of 1846 to 1860, several cases of the illness occurred near Broad Street in the Soho district of the City of Westminster, London, England. This preceded 'germ theory' as a cause of disease, and at that time it was not known that bacteria in the water caused cholera. John Snow had mapped out the cases in the Broad Street area and came to the conclusion that the pump was involved,[2] even though his evidence was not watertight. In order to stop the disease from spreading, he had the handle of the Broad Street pump removed. While few believed him, the move by Snow effectively ended Soho's cholera outbreak. This historical example is taught to all students of public health to exemplify the need to take public health action even if the evidence is incomplete. Even though I subscribed to this approach, I had a somewhat higher bar for the evidence needed for action than that set in 1854 by John Snow. And the information behind masks just wasn't there yet.

As the MAC continued to delve into the issue, I received a timely message from Professor Max Price, a public health doctor and former vice-chancellor of the University of Cape Town, asking whether we would be making a recommendation on the topic soon. He was strongly in favour of masks. I felt that he could make a valuable contribution to the work of the MAC in this area. The only problem was that we did not have a mechanism to involve non-MAC members in the MAC activities. With the assistance of the MAC secretariat, I established a working group on masks to accommodate views on the subject from Price and other experts who were not officially part of the MAC. The thinking was that masks could help to prevent the spread of respiratory or smaller aerosol droplets, which are released by people when they talk, cough or sneeze. It might also serve as a reminder to the wearer not to touch their face and risk contamination through contact of the hands with the mouth, nose or eyes. Price argued cogently for the use of masks, but MAC members fell on both sides of this debate. The MAC's in-house expert on masks for infection control was Professor Shaheen Mehtar. She is an infection prevention and control specialist and served as chair of the Infection Control Africa Network, in which capacity she also served on the WHO committee reviewing the evidence on masks. We were fortunate to have someone from the MAC right at the heart of where the masks debates were occurring in the WHO. She was cautious about masks initially but played a key role in the advisory that recommended masks. Opinions in the MAC were quite varied, showing views on both ends of the spectrum as a result of the lack of clear or compelling evidence for masks.

If the MAC was to support the idea of masks, we felt they would have to be cloth masks because all supplies of medical masks available in the country were desperately needed by health care workers, and worldwide demand for medical masks had placed a premium on them. But how effective were cloth masks? A 2015 Vietnam study published in the *British Medical Journal* showed that cloth masks were substantially inferior to medical masks in the protection they offered, and in some cases, as they dampened with prolonged use, could arguably be worse than wearing nothing.[3] Under those circumstances, was it wise to promote them? And would South Africans agree to wear them?

Days went by and still no final decision had been reached in the MAC. We were missing a piece of the puzzle, something that would give us an evidence-based nudge. It came in the form of a scientific paper titled 'Respiratory virus shedding in exhaled breath and efficacy of face masks' published in *Nature Medicine* on 3 April 2020.[4] The three-year study on the impact of masks in influenza prevention involved 246 patients in a Hong Kong hospital and, by coincidence, included patients who had been admitted with SARS-CoV-2 infection. It showed that face masks significantly reduced the detection of coronavirus in the exhaled breath of Covid-19 patients. While 30% to 40% of 10 patients without masks had coronavirus in their exhaled breath, none of the 11 Covid-19 patients with masks had coronavirus in their exhaled breath. Through lowered amounts of exhaled coronavirus, wearing a mask should reduce the spread of the virus from individuals with the virus. The masks also reduced exhaled influenza virus, though to a lesser extent.

As soon as I saw that paper, I knew that we could now more confidently take a position – even one that was not supported by the WHO. That same day, I sat down and knocked out the draft advisory, which was then sent to all the MAC members for their comments. The advisory was finalised and submitted to the Department of Health six days later, on 9 April. Mkhize wasted no time; at his daily briefing the following day, he made the announcement that everybody should acquire cloth masks but emphasised that it was another tool in the existing anti-Covid-19 toolkit to be used together with – and not instead of – handwashing, sanitising and social distancing.

The wearing of masks in public became mandatory (as opposed to recommended) in South Africa on 1 May 2020 as the country moved into Level 4 lockdown. By that stage, most South Africans were wearing them anyway and there was a high level of compliance. Thankfully, none of the politics attached to masks that was building in the US seemed to be evident in South Africa, though Twitter (a platform I was now forcibly becoming more familiar with) had lots of comments about masks being part of our government's strategy to control the people, a grouping that unfortunately only became more vocal as the lockdown measures continued, in spite of the growing evidence. But here, once again, comes a lesson from John Snow. In the face of constant naysayers, Snow continued to stand his ground and compile more data around the water contamination.

Our early uptake of masks in South Africa was vindicated about two months later when, in early June 2020, the WHO updated its guidance to recommend that governments ask everyone to wear cloth face masks in public. Since our recommendation, evidence had continued to grow to support their use. In 2022, a meta-analysis of over 20 million people, covering 92 regions across six continents, was published in the *Proceedings of the National Academy of Science*,[5] showing that masks had reduced the transmission of SARS-CoV-2 by 19% overall, providing some of the most compelling evidence that masks did work in preventing the spread of SARS-CoV-2. I believe that the use of masks made a vital contribution to the suppression of Covid-19 spread in South Africa and I am proud of the MAC's role in providing this advice in the face of uncertain evidence. Sometimes it is worth it to be less stringent in the call for evidence if it means saving lives, which I have no doubt we did. Still, there would be many more hard calls to make in the future and the MAC still had a lot more to do.

On the day that the MAC's advisory on masks was finalised and submitted, I received a message from the Minister of Health's office. They asked me to do a short presentation with the latest information on Covid-19. I wasted no time in preparing some slides that afternoon and was ready to do a presentation by the evening.

By the end of my preparation, it turned out to be a bit more than just a simple update. I felt it was important to not just talk about the virus on its own but also put forth some ideas for how South Africa could deal with Covid-19 more comprehensively. In any situation of uncertainty or where the challenges are significant, people tend to ask: 'What's the plan?' It was clear to me that the South African public needed to know what the plan for Covid-19 was. So, I proceeded to develop and explain an eight-stage national Covid-19 response plan.[6] Many of its measures – certainly the first four stages – were already being implemented.

Stage 1 was 'Preparation' and included community education, the setting up of laboratory capacity, and surveillance. Stage 2 was 'Primary prevention' and included the implementation of measures such as handwashing and social distancing, the closure of schools, reduction of gatherings and closing of borders. Stage 3 was 'Lockdown', which involved intensifying the curtailment of human interaction so everyone who was infected became a 'dead end', unable to pass on the virus. Stage 4 was 'Surveillance and active case finding'. This was a unique component of the South African response and was far more proactive than many other countries' responses. Already, the Department of Health had despatched 28 000 community health care workers who were going door to door in vulnerable communities screening and testing for cases.

Stage 5 was the 'Identification of hotspots', to look at where cases were occurring at a rate that was higher than expected. Stage 6 was 'Medical care for the peak', including monitoring the case load and capacity; managing staff exposures and infections; building field hospitals for triage; and expanding ICU bed numbers, ventilators and oxygen supply. Stage 6 was the subject of particularly intensive planning on the part of the government and medical personnel. We were concerned, for instance, not only about the capacity of our health care systems but also about equitable access to health care facilities. This was motivated by the disappointing picture coming out of the US, which showed the disproportionate burden of disease among black and Hispanic people, who had less access to quality health care. We were also concerned about what Covid-19 might mean for the 2.5 million South Africans living with HIV but not on treatment, as well as those with TB. We were also aware of the fact that the Covid-19 pandemic peak in South Africa was likely to coincide with the annual influenza season, which might mount an even bigger health care challenge than expected. This convergence of factors meant that health care facilities had to be ready to provide equitable access to services when the wave was at its highest point.

Stage 7 was 'Bereavements and aftermath', which included expanding burial capacity, regulations on funerals, and managing psychological and social impacts of the pandemic. Stage 8 was called 'Ongoing vigilance'. I illustrated the need for vigilance through a graphic of firefighters putting out small forest fires in order to avoid a raging inferno. This stage included a range of measures to ensure that we stayed one step ahead of the virus.

This Covid-19 plan slide took quite a while to prepare, but I felt it was time well spent as it drew upon the available evidence and dealt with

South Africa's unique challenges. I sent it off to some colleagues for their comments and feedback – it received strong support. I was particularly reassured when Yogan Pillay wrote back saying that he supported this approach. Putting this slide to bed was key, as it then allowed me to focus on what I needed to include in the update that the minister's office requested.

I knew I needed to make a slide-set that was not academic, but just the use of slides in the first place made it more like an academic lecture than a lay presentation. However, slides help to graphically illustrate the point being made verbally and so I seldom do presentations without slides. The way to do a non-academic presentation with slides is to ensure that the slides are not too technical but provide the available scientific information simply with just key words and easy-to-interpret graphics. After all, I was trying to ensure that everyone listening would be able to understand the pandemic. This would not be an easy task and so I settled down to some hard work on preparing a slide-set that would be *educational* without being too technical, *enlightening* without getting bogged down in the details, and *forward-looking* without sugar-coating what lay in store.

CHAPTER 8

'Next slide!'

Even with over 20 000 Twitter followers, I remain hesitant about social media. Regardless, I put my slides there because I felt that people should have access to the information to help them make their own decisions.

'*Prof Karim*' was trending on Twitter on the evening of Monday, 13 April 2020, and for part of the following day. Overnight, I had become a household name and the public face of the South African Covid-19 response. Over the following several months I faced an unprecedented and sustained surge in interest in my knowledge and views on Covid-19. It transformed my life.

I learned that my name was trending from my eldest daughter Safura. She and her two siblings Aisha and Wasim – all of them digital natives – had been back in the family home in Durban since just before the start of the stay-at-home lockdown. Now they were excitedly awaiting my return from the National Command Centre where I had taken part in a two-hour live prime time television briefing on Covid-19. My children seemed to think the Twitter issue was a big deal. Not being a social media user myself and entirely unversed in the terminology that goes with it, my bemused retort to their enthusiasm was: 'Trending? No, no … I'm just wearing my usual clothes …' Needless to say, I had to put up with more than a little eye-rolling.

Looking back, that minor linguistic mix-up was a signal not only of my ignorance about social media; it presaged a bigger failure to fully grasp the significance of my presentation in the hearts and minds of a South African public that was becoming increasingly anxious and impatient after 18 days of the stay-at-home lockdown, especially since they had just received news that the lockdown was to be extended by a further two weeks. When the stay-at-home lockdown was first announced by the President on 23 March and implemented three days later, people had, by and large, accepted the need for the nationwide lockdown and were generally supportive of the government's decision to impose it.

Many had watched the chaos and devastation the virus had wrought in Europe earlier in the year, especially in Italy, and were now following its early impact in the US. People were justifiably fearful. If first-world countries struggled to manage the virus, how would South Africa cope? Health care facilities in South Africa were struggling to cope before Covid-19, corruption and incompetence was rife, poverty was endemic and existing disease burdens were high – it didn't seem like we had a strong defence.

However, after almost three of weeks of being confined to our homes and in the wake of the recent extension, attitudes towards the restrictions were starting to shift, and uncertainty, doubt and frustration were creeping in. Where was this deadly virus? Did it warrant such drastic action? And how long were people expected to put their lives and livelihoods on hold for something they couldn't even see?

When they tuned in at 7pm on Easter Monday 2020 for a briefing on the 'Technical aspects of Covid-19', hosted by the Minister of Health, South Africans were looking for answers.[1] The time was ripe. If my presentation had come a week or two earlier, or a week or two later, it might not have had the same impact. But at that moment, people had a pressing need to know what was going on. Importantly, as it turned out, they also needed to know that those in charge had someone who knew what was going on, and that decisions were not being made without good reason.

To his credit, President Cyril Ramaphosa recognised this state of play when he asked me to address the South African public and told the Health minister to organise this via a live TV broadcast to take place that evening. 'Everyone deserves to hear this,' he told me after I had given him a version of my presentation earlier in the day in an online link-up to Pretoria.

That my presentation hit the mark with the public was partly because of the extraordinary process behind its compilation. It was the product of a rapid series of revisions, refinements and improvements over the course of a frenetic four-day period, during which time I delivered the presentation six times in total – four times in various high-level government forums, once to President Cyril Ramaphosa, and eventually to the South African public live on television.

All sessions were conducted online but that didn't render the episode any less intense. It was a highly pressured experience. Each time I completed one presentation, it would be followed by questions from those to whom it was presented. This kept me on my toes and helped to identify gaps in the information and guide the process of honing the contents of the PowerPoint slides. The end result was that each presentation was better than the last.

The first four presentations were conducted from my home office, which I had set up in a section of my living room during lockdown. We have an open-plan set-up, so the sound of me in a virtual meeting tends to carry beyond the vicinity of my desk. This only became fully obvious to me when my family members told me that the Easter weekend of April 2020 will forever be associated with the sound of me calling out two short words: 'Next slide!' In many of the presentations I gave that Easter weekend, I had no control over the slides; there was a third party involved in moving the slides along in tandem with my commentary. So, at home and even beyond, 'Next slide!' came to capture the prevailing zeitgeist.

The first iteration of the slide show was delivered to Health Minister Zweli Mkhize, Deputy Health Minister Joe Phaahla, and Acting DG Anban Pillay on Thursday, 9 April. Given the make-up of the audience, it didn't need to be particularly lengthy and comprised only three or four key slides depicting trends in the epidemic. After that, the minister asked me if I was available to participate in a Zoom meeting to brief the Parliamentary Portfolio Committee on Health the following evening. The briefing was aimed at reflecting the progress the department was making in dealing with Covid-19 in the midst of the stay-at-home lockdown. My task was to provide an update on the state of the pandemic and, as expected, the minister asked me to prepare a few slides. Because it was the Easter weekend and I did not want to take away the first real break that the MAC members had, I didn't feel it would be appropriate to call yet another emergency MAC meeting just for a presentation and so I proceeded to develop the presentation, consulting some of the MAC members as I went along.

I got to work, drawing on my CAPRISA colleague Dr Cheryl Baxter, a senior scientist in my office who is an ace at making graphic slides. She collated updated data and graphics and put together some more slides, which I believed contained relevant information and captured the trends and trajectory of the pandemic. I recruited Quarraisha to help me with the slides as the task needed more time than I had. Quarraisha makes great slides as well and she knows that I take a lot of pride in my PowerPoint presentations, which are usually an essential part of the lectures and papers I am invited to deliver around the world. I find the combination of graphics and illustrations, graphs and text in bullet points very useful to any audience trying to understand complex scientific concepts. Each element on a slide has to be chosen or designed very carefully to achieve maximum clarity. Also critical is the sequence of the slides as they need to flow and build up the story in layers. The collection of slides Quarraisha and I put together for the Portfolio Committee was specifically tailored to their needs – a somewhat technical affair containing statistics about local, regional and global infections; figures on contact tracing in South Africa; hospitalisation and testing; and hospital preparedness and mortuary capacity. I recently saw that the original PowerPoint presentation – all 35 slides – is still on the Parliamentary Monitoring Group website.

The meeting was attended by provincial Health ministers (referred to as MECs) along with their heads of department (HODs). The interim head of the NICD, Professor Lynn Morris, was present. A long-standing colleague who is a leading researcher in reproductive health, Professor

Helen Rees, was attending in her capacity as board chair of the South African Health Products Regulatory Authority (SAHPRA). There were also journalists also in attendance.

At the end, I was struck by how much the members of the Portfolio Committee seemed to appreciate the input, how engaged they seemed to be with its contents and the extent of their questions. It occurred to me, based on their feedback, that there were still some gaps in the general understanding of the pandemic. It also occurred to me that there were too few people out there with the requisite expertise who were taking the time to describe the global pandemic in any detail and explain where our country stood in relation to it.

Following the Portfolio Committee briefing, the minister asked me to present to two more government bodies the following day: the National Joint Operational and Intelligence Structure, commonly referred to as NATJOINTS; and the social services cluster ministers. Naturally, I agreed, and got back to fine-tuning my slides, adding more information. I had decided that if people really wanted to understand the epidemic, a few more details would not go amiss.

Chaired at the time by Secretary of Defence Dr Sam Gulube, whom I knew from his days at the MRC, NATJOINTS is the national co-ordinating structure of the country's security and law enforcement groups. When Covid-19 struck, it was tasked with co-ordinating the government's daily response to Covid-19. There were about 40 people on the NATJOINTS call. The committee has its own protected non-commercial software, known as TE Desktop, for video-conference calls, and it is highly secure. I couldn't actually tell the identity of all of the attendees, but I remember noticing National Prosecuting Authority head Advocate Shamila Batohi and the head of the South African Revenue Service (SARS), Edward Kieswetter, among the participants.

At the end of my presentations, there were again many questions, which I dealt with systematically. When the DG of the Department of Science and Innovation, Dr Phil Mjwara, indicated he had a question and then proceeded to ask why his department's logo was not on the slide alongside that of the Department of Health, I took this as a sign that he recognised the worth of my slide show, that it was likely to be widely viewed, and he wanted to capitalise on the visibility it offered to the relevant government departments.

NATJOINTS members declared themselves to have gained a firmer grasp on the epidemic, which was precisely the intention. I used their questions after the call ended to identify areas where I needed to be more expansive or, conversely, more precise or concise. In the end, the overall presentation became slightly shorter. I applied the same process of revision when I presented it later that same day to social cluster services ministers, who fall within the health sector, using the useful feedback I'd received to make further refinements.

The next day was Easter Sunday, and it came with a welcome brief hiatus in the presentation circuit. But the frenetic pace of that Easter weekend was far from over. On the morning of Easter Monday, I received a message from the Health minister's chief of staff, Advocate Sibusisiwe Ngubane Zulu, to say the minister wanted me to make another presentation – this time to President Ramaphosa. 'At the command centre,' she said. Zulu is a senior lawyer and had even served as a judge; it was not surprising that she had an air of authority about her.

'Yes, sure,' was my response, 'but how?' My first thought was that I would have to travel up to Pretoria, where I understood the National Command Centre to be. But during the stay-at-home lockdown, travel by air had been shut down and I wondered if it meant an impromptu road trip. Zulu explained that there was a command centre in Durban, actually in Sydenham, about five minutes from my home. Mkhize was already there waiting for me. I grabbed my laptop and off I went.

The command centre is a massive military complex. I wasn't aware of its existence until that Monday, but I had no trouble locating it. I was ushered into one of the boardrooms, where Mkhize was waiting. He told me I would be presenting to the President at midday for about 15 to 20 minutes. I realised my 30-odd slide show was far too long for that time frame and that it would have to be reduced to around 12 slides.

Again, I got to work, selecting those slides I thought most relevant and best captured the situation in South Africa at that time.

Once they were ready, the slides first had to be sent to the President so that he could view them as I spoke to them on our call using TE Desktop software. Again, someone at the other end would be controlling them. The trouble with that military building was that, once inside, there was no cell phone signal and sending data electronically was not a simple matter. Eventually, we were set up and at noon, as scheduled, I delivered a 20-minute presentation to President Ramaphosa. When I had finished, he asked a few questions. Then he said I needed to make the presentation again, this time to members of the National Coronavirus Command Council – which comprised members of the cabinet who were in charge of the government's Covid-19 response.

Of course, I agreed, but suggested that a more detailed presentation might be more useful for people to understand the full picture. It was then that the President said that the South African public also deserved to see the presentation straight after the command council. I was impressed by his overall approach and was ready to proceed. However, I suggested to Mkhize that a public presentation would benefit from the participation of three experts to comment on my presentation and provide different scientific perspectives to mine. I explained that in science, contestation about what the evidence is indicating can vary and that it is important to get multiple views. Hearing the comments of other experts would give the public a better understanding of what was or wasn't being contested in our understanding of the pandemic. He liked this approach.

It took me only a moment to come up with three suggestions. I knew that I needed to identify individuals who were accomplished scientists, would know the epidemic in South Africa well enough to comment at short notice and would not hesitate to share their interpretations and views of the epidemic, even if they differed from mine. I suggested Professors Koleka Mlisana, Glenda Gray and Brian Williams. Mlisana was the first choice because she had a thorough grasp of daily Covid-19 testing and cases as head of research at the NHLS, Gray for her knowledge of viral transmission and vaccines and Williams, a South African epidemiologist based in Geneva, for his international perspective. Both Mlisana and Gray were also members of the MAC. Williams is one of the world's leading authorities on infectious disease mathematical modelling and an expert on epidemics from his role at the WHO's tuberculosis control programme until his recent retirement. I knew I could call on him at a few hours' notice because we were in regular contact. When I am in Geneva to chair a WHO Scientific Advisory Committee or a UNAIDS Scientific Expert meeting, I usually have dinner with Williams and his wife, Dr Eleanor Gouws, who was my PhD student and is now a senior statistician and project officer at UNAIDS. Williams and I have had some fierce debates on epidemic control during those dinners, while Gouws is at pains not to take sides.

I quickly shot off an email to each of them, asking if they could be available for a televised Zoom video conference at 7pm, after which they would be required to comment for about five minutes on my presentation. I followed up my emails by calling each of them (standing in the garden to get cell phone signal) to confirm their availability and to explain the format of the media briefing. Because it was a live broadcast, there was no room for any mistakes. All three of them were happy with the arrangements but, understandably, said they needed to see a copy of my slides beforehand. I quickly got down to work on a revised set of slides. By now it was around 1pm and I had about two hours before I was to brief the command council.

I was so caught up in the process, I didn't eat lunch. That is unusual for me as I prefer to eat at mealtimes to avoid snacking. The minister's lunch had been prearranged and was brought in for him. No meal had been prepared for me – my presence was unexpected, at least by his staff. They offered to go out and buy something for me, but I was too busy to eat.

My 3pm appointment with the National Coronavirus Command Council came around quickly. In total, my presentation to them took about 45 minutes and I became concerned that it was far too long for a television briefing. I would have to relook at the slide collection – again.

After my presentation, the questions from the command council were coming in thick and fast and I was running on pure adrenalin. I was writing so fast that my index finger was starting to ache – I have a habit of writing down an abbreviated form of each and every question with the name of the person asking it so that my response can be directed appropriately.

The question-and-answer session lasted for over an hour and ranged from queries about bat coronaviruses to diagnostics and testing. I was kept on my toes. I was struck by the strong engagement in the process. I felt I had to do my best to help all of them understand the epidemic as deeply as possible in the time we had. There was strong support in the command council for the public broadcast.

My part of their meeting ended at around 5pm. By this time, I was seriously flagging. I left the building to phone Quarraisha and asked for help. 'I'm going on live TV soon, I still have quite a bit to do, and I am hungry – I need your help,' I said. 'And please bring me a jacket and tie.'

While I waited for Quarraisha, I popped my head into the main venue at the command centre, from where I was told the broadcast would take place. It was a huge and daunting space with multiple television screens along the walls and three big screens in front. As I exited the hall, I was very happy to see Quarraisha and gratefully took a few minutes to eat the roti-and-curry rolls she had brought with her. With no time to waste, I then worked on the slides with Quarraisha's help. I then sent the new version to Mlisana, Gray and Williams and followed up with an email to check that they had the slides and would be ready to comment later that evening. In response to their queries, I made a few more changes to the presentation for clarification.

At around 6.55pm, the slide show, officially titled 'SA's Covid-19 Epidemic: Trends and Next Steps', was ready in its seventh iteration and I was feeling confident that it was probably the best version of itself. Almost every slide had been edited multiple times to make each one easy to follow and understand. I had split it into two parts – Part 1 was on 'The Coronavirus Pandemic' and Part 2 was on 'South Africa's Covid-19

Response'. It now comprised 34 slides and it followed my standard format, which meant that the presentation starts by outlining what I am going to say, then proceeding to say it with the supporting data, and ending off with a concluding slide that summarises what I have just said, so that the take-home messages are clear. All my talks follow this format – I find that it makes it easier for the audience to follow if they have an outline up front and then know where I am in the sequence that I am covering in my presentation.

Since the chief of staff, Sibusisiwe Zulu, was going to manage the Zoom aspect of the presentation, it was time to send the file to her. It was her responsibility to control the slides, in sync with my verbal explanations. Sending the presentation to Zulu seemed to take forever. I went back into the garden outside to get a stronger signal to speed up the process. We were running out of time. Eventually, it went through. I shut down my computer and hurried off to my designated seat in the main command centre venue, next to Mkhize. Ms Nomagugu Simelane-Zulu, the KwaZulu-Natal MEC for Health, was seated on his other side.

The room was packed with reporters and three national news television crews: SABC, eNCA and Newzroom Afrika. Even though they were socially distanced, it still seemed like a lot of people. The Government Communication Information System had sent out a media advisory earlier in the day, announcing the public briefing, and interest was clearly high.

During the entire episode, Zulu had been a model of calm and efficiency. I had been consistently impressed by her ability to handle the pressure of putting the briefing together and dealing with the technological challenges it presented. However, just at the point at which the Zoom meeting was due to begin, she came up against an unforeseen hurdle: the online meeting was oversubscribed. It could only accommodate 500 and, by the time we were ready to start, the three experts scheduled to comment were outside in the virtual waiting room unable to enter the meeting.

I thought that we should start on time and figure out how to bring them into the Zoom while the presentation was under way, but Zulu was having none of it. She announced to everyone that she was going to cancel the Zoom meeting and reopen it afresh, so all participants would need to log on again. At this point, Quarraisha was sitting next to her. Her job was to help find the people who needed to be in the meeting and bring them in first. These included the three experts, but there were also some ministers and media representatives who needed to be given preference. Once that was done, the door was reopened, and we were quickly back at maximum participant capacity.

By now it was 7.25pm and we had lost almost half an hour, but Zulu was not showing any signs of stress. She proceeded in her systematic manner, and we kicked off at around 7.40pm with opening comments from Mkhize. He announced that the briefing would be an hour long. Then he continued, as he did every day, to provide the latest Covid-19 statistics. On that day, the number of positive cases in South Africa stood at 2 272, with 99 new cases in the last day. The death toll stood at 27, with two deaths occurring over the previous reporting period.

It was an important moment. Mkhize leaned over as he introduced me, handing the baton over – it was time to start my presentation, the first that I had ever done on national television. About 15 minutes into my presentation, our collective inexperience in using virtual conferencing platforms for events, and filming such events, tripped us up again. When I was on the 13th slide, the minister told me to stop. Seconds before, I had noticed Zulu gesticulating to the minister, but without understanding the problem, I had simply carried on. I later learned from Quarraisha that it had become evident to Zulu and to her, from comments in the chat section on Zoom and social media, that the TV cameras were trained directly on me rather than on the slides to which I was speaking. None of us at the venue, including the television crews, had realised this because we were literally surrounded by multiple screens showing us the slides. But it meant that despite my intermittent calls for 'Next slide!', a call to which Zulu was diligently responding, none of the slides were being seen by the audience watching on television at home or via social media sites.

After telling me to stop, Mkhize asked the TV crew to focus on the slides rather than the speaker … and then we started the slide presentation again from the beginning. By now I was extremely familiar with the material. It was the seventh time I had delivered some version of the presentation (excluding my having to repeat the first section of the final version) and I think I could have done it blindfolded. Based on years of experience, I usually have a good feel for the way a presentation is going and being received during delivery, and my assessment that evening was positive. Having said that, I must admit to being relieved when I reached the point at which I could hand over to the three experts for their comments. As I had expected, each of them made an important contribution. Their input gave me a short reprieve before I faced questions from the public.

The questions from the public and media were a mixed bag and largely reflected the genuine need for information. They included the value of wearing cloth masks; the government's strategy to deal with socio-economic fallout; protection of health care workers; testing; and possible reasons behind the South African epidemic's trajectory that was different from the UK. During question time, Quarraisha was still sitting with Zulu, where she was helping to screen the questions, select those that represented areas of high interest, and then pass them on to Zulu, who could then pose them to the panel in a structured way.

Mkhize finally closed the live briefing by describing it as an opportunity to provide 'a glimpse of the science' that the government is drawing upon. Being a medical doctor himself, Mkhize was at pains to emphasise the importance of evidence in assisting the government's response to Covid-19, and I think his leadership during the first year of the pandemic, notwithstanding the circumstances that later led to his resignation, helped to establish a healthy relationship between science and politics in South Africa. He respected scientists, even when they differed from him and openly challenged him.

At that point, it was around 10pm and I had been in the command centre in Sydenham for well on 12 hours. One final technological glitch still lay ahead. On some of the recordings available online, you view a recording of the event that shows me and the two ministers standing up with some relief from the main table where we had been seated for nearly two-and-a-half hours. I take off my jacket, glance at my watch and, forgetting that I am still wired up to the mic and unaware of the rolling cameras, I say: 'So much for the one-hour session!' It could have been worse, I suppose.

The adrenalin that had been sustaining me over the course of that day and the build-up to it started to drain away. I suddenly felt very tired and needed to get home for dinner and some rest. Several people stopped me on the way out to express their appreciation for the presentation but having engaged with the information so closely over the past weekend, I think I had lost some perspective and had little understanding of its import.

It was only on my arrival back home that I started to realise that the briefing had been a big hit. Safura excitedly showed me the deluge of tweets. People seemed genuinely grateful for my input. I was described as a 'national treasure' in several tweets. Judging by the comments, people seemed to have listened very carefully to what I said and absorbed it.

Safura said that if I didn't create my own Twitter account, someone else was going to set up a fake account in order to capitalise on all the traffic I was generating. It was all a bit much to think about at that late hour, but I gave her permission to set up a Twitter account on my behalf. It obtained a blue tick almost immediately, which I learned meant that it was authenticated, and overnight I attracted over 12 000 followers, with that figure rising quickly over the following day to reach 18 000 and over 20 000 a further day later.

My enduring suspicion of social media in all its forms is because I am cautious of free software – someone *is* paying. We are all aware that companies like Google, Facebook, Twitter and others sell their access to users and their user information to become some of the world's richest companies. It seems that many people are happy to give their personal information away freely to social media platforms. So, even though I was not keen on my personal information being in the hands of a social media platform – I capitulated and set up the Twitter account, but I drew the line when it came to Facebook. To this day, I still treat Twitter with a great deal of caution and only rarely do I ask my daughter to tweet on my behalf.

In any event, I was now on social media, and I made my first tweet that evening shortly after the account was created. It was fitting then that what I chose to share was the slide-set from my presentation – the slides were in high demand by media outlets and requests were coming in fast to both the Department of Health and my communications manager, Smita Maharaj. Clearly, the hours and numerous revisions that had gone into crafting each slide had paid off. I felt that people should have access to the information to help them make their own decisions. I went to bed that night exhausted and oblivious of the requests flooding my inbox, blissfully unaware of what this presentation had started.

CHAPTER 9

Knowledge is power

*Building on the inclusive approach, I set out to convey the idea that
all of us – black, white, old and young – were all facing this viral
threat; we were all in this together and a united response was
the best way forward.*

I had just completed the Easter weekend, which started out small by
giving an update to the Department of Health and ended on a bigger
stage, being broadcast live to the South African public simultaneously
on all three national news channels, radio and on social media. I had not
informed my CAPRISA staff about the series of presentations or the live
television briefing because they had taken place over the Easter weekend
and because things had moved so quickly. Regardless, almost all had
watched it on television. Early the next day, Smita Maharaj wasted no time
in getting me on the phone. She had been caught off guard when she had
seen me the previous evening alongside the minister in the live television
broadcast. Maharaj burst out, 'I am being inundated with requests from
local and international media for copies of your presentation and for
follow-up interviews. And this went on right through the night!'

Maharaj took on the complex task of finding a judicious approach to
dealing with the very long list of interview requests that simply kept on
coming over the following days, weeks and months. There were also invitations to participate in briefings and webinars. I quickly gave over the
decision-making to Maharaj, who is much better than I am at such matters and got into the habit of preparing for a typical day marked by radio
interviews in the mornings, webinars, MAC meetings and print media

interviews during working hours, and television interviews towards evening. The next day, it would begin all over again.

Before that eventful Easter weekend, I was already doing interviews for national television and radio on the issue of Covid-19. I had a regular evening slot on Newzroom Afrika, a five-minute update on Covid-19 every weekday. There had also been some interest from local and international print media before the virus was even reported in South Africa, but nothing could compare with the level of interest shown after the 13 April presentation.

Reports from media monitoring services provide some impression of the general tectonics: according to Newsclip, my overall clip print and broadcast count increased by 652% from 1 January to 30 September 2020 compared to 2 April to 30 December 2019. According to Meltwater, there were 2 246 articles in local online media and 1 104 articles in global online media between 1 January and 30 September 2020 that mentioned or featured me in some way. If this is averaged out, it translates to an online article every two hours over that nine-month period.

My pre-Covid-19 visibility as a scientist was already relatively high. In 2017, I was placed in a *South African Journal of Science* article among the top five of publicly visible scientists in South Africa as ranked by members of a science-media panel made up of journalists across all local media.[1] Now I also had a profile among ordinary members of the public. Often when I was out at the supermarket, at the petrol station filling up my car, or walking with Quarraisha along the Durban beachfront, people would recognise me, even though I was wearing a face mask – and often a baseball cap as well. Many of them would go out of their way to greet me.

The Easter Monday presentation – and its delivery – enjoyed the benefit of a great deal of preparation, practice and fine-tuning over the course of an intensive few days. It was designed to convey complex epidemiological information as clearly as possible. However, it contained within it something that went beyond mere information. Since that day, I've often had cause to wonder exactly what made the presentation so impactful. Why did it resonate so strongly with the public?

On reflection, I've had to conclude that there were many reasons. One was the sense of reassurance and empowerment it provided. Having lived with the virus for over two years and having become more complacent about it, it is easy to forget how much trepidation Covid-19 brought with it, particularly in the beginning when we were relatively ignorant about its real nature and impact, and lockdown was a foreign concept for most of us. I was reminded of the famous aphorism attributed to Francis Bacon: *knowledge is power*. Under the circumstances we faced, knowledge of the virus and our national response gave people power over their own fears, fears that often emanated from feelings of vulnerability and powerlessness related to the unknown.

I think people also found it reassuring to know that there were scientific and medical experts out there who knew what was going on and were leading from the front. I think people actually surprised themselves by the level of pride they felt in the South African scientific expertise on display during that briefing, not just in me, but in the expert commentators and more broadly on the scientific fraternity who served on the MAC. The MAC was now on a pedestal, transformed from its backroom role and thrust into the eye of the public through the media.

The presentation also had the effect of bringing people onside. In itself, the broadcast was a signal that the government and the scientists were sharing as much information as they had about the virus. We were taking the public into our confidence, as Mkhize would say from time to time. The fact that my presentation did not shy away from technical epidemiological concepts and terminology also helped to create the (correct) impression that we did not think the average South African was not intelligent enough to understand it. When the President had told me earlier, 'Everyone deserves to hear this,' I heard his words as a signal of transparency and respect for the people. Building on this inclusive approach, I set out to convey the idea that all of us – black, white, old and young – were facing this viral threat; we were all in this together and a united response was the best way forward.

Another reason for the impact of the briefing was probably its novelty:

never before had we sat down as a nation to listen to scientists on an issue of such importance. It became more common as time passed, but at that stage I think people found the concept quite fascinating. If I had been asked anytime pre-Covid-19 if a 45-minute slide-set presentation, typically presented at a scientific conference, would go down well on television, I would have said the idea was crazy – everyone would be asleep or would have changed the channel within five minutes.

Finally, I think the timing of the broadcast was significant. People were in a kind of limbo. Life was literally on hold and there was a great deal of uncertainty about what the immediate future might look like. I happened to be in the right place at the right time, and I had the kind of information people were looking for. Until then, they had picked up bits and pieces of information from various sources about the epidemic – there was certainly a great deal of information available – but they had not yet had the benefit of having it all pieced together into a full story, one that reached back into the recent past, gave an informed but accessible scientific overview of the present, and offered some idea of what shape the short-term future might take – a sort of beginning, middle and end.

I began my story in the wet market in Wuhan in November 2019, where it is believed (but not known definitively) that pangolins infected with a bat coronavirus may have facilitated the infection of human beings. The pangolins theory lost favour over time and transmission directly from bats to humans was being recognised as a possible option in the third year of the pandemic. I traced the spread of the novel virus to South Africa via a small group of travellers and explained its subsequent growth within our national borders via community transmission. Given the frequent comparisons taking place then between Covid-19 and influenza, I tried to stress the virulence of the novel virus and the rapidity with which it was likely to spread in the absence of any natural immunity.

Like any science, the field of epidemiology comes with its own unique terminology and so it became necessary for me to explain concepts such as 'exponential growth', 'community transmission' and 'reproduction number', all of which were critical to the process of tracking, measuring and controlling the virus spread. It was necessary for people to understand these terms if they were to follow the rest of the story.

I was pleased to be able to give people some good news: the curve was starting to flatten. After hitting a peak of an average of 110 daily cases in late March 2020, the curve's trajectory had started to plateau, and we were then reporting 60 to 70 cases per day. The decline in the infection rate occurred at just the right time, taking incubation period into account, after the declaration of our state of disaster and subsequent stay-at-home lockdown. When compared with the sharp rise in case numbers we were seeing in other countries, like the UK, for example, our epidemic seemed to be quite different, with a trajectory that had started flattening out on 26 March 2020, while those of other countries continued to rise. It was hard to argue that the timing was just coincidence and not further evidence that the altered trajectory was a consequence of the restrictions of the state of disaster.

Even against so-called 'successful countries', such as South Korea, Japan and Singapore, we were showing very encouraging results. In the interests of transparency and as an opportunity to shine a light on some of the scientific debates taking place behind the scenes, I offered three possible reasons for this decline: insufficient testing; low uptake of testing – especially in poor communities; and successful early mitigation measures by government. I showed how the available evidence pointed to the last mentioned as the best explanation among all three: the public health measures and restrictions were working, at least partially, to reduce community transmission, in the process buying us valuable time to prepare our health systems.

I must add that this was not a universally accepted interpretation of the data. Even within the MAC, there were a few scientists who argued that the South African trajectory was not unique and that the curve would have flattened anyway without any interventions by government. No evidence was forthcoming to explain why the epidemic would naturally flatten without interventions in South Africa but not elsewhere. It was almost impossible to prove the causal relationship between the restrictions and change in trajectory from a scientific perspective, but the gist of their argument that the curve would have flattened naturally was that government interventions could not and should not be given credit for any slowdown in infections. These kinds of differences of opinion came to characterise the discourse around the Covid-19 response and I viewed them as part and parcel of healthy, robust debate, but always returning to what the evidence was telling us. I was used to robust debate and differences of opinion as they are also commonplace in AIDS, just without Covid-19's strong political overtones.

Not all the news I delivered that evening was good. Despite the flattening of the curve, it was unclear as to when the stay-at-home lockdown should be lifted; there were fears that an abrupt return to normality might undo the gains made. I showed how we were tracking current lockdowns in India and China in order to understand the benefits and limitations of their lockdown experiences. At the time, there were also real concerns about the possibility of transmission surges in high-density urban areas such as greater Johannesburg, Cape Town and Durban. The burning question remained: when would the lockdown end? Speaking to a slide titled, 'What should we do this week?' I argued: 'Monitor community transmission.' We could use the trends in case numbers, as a proxy for the reproduction number (R_0, which is said as R-nought) to guide our next steps and inform the process for the lifting of lockdown. If data from the coming week showed the average daily case numbers to be above the expected threshold, then the lockdown would need to continue. However, if we saw daily increases within the expected range, this would open the door to an easing of restrictions.

Then came my 'difficult truth' slide, which announced that despite the early successes produced by our proactive approach, South Africa would not be able to escape the pandemic. Our country was unlikely to escape an exponential spread of infection – unless it had a special protective factor, or 'mojo', that did not exist in any other population in the world. It was a highly attractive prospect but a very unlikely one. In fact, it was so unlikely as to be not worth considering. While the lockdown had bought valuable time for our health system to prepare for a peak in cases and take advantage of the improvement in both testing and treatment, based on what we had seen of the virus spread around the world, a growth in infections was inevitable.

In the wake of this sombre news, I emphasised the benefit of having gained extra time to prepare for the peak of the epidemic before cases started to present clinically and hospitals were overrun, which had been the experience of a number of countries around the world. Field hospitals were making good progress in Cape Town and elsewhere, I explained. In order to give people some idea of what the future held, I continued to outline the subsequent stages of the national plan, using the detailed slide I had prepared showing the eight-stage national Covid-19 response plan. My illustration of the need for vigilance through a graphic of firefighters putting out small fires to prevent a serious forest fire was a big hit. Several people sent me messages about this series of three graphics.

Elderly people were a particular concern. I had given some thought to a partial voluntary lockdown for older people until the end of September 2020 – or whenever the epidemic had subsided sufficiently, and it was considered safe for vulnerable people to re-enter society. I put this option of a voluntary stay-at-home lockdown for the elderly until September onto a slide. It was gratifying to know that people had listened closely to the content of my presentation. In September that year, I received a number of messages from senior citizens asking if they could go back to the hairdresser and bridge classes!

Two negative repercussions of the presentation emerged a few days later.

The first was the way the media demands really impacted on my time management – I found that I was being taken away from important tasks and there was not a lot of time beyond the MAC and media commitments. Maharaj considered all media requests seriously, but I could only manage a fraction of the interviews, referring the remainder mostly to MAC colleagues. The MAC came first. I had put aside my HIV and TB research to focus on Covid-19, so my priority lay, as it always had, with devoting my time to the science. Media appearances and interviews were secondary and had to be fitted into my schedule around my responsibilities to the MAC. While I initially thought of media as an extension to the work I was already doing to communicate science, it was becoming apparent that this was not always the case. Research was clear cut – I knew what I was trying to achieve. But media interviews were disparate, and it was not always discernible if I was fulfilling my role in educating and informing the public. My life had taken a momentous turn, veering suddenly off its well-lit, familiar research highway and onto a bumpy, unclear track with an uncertain destination.

The second negative repercussion was the growing confusion in the eyes of the public about my role in providing science advice. Scientists do not tend to exist in the spotlight. Our work is built on decades of working quietly behind the scenes. It is precisely for this reason that the attention I received following the Easter weekend presentation was baffling, and its impact came as such a surprise, even to me. The problem with becoming so prominent in the public eye overnight was that not everyone was able to grasp exactly the distinction between providing scientific advice on the Covid-19 response and making decisions on the next steps in the Covid-19 response. This was exemplified in the comment by a newspaper columnist, two days after the presentation, referring to me as the 'guy running the fight against the coronavirus'.[2] The conflation between giving scientific advice and deciding policy (being in charge) became widespread and it continued to manifest in various ways throughout my term on the MAC. In my mind, I can pinpoint its origins to that landmark public briefing that inadvertently placed me on a podium and gave me the appearance of the person who was calling the shots. Despite perceptions to the contrary, my purpose has always remained the same, as it had been even before the advent of Covid-19 or the MAC: standing up for science.

From reluctant medical student to pandemic science adviser

CHAPTER 10

Formative early years in science

From medical student to epidemiologist and virologist over the past four decades, I gained experience through hard work on the ground to understand how viruses were spreading, causing epidemics and what it took to stop them.

In the aftermath of the Easter Monday presentation, several journalists asked me about how I came to know all about viruses and pandemics. There is no simple answer to this question. It takes many years of hard work and experience studying virology, epidemiology and epidemics – and past experience in dealing with epidemics is key. There is a long history behind my interest in solving problems. My fascination with viruses and how they spread goes back more than four decades to my early years.

Growing up, I idolised Isaac Newton in school and marvelled at his amazing contributions to science. My fascination for science was heavily influenced by my high school maths and physics teachers, Mr Ashik Hansraj and Mr Cassim Seedat. Both of them played a significant role in fostering my love of all things analytical and scientific. Their influence permeated not just my eventual career path but also the decisions I've made in my life. During my high school years, I was always a top maths and physics student. I was also confident about my ability to understand problems and find solutions. Not being able to do so would result in days of introspection. If I didn't get 100% in my tests, I would continue to mull over the answer that had eluded me: *Where did I go wrong?* Simply knowing the solution was not enough; I needed to figure out how to get there and how to avoid repeating my mistakes.

My obsession with problem-solving and strength in maths and science made engineering seem like the obvious career choice for me. When the time came to apply to universities, engineering was my degree of choice. But it was 1977 and under South Africa's apartheid regime, with universities segregated according to race, there were limited options available to a black student of Indian heritage such as myself. I had to keep as many of those options on the table as possible. So, during my matric year, I applied to a number of engineering faculties – and medical schools as a backup.

White students were able to choose from a range of well-resourced universities that offered a full range of programmes. African, Indian and Coloured students, who were collectively referred to as 'black' students, on the other hand, were expected to attend institutions known colloquially as 'bush colleges', universities of inferior quality that catered for particular racial and often ethnic groups. A handful of African, Indian and Coloured students were accepted at whites-only universities but only by dint of 'ministerial permission'.

There was no guarantee that I would fall into that category and even if I did get accepted, there was the problem of money. How would I pay the university fees? My father had a job in a factory that brought in enough to keep the family afloat, and I used to help out after school by serving behind the spice (masala) counter at a general dealership run by my uncle. It was enough to support our family of five, but university fees were a bridge too far. The only hope I had was to secure a scholarship or a loan.

When the news came that I had been accepted into the engineering programme at the University of Durban-Westville (UDW), a university founded to cater specifically for Indian students, it was bittersweet. I had been accepted based on my academic results, but there was no scholarship on offer. I decided to start classes anyway – in the hope that a scholarship might still be forthcoming – and attended lectures in the Engineering Faculty for the first three days of the academic year. I did not actually register as I did not have the fees needed. I spent those days anxiously awaiting some word about my scholarship application to a local engineering company. At the end of my third day of engineering classes, I finally received a letter, but not the one I was expecting. The University of Natal's Medical School was offering me a place among that year's undergraduate medical student intake – and it came with a full scholarship of R1 200 per annum.

The Natal Medical School was established in 1951 as a faculty for only African, Indian and Coloured students. It was referred to as UN-B – University of Natal Black division. Even though it was part of a whites-only university, the medical school did not accept white medical students. It was a complicated and anomalous situation within the broader context of grand apartheid, but the training provided at the school was comprehensive and rigorous. It trained a generation of talented black medical students, many of whom went on to occupy senior leadership positions throughout the country and within the first democratic government. The scholarship I received turned out to be funded by an organisation known as the Indian Centenary Scholarship Trust and I would only need to pay the money back to the trust after my internship (six years down the line).

After just three days, I left engineering and started my medical degree, though with some reluctance. The truth is that if I had received a scholarship for engineering, I probably would have stuck with it. I had begun to enjoy the work at UDW for that brief period, but my life would have looked completely different, and I have no regrets about the way it has turned out.

As a medical student, I would present myself every month to the school cashier to receive my monthly allocation of R74 to pay fees and other expenses, including my daily bus fare from our family home in Chatsworth. I enjoyed medical school, but it took some time for me to develop a real passion for it and I was neither the best nor the most conventional of students. I spent a lot of time playing table tennis and if I went to one lecture a day that was quite a lot. Dr Nesri Padayatchi, who was one of my peers at medical school and served as deputy director of CAPRISA, would often facetiously comment that I was studying medicine 'by correspondence'.

One of the problems I had was that I tended to drift off in many of my lectures; to me they didn't seem to be the best way to hold my attention or to learn. Given my ability to absorb large amounts of information through reading, I found it much easier to simply read the textbook, memorise its contents in preparation for the examinations, and be done with it. This approach worked very well in most subjects, but it was not bulletproof. I failed anatomical pathology in my third year because I simply could not bring myself to study for the exam. Fortunately, I qualified to sit a supplementary examination, which I managed to pass. It was the only course I had ever failed in my life and the experience left me feeling a little rattled. There were reasons for that singular slip in third year: it was 1980, the year of school boycotts, and I had immersed myself in anti-apartheid student politics. I had also started to study computer science and statistics – both being my abiding passions – through correspondence with the University of South Africa, alongside my medical degree. My life was admittedly 'all over the place', as they say.

These were not the only reasons for failing anatomical pathology. On reflection and after consulting with the head of the department, I realised I had been complacent about the subject – but the truth was that it did not hold sufficient interest for me. I realised I had never entirely committed myself to medical studies, possibly because the prospect of general practice just failed to capture my imagination. Luckily that would soon change. A turning point came when, in the course of my political activities, I met Professor Hoosen (Jerry) Coovadia, a world-class clinician-scientist in the Department of Paediatrics, who served in the leadership of the Natal Indian Congress, an ANC affiliate. In addition to a shared political outlook, Coovadia and I got on well intellectually. I used to go to his office and eat my lunch with him on a regular basis. He treated me more like a son than a mentee, but he was also a committed and inspiring academic mentor. Coovadia was a creative thinker whose mind was always coming up with new ideas for research projects. Listening to him and watching him work, it started to dawn on me that there existed an exciting alternative path to general medical practice: medical research. Pushing the boundaries of knowledge and having an impact on the world of science appealed to me enormously and Coovadia was the best mentor I could have found to guide me on that path. I ended up writing my first academic paper with him, while I was a third-year medical student.

During my third year, I also developed a fascination for viruses; not just viruses themselves, but their capacity to spread and cause mayhem among human populations. I remember attending what must have been one of my first lectures in virology in 1980, where Dr Isobel Windsor, then head of the Department of Medical Virology and Virus Diagnostic Laboratory at the University of Natal Medical School, put up an electron-micrograph picture of what to me looked like a sputnik satellite. On the board, she laboriously wrote out the word: *Icosadeltahedron*, which is the descriptive term for the shape of the virus.

My 'sputnik' turned out to be a picture of a bacteriophage, a virus that infects bacteria, with its classic icosahedral head atop a tail sheath and fibres. Next came the helical Tobacco Mosaic Virus, the first virus ever to be identified by scientists. Windsor had done her PhD research on Tobacco Mosaic Virus. I found myself intrigued by their shapes but more especially by what their shape revealed about their ability to infect, to replicate, and to spread. It seemed to me that viruses were pieces in a much larger, more fascinating puzzle. That larger puzzle turned out to be epidemiology.

After graduating with my medical degree in 1984 and completing my internship at the King Edward VIII Hospital in Durban, I started research work at the Research Institute for Diseases in Tropical Environment at the Medical Research Council (MRC) in 1985, where I had secured a one-year post-intern scholarship. Ironically, my office at the MRC was located in a building that was demolished to make space for CAPRISA in 2002. In fact, my little post-intern bursar's office used to be on the same site where the CAPRISA boardroom currently sits. In the mid-1980s, the MRC was then still under the leadership of its founding president, the formidable Professor Andries Brink, who was also co-founder and Dean of the Stellenbosch University Medical School as well as personal physician to former South African president BJ Vorster. Brink, a cardiologist by training and a perfectionist by nature, was not a man to be trifled with and he led the MRC with authority for nearly 20 years. When I met him in 1985, I had little notion that 27 years later, I would be stepping into his shoes as MRC president. At that time in my career, my focus was less on leadership than the idiosyncrasies of a highly infectious, partially double-stranded DNA virus: the hepatitis B virus, which was causing liver disease, mostly among children in southern Africa.

My focus on the epidemiology of hepatitis B originated through a suggestion from Coovadia. He was working on a hepatitis B project, which focused on its relation to nephrotic syndrome and kidney disease. But that was not where my interest lay. My public health instincts were gaining traction and I was keen to understand more about the pattern of disease and the factors behind its spread, specifically in vulnerable black communities. As a site for my research, I chose what is known as a 'place of safety' or children's shelter situated in Umlazi, the largest black township in KwaZulu-Natal. The place gave shelter to children of all ages who were either fleeing abuse, who were orphaned, or who were wards of the court because they were too young for incarceration. While it was not technically a prison, the children were compelled to stay on the premises.

Compared with other urban and rural settings, levels of infection in the shelter seemed to be abnormally high epidemic levels. Transmission of hepatitis B virus is caused by exposure to infectious blood, so it can be transmitted through sexual contact, blood transfusions and the use of contaminated needles. Like HIV, it can be transmitted vertically, from mother to child during childbirth. None of these textbook modes of transmission seemed to apply in the case of the Umlazi children's shelter. I wanted to investigate the possibility that community transmission might be happening through the not inconsiderable population of mosquitoes that infested the place. So began my first epidemic investigation, all the way back in 1985.

Together with my research colleague Dr Alida Fouche, who was doing her own research on malaria mosquitoes, we collected mosquitoes from the Umlazi site and analysed any human blood they were carrying.[1]

Fouche had developed a nifty gadget to collect the mosquitoes without killing them, which proved very effective. It took us about six months to get the results. Ultimately, we couldn't prove that mosquitoes had caused the outbreak, but the findings still pointed to something interesting. Part of our research, published in the *International Journal of Epidemiology*,[2] confirmed a higher rate of infection among the children and highlighted some gaps in our understanding of why this venue was home to a localised hepatitis B epidemic. Even if mosquitoes did not actually transmit the disease, our research had opened the door to the possibility of using mosquitoes to track the spread of the virus, which is an important part of epidemiology. Still determined to learn more about the virus, I did further research on the contribution of ritual scarification and ear-piercing to the spread of hepatitis B, helping to improve standards of hygiene and awareness of the need for effective sterilisation techniques. I followed this up by conducting studies on other hepatitis viruses as well.

After my year at the MRC was up, I was keen to specialise, and to deepen my understanding of viruses. I joined the Department of Microbiology at the University of Natal as a registrar in 1986. I spent most of my time in the Department of Virology, which was a sub-department of Microbiology at the time, as I was simultaneously working on my PhD on hepatitis B virus. While in this position, I had my first encounter with another virus: HIV. In between doing research and lecturing, I worked alongside Windsor in the viral diagnostic laboratory, providing HIV test results to patients. HIV, which had been identified only two years earlier, was understandably a source of great interest to virologists and epidemiologists and its spread in South Africa was being closely monitored. As a post-intern bursar at the MRC, I had already delivered my first lecture on HIV at McCords Hospital at the invitation of Dr Helgar Holst, who was hospital CEO at the time. During this period, alongside my studies on hepatitis viruses, I developed a growing interest in HIV, although I was a long way off from establishing myself as a researcher in the field.

It was during my time in the Department of Virology that I came to a realisation about my future professional path: I was most excited by studying the combination of virology and epidemiology, through research on the spread and containment of viral infections. While I deeply appreciated the experience of doing my own laboratory research and learning how a laboratory worked, I knew that being confined to a laboratory was not something I wanted for myself in the long term. My sights were on a bigger picture, a broader horizon. The nexus between virology and epidemiology felt like a much better fit.

There was another important development that year. Thanks to an expensive piece of laboratory equipment, I got to meet my future wife – Quarraisha. Her research, which she was doing in the Department of Haematology, required the use of an ultra-centrifuge, which was only available in the Department of Virology – the exact place I happened to be working. Since I was nominally in charge of this equipment and my office was very close to it, it provided the opportunity for us to meet. It turned out that we shared many of the same interests in research and the potential of public health as a tool in addressing social inequality. The following year, 1987, we both had an opportunity to study public health and epidemiology at the School of Public Health at Columbia University in New York – and we seized it with both hands. I went first in mid-1987 and came back to South Africa at the end of the year to get married. We then went together to New York to study at the beginning of 1988.

I had received the funding to do my master's in epidemiology through a Rockefeller Foundation fellowship. Luckily, the terms of this fellowship were quite flexible in scope, allowing me to pursue a wide range of academic endeavours. I had gone to Columbia University thinking my focus would be on the epidemiology of hepatitis B, but instead a world of other possibilities opened up to me. In addition to epidemiology, I had the opportunity to study health economics through a joint London School of Economics and London School of Hygiene & Tropical Medicine programme in the UK, and later I visited the US Centers for Disease Control and Prevention in Atlanta, where I learned about methods of epidemic investigations.

To say that Columbia University represented a seminal year for us is almost an understatement. As soon as we set foot into the School of Public Health, the topic of talk was HIV. Almost every week there would be three to four lectures on HIV by eminent scientists. New York felt like the epicentre of HIV scientific developments at the time. In addition, the number of people dying from AIDS was rising and there was a vocal activist movement pushing for HIV-research-related policy change. It was fascinating and inspiring. And my focus was growing firmly on HIV.

At that stage, not much was known about HIV treatment. It was still very early days, but treatment trials had started. I remember attending, among many great lectures, one delivered by oncologist Dr Samuel Broder from the NIH's National Cancer Institute. He described the trials, which had started in 1985, that had led to the discovery and development of AZT as the first treatment for AIDS. Broder led the study in a collaboration with scientists at the Burroughs-Wellcome Company (now GlaxoSmithKline).

During that lecture, I felt like I had found my element. Eager to learn more, I attended as many other lectures and talks as I possibly could.

The opportunity to study at Columbia University at that particular time in the history of HIV science was a highlight of my life. It was a deeply formative period. We were at the cutting edge of HIV science and research. We were also meeting both current and future leaders, people who would be part of a vital global scientific network, upon which we could draw while conducting research in South Africa. One of these people was Dr Thomas Frieden. Frieden reached me by telephone one day and asked if I would agree to be interviewed for a news article he was working on about apartheid in South Africa. He was then completing a residency in internal medicine at Columbia-Presbyterian Medical Center. It was a memorable meeting. He later became the director of the US Centers for Disease Control and Prevention and was a former commissioner of the New York City Health Department.

During our time at Columbia, both Quarraisha and I benefited from the mentorship of Dr Mervyn Susser and his wife Dr Zena Stein, a research duo from South Africa. Susser was a founding director of the Gertrude H. Sergievsky Research Center in the School of Public Health at Columbia

University. He and Stein were among a group of epidemiologists who were working to fight the HIV epidemic in the US, but they also had a keen interest in HIV-related developments back in South Africa. It was an interest that Quarraisha and I were looking forward to continuing upon our return to the country after graduating.

When I returned from New York at the end of 1988, I took a position of registrar again, this time in the Department of Community Health at the Faculty of Medicine at the University of Natal. Given the choice to continue my training in virology or specialise in community health, I had opted for the latter. My New York experience had left me with little doubt about where my professional future lay and it was definitely public health. Going back into a laboratory to complete my studies in microbiology with an emphasis on virology (a specialist qualification in virology was not then available in South Africa) felt like a step backwards when compared to the prospect of unravelling the mysteries of the HIV epidemic *on the ground*.

I was now firmly committed to studying the epidemiology of viral infections. I realised that my true calling lay not in serving the individual patient, but in serving the community as a whole. Helping to ensure that people were healthy at community level required a different approach, one that combined my love of science and intense curiosity with a commitment to social justice and equity. Through a combination of virology and public health I felt I was more able to serve as an agent of social change.

As part of my registrar training in community health in 1990, I worked with Dr Fiona Robinson at the Durban City Health Department, trying to understand how the TB epidemic was continuing to grow in Durban, and how we could improve TB contact tracing to change this trajectory. In all of my investigations I was utilising my training in epidemiology and honing what I had learned at Columbia University.

In 1992, I graduated as a specialist in community health (now referred to as public health medicine), but I regretted not going back to complete my remaining 18 months of virology training. That changed in early 2022, when the Colleges of Medicine of South Africa conferred on me the Fellowship of the College of Pathology in Virology, effectively making me a specialist in virology as well. Now I get to say I am officially a card-carrying virologist and can enjoy practising both my specialties, public health and virology, daily in my work on HIV and Covid-19.

As I walked up to receive this honour at the college graduation ceremony in Cape Town, my mind wandered back to my first experience of investigating a large community epidemic of a virus, which came from a measles outbreak in KwaZulu-Natal in the early 1990s. Again, working with Coovadia as my mentor, I visited several clinics in the province to investigate why the virus was spreading despite compulsory measles vaccination. Measles vaccination is mandatory for one-year-old babies, but vaccination coverage in this group was quite low in this community. I then studied the operational challenges of vaccination that might explain why so many children were slipping through the net and not getting vaccinated. Among my observations was a lack of adequate refrigeration for the vaccine. The WHO recommends that measles vaccines be stored at a constant temperature of between 2–8 degrees Celsius. My research showed that many clinics did not have refrigerators that were working and those that did work were not dedicated to the storage of the vaccine – they were also being used by staff to store their lunch and other perishables, which compromised the storage conditions for vaccines. When asked to publicly comment on the findings of the investigation, Coovadia came down hard on the Department of Health for failing to address poor vaccination practices at clinic facilities. It was the apartheid era and the whites-only National Party was in power, although its stranglehold on the country was waning in the wake of the release of Nelson Mandela in February 1990. There was a great deal of justified sensitivity around the fact that most of the children being adversely affected by inadequate facilities at state clinics were black. Coovadia is not one to mince his words, particularly on the issue of social injustices, and his comments were a classic case of 'speaking truth to power'.

His comments came to the attention of the Minister of National Health and Population Development, a position then held by Dr Rina Venter, a former social worker and the first female member of cabinet in South Africa. Venter's office called Coovadia and asked him to meet at her office at the parliamentary buildings in Cape Town to discuss the issue. Since I had done most of the research, I was asked to accompany him, and so the minister's office arranged for both of us to fly to Cape Town. Our meeting with Venter was something of an eye-opener. I was expecting someone who embodied the closed-mindedness and race-driven thinking of the National Party that she represented. Perhaps we were expecting a more defensive response from a direct political opponent, but in fact Venter seemed sincerely interested in identifying the key problems and working towards their solution. I think, despite his political views, Coovadia was also impressed with her. She committed to addressing the refrigerator problem in the clinics and listed practical steps towards doing so. As we walked out of the parliamentary precinct and made our way back to the airport, I had the impression of having met someone who was committed to dealing with the problem we had identified through our epidemic investigation. And, despite our differing political views, it felt rewarding to be part of that process.

Excellent research in its social context became an important driver for me. I was poised at the edge of a life-long career in medical research and epidemiology, and our country was emerging from decades of apartheid, a system fundamentally premised on inequality. I understood that apartheid would leave a large footprint of inequity that would be evident in all spheres, including human health. Part of my responsibility was to do what I could to address this inequity, with particular emphasis on the disproportionate burden of infectious diseases in disadvantaged communities.

Over the next few years, I was drawn into national disease control efforts, specifically through my participation in the National Advisory Group on Immunisation (NAGI) and the South African Polio Expert Committee. The NAGI was set up in 1993 to advise the government on vaccines under the chairmanship of South Africa's leading virologist and vaccine expert, Professor Barry Schoub. Both Coovadia and I served on the NAGI at its inception. I took over as chair of the NAGI in 1997. At the time of the NAGI's formation, one of the biggest pandemic threats was perceived to be influenza. South Africa was not alone in this concern: governments around the world routinely monitor outbreaks and develop contingency plans for influenza pandemics. By now, I had been involved in investigating and implementing control measures for more than a few viral epidemics and I had learned that preparedness was going to be key in looking at the potential of an influenza pandemic. This is a lesson I have continued to carry with me. During my time on the NAGI, we reviewed plans for influenza pandemic preparedness and took steps to stockpile Tamiflu. The National Institute for Virology, under Schoub's leadership, had established surveillance for influenza strains and we reviewed the results regularly as part of our influenza pandemic preparedness.

One of the accomplishments of the NAGI that I am proud of is its role in the introduction of the hepatitis B vaccine in our country. The NAGI investigated and recommended the introduction of universal hepatitis B vaccination in South Africa. Since I had done my PhD research on hepatitis B, I was very well versed with the science involved with the hepatitis B vaccine. This vaccine was successfully incorporated into the country's routine Expanded Programme on Immunisation schedule in 1995.

A year later, in 1996, I was appointed to chair the South African Polio Expert Committee. This committee was given the mandate to undertake the steps towards our country being declared polio free as part of the global polio elimination programme. The tasks included undertaking investigations to identify potential local hotspots for transmission of polio and co-ordinating national efforts to investigate each case of paralysis to assess if it could have been caused by polio or even by the polio vaccine (known as VAPP – vaccine associated paralytic poliomyelitis). The Polio Expert Committee eventually declared South Africa polio free in 2019.

Each new role I took on came with a new set of lessons and I was slowly learning about the different facets of science. Over the course of about four decades straight after I finished medical school, I gained experience in conducting research, providing science advice and implementing public health measures on epidemics. Managing public health outbreaks was becoming my area of expertise, whether it was a small, localised hepatitis B outbreak or a large community measles outbreak. I had done the hard work on the ground to understand how the viruses were spreading, what was causing these epidemics, and what could be done to stop them. All of this meant that when the time came, I was primed to take up the bigger challenge of the global HIV pandemic.

CHAPTER 11

Lessons from AIDS

In my years of AIDS research, I learned that major scientific discoveries require excellence, perseverance and resilience, while being willing to listen to and engage with differing viewpoints, and defending science when it is under the kinds of threats that AIDS denialists posed.

Upon returning from New York at the end of 1988, both Quarraisha and I were ready and excited to tackle the biggest epidemic challenge of our time – AIDS. Little did we know that this journey would lead us to several important scientific discoveries. Scientific discoveries are sometimes glamorised by the media as overnight breakthroughs. In reality, they are the product of painstaking, prolonged, meticulous and often tedious work. Mistakes are made and failure is frequent. In the 30-plus years that Quarraisha and I have been doing AIDS research, we made research progress and important discoveries, but there were also considerable obstacles, challenges and failures that we suffered along the way. After all, AIDS was much more than a viral disease. It was interspersed with politics, activism, exciting science and challenges at every turn.

In 1990, while I was completing my registrar training in community health, Quarraisha had joined the MRC and, working with Dr Malcolm Steinberg, she created the MRC's AIDS Research Programme in Durban. In 1992, as a newly minted public health specialist, I was recruited by Professor Walter Prozesky, MRC president at the time, and Dr Derek Yach, MRC Group Executive for Research, to take up a position of senior epidemiologist in Cape Town at the Centre for Epidemiological Research in South Africa (CERSA) – at the time the largest MRC research unit in the country. Within a year, aged 33 years, I was appointed Director of CERSA, a position I held for about a decade, until 2001. As part of an MRC intra-mural restructuring exercise, the MRC's existing AIDS research programme, which was being led by Quarraisha at the time, was incorporated into CERSA. Quarraisha and I were now formally working together on AIDS research in the same research unit.

In the early 1990s, we conducted one of the first large community-based surveys to assess the scale of the HIV epidemic in rural KwaZulu-Natal.[1] This study set us on our path in HIV research, as it provided empiric evidence of the high rates of HIV infection in young women driven largely through sex with older men. This was a major finding as it laid the basis for prioritisation in prevention, where the focus would now be on protecting young women. It was a game-changer for both Quarraisha and myself as it allowed us to better understand the community dynamics at play and what was behind the high rates of local HIV transmission.

But it wasn't all positive. Our early findings about the significance of age-disparate sex in spreading HIV were challenged over time by other groups whose studies showed different results. We had to defend that initial finding repeatedly, an important process in scientific discovery. The debate around our 1990 finding was finally laid to rest about 25 years later, when we did a really large community-based study of HIV transmission. In an analysis led by our colleagues, Professor Ayesha Kharsany, senior epidemiologist at CAPRISA, and Tulio de Oliveira, they used phylogenetics to provide empirical evidence for the 'Cycle of HIV Transmission', showing young girls are most often infected by men about ten years older.[2] These findings were rapidly adopted by UNAIDS and were the basis of the 2016 UNAIDS Report on the 'Life-cycle approach to HIV'.[3]

This UNAIDS report has been used by several African countries for national policy-making and planning. For example, the first objective set in the South African National AIDS Plan is to break the 'Cycle of HIV transmission' through reducing HIV incidence in young women. There were at least two important lessons we took away from this experience. Firstly, that science is a domain of contestation and interpretations of the same data can legitimately vary. This does not make one party right or wrong; these are just differing views on the path to discovering the truth. Thus, we learned the importance of listening to and acknowledging alternate views. Secondly, we learned that our scientific findings have to be rigorous so that they can withstand multiple challenges and the test of time. This has become the essence of our approach in science – to continually strive for excellence with no compromise.

For almost 20 years after we first published our community-based epidemiological data in 1990 showing the vulnerability of young women, the only prevention options available to them were abstinence, behaviour change, condoms (male and female) and medical male circumcision. We asked ourselves which of these were actually tools for girls and young women in Africa, where most were likely to have only a few years of formal education, limited economic opportunities, and were likely to be dependent both economically and socially on men for their well-being. How could these young women realistically be expected to negotiate with their (older) male partners about behaviour change or circumcision? The answer was self-evident: they could not.

For many researchers in the field, including us, the solution lay in vaginal gel microbicides, which would alter the conditions in the vagina to make it inhospitable to the virus. Quarraisha and I did our first microbicide trial in 1993.[4] After that initial study, we conducted several other microbicide trials. All of our trials, and the many trials conducted by others, consistently failed to show positive results. At the peak of our frustration, in 2003, we changed tack to focus on antiretroviral drugs for prevention, and specifically a new drug called tenofovir. Could this drug be used in a microbicide vaginal gel to prevent infection of women during sex – in other words, a pre-exposure prophylaxis – and could it do so safely? In May 2007, the CAPRISA 004 trial got under way to answer this question.

Just as we were starting the trial, an article appeared in *Nature*, which declared our trial 'doomed by design'.[5] It reflected some of the scepticism among peers and colleagues in the global microbicide field, particularly those in the UK and US. Once again, our research was under attack for not being scientifically valid and we had to defend it. We were not immune to the criticism, but we were confident of our position. We engaged respectfully with the concerns raised about the design of the research but held our ground. We were vindicated when a meeting of all the major microbicide scientists, including most of our critics, agreed that our study was scientifically valid and should continue.

Our commitment and perseverance paid off. Three years after the *Nature* article appeared, and 18 years after we first embarked upon the microbicide research path, we were able to announce positive results of the CAPRISA 004 trial at the 18th International AIDS Conference in Vienna, Austria, on 20 July 2010. Tenofovir gel, applied before and after sex, reduced HIV incidence by 39%. This protection went up to 74% where high levels of the gel were detected. We now had proof-of-concept that an antiretroviral agent can prevent sexual transmission of HIV in women. In the same trial we also discovered that the gel reduced genital herpes infections by as much as 51%.

The announcement of the CAPRISA 004 results was greeted by a standing ovation at the Vienna International AIDS Conference, a reaction that had never previously been seen in these usually sepulchral scientific meetings. The results made front-page headlines in leading newspapers globally, including *The New York Times*, *The Washington Post* and *The Wall Street Journal*. The findings were ranked by the journal *Science* as one of the Top 10 Scientific Breakthroughs of 2010 and our research was featured among *The Lancet*'s 'Paper of the Year' in 2010. They were heralded by UNAIDS and the WHO as one of the most significant scientific breakthroughs in the fight against AIDS. Subsequent to our findings, a range of studies of tenofovir as oral pre-exposure prophylaxis (PrEP) announced positive results, leading in 2015 to the WHO's global guidelines for the use of oral PrEP containing tenofovir for all those at high risk of HIV infection. These guidelines were implemented in South Africa in 2017.

The next stage of research, over the last five to seven years, has been spent unravelling a very complicated equation involving the vaginal microbiome, HPV and genital inflammation – all of which are working in different ways to affect susceptibility to HIV infection. In each microbicide study we did in 18 years of research before the momentous CAPRISA 004 trial, where we repeatedly failed, we learned something new and vital in the fight against HIV. Each set of findings from our studies created an opportunity for us to improve on existing technologies targeting the reduction of HIV infection in women, until we succeeded.

More than 30 years later, why are we still on the same path, namely, the search for technologies that can protect women? Unfortunately, young women still bear the brunt of the HIV epidemic in Africa. The problem has not been fully solved and we still have much work to do. While significant, the implementation of oral PrEP in the form of a daily tablet has not solved the problem of infection because of the difficulty women have in taking the drug on a regular basis. And so, we have now trained our efforts on long-acting formulations, technologies that empower women and which they can use without having to think about them on a daily or even weekly basis.

The HIV-prevention research path has been marked by a number of challenges and consecutive decades of hard work and perseverance. It has been a slow process, but Quarraisha and I are grateful to have been at the centre of a number of major scientific breakthroughs that have contributed to changes to global and national policy around HIV prevention. These years have brought many important lessons for us; the importance of doing scrupulous research that can withstand critique, being open to other points of view in science and, most importantly, perseverance in the face of adversity. But HIV taught me much more than science. It was also a test of character and fortitude in the midst of controversy in a complex political terrain.

By the time that President Thabo Mbeki came into office in mid-1999 and started publicly questioning the link between HIV and AIDS and finding support for his view from scientific dissidents, I was leading the MRC's AIDS research and was one of the faces of HIV/AIDS research in South Africa. Hence, I was being called on frequently to counter the

President's position through the media.

Coovadia and I, together with several others, were outspoken critics of the AIDS denialist position, which translated directly into delayed access to life-saving drugs, not to mention confusion and fear in the minds of the public. The landmark 13th International AIDS Conference held in Durban in July 2000, with Coovadia serving as the official conference chair and me as the scientific programme chair, were lightning rods for public interest in the issue as well as government opprobrium. Quarraisha was also involved in her capacity as head of South Africa's AIDS Control Programme and a member of the International AIDS Society's governing council.

When he opened the International AIDS conference, Mbeki doggedly stuck to his denialist stance, emphasising the link between poverty and AIDS, saying nothing about HIV-prevention plans, particularly with regard to mother-to-child transmission, which was a big issue at the time. Overwhelmed by the tide of scientific evidence and pro-treatment activist opinion at the conference, then Health Minister Manto Tshabalala-Msimang summoned both Coovadia and me to an audience with her on the eve of the first day of the conference. In a hotel room in front of several provincial ministers of health she berated us harshly and accused us of being unpatriotic. She was particularly upset with Justice Edwin Cameron's opening speech and derided the Durban Declaration, a statement by over 5 000 scientists released at the start of the conference, providing the scientific rationale for why HIV is the cause of AIDS.

How could we oppose the government at an international conference? she shrieked. Coovadia, who had spent most of his life actively fighting against apartheid and working to secure democracy that led to the ANC-led government, of which the Health minister was a part, was having none of it. He reminded Tshabalala-Msimang that during the height of apartheid he had been risking his life at the frontline. 'They bombed my house, not yours,' he said. Tshabalala-Msimang was furious. Turning to both of us, in a not-so-veiled threat, she said: 'You are here today, but tomorrow, all your friends will be gone and then there will be me. And then there will be you.'

It was a key lesson about the need to stand one's ground in the face of political pressure. In any event, we were very secure of our ground as scientists. Together with several of our country's leading scientists, I had been dealing with the political pressure of the controversial South African Presidential AIDS Advisory Panel set up by Mbeki to discuss whether HIV exists and whether it causes AIDS. It was a difficult time for us as scientists as we had to debate the underlying science of HIV with the AIDS denialists, who were led by a prominent US scientist, Dr Peter Duesberg, and his colleague, Dr David Rasnick. I had to learn to counter denialist 'anti-science' with rational scientific arguments. During these debates I learned how true Brandolini's asymmetry principle was: 'The amount of energy needed to refute bullshit is an order of magnitude bigger than that to produce it.'

Some 22 years after the Mbeki AIDS panel, Rasnick resurfaced in a South African legal hearing, arguing that Covid-19 was not a new disease and that it was not caused by SARS-CoV-2. It seems that the denialists recycle themselves with each new pandemic. Once again I came to appreciate Brandolini's law – that the effort of debunking misinformation is much more onerous in comparison to the relative ease of creating it in the first place. It really is a lot of work to put together rational arguments in responding to nonsense!

Predictably, we came under enormous pressure for opposing the President on the AIDS issue. There was no way we were going to back down and deny what we knew to be true about HIV and its causal links to AIDS. And so, we developed our resilience in dealing with the challenge of politics vs science – and we did our best, in dealing with those in authority who wanted an alternative narrative and reality, to ensure that science carried the day. It served to alert me to the dangers and reality of political obfuscation during times of crisis. One could not escape the reality that we were essentially arguing about ideology and beliefs while a deadly epidemic – for which there was a promising treatment – was raging around us.

In hindsight, it is easy to be struck by the parallels between our situation then and the situation the US found itself in 20 years later with Covid-19 under the Trump presidency. By calling Covid-19 the 'Chinese virus', President Trump actively encouraged the view that Americans were under siege by a foreign threat. He also initially kept saying that the virus would go away and denied its significance instead of confronting the problem. This kind of misrepresentation seeks to blame others or pretend the epidemic is not really a problem and goes hand in hand with all kinds of misinformation, which in turn spawns conspiracy theories. In my experience, conspiracy theories are often a distraction deliberately designed to draw attention away from a much bigger problem – a problem that leaders sometimes feel impotent about or incompetent to solve.

From that aberrant Mbeki Presidential AIDS Advisory Panel, I took the lessons I could: valuable experience about how to engage, at a highly adversarial level, with a group of scientists with divergent (mostly nonsensical) views. There was no way to achieve common ground with AIDS denialists, but the skills that came out of that experience were valuable, nevertheless. They have served me well in my participation in and leadership of various high-level panels and committees, and, of course, in dealing with Covid-19.

Most important of all, however, I gained experience in defending science.

CHAPTER 12

From AIDS to Covid-19

*Extrapolating from HIV to SARS-CoV-2 needed an understanding of
how coronavirus biology is different – an essential step to
extrapolating a pandemic endgame.*

When he included Quarraisha and me in his 'Heroes in the Field' list in December 2020, Microsoft founder and philanthropist Bill Gates wrote that it was unfortunate that much of our focus on HIV/AIDS research had been diverted to helping guide the Covid-19 response in South Africa.[1]

'On the other hand,' he said, 'it is a reminder of how fighting old diseases like HIV helps the world prepare for new ones like Covid-19. Investing long term in programs like CAPRISA – or work on polio or malaria – not only prevents deaths and disability from specific diseases, it also strengthens the overall field of global health. So, when a pandemic comes along, we have a network of experts like Quarraisha and Salim ready to pitch in …'

Gates was correct. Quarraisha and I have been fighting the 'old disease' of HIV for over three decades – both as a couple and as part of a bigger team at CAPRISA and beyond. Our life-long experience in infectious disease also put us in a prime position to tackle new global pandemics. But it had been a long road to get there.

Until Covid-19, there has never been a full-blown pandemic affecting humans that has been caused by a coronavirus. At any given time, there are hundreds of coronaviruses in circulation, mostly within animal species, although they have the potential, under certain circumstances, to jump to humans in what is known as a 'spillover event'. Since their discovery in the 1950s, four human coronaviruses had been identified as the cause of a range of respiratory infections, including the common cold. They include Coronaviruses 229E, NL63, OC43 and HKU1.

In the past 20 years alone, we have discovered three more – SARS, MERS and SARS-CoV-2 – all of which are far more serious than their common predecessors. As most experts have noted, including Peter Piot in a 2021 Gairdner seminar, while pandemics have been around for centuries – largely precipitated by encroaching human settlements – we have recently been seeing more of them, and local outbreaks now have a higher risk of spreading globally owing to increased travel, climate change and a host of other factors relating to the impact of human activities on the planet that have disrupted the ability of humans to live in harmony with their environment.

When SARS appeared in China in 2002, I had taken a keen interest in its emergence and trajectory and anticipated it would become a global pandemic. I remember discussing the matter with Dr Margaret Chan, when she was Director-General of the WHO, as she had been the Director of Health in the Hong Kong government when SARS first broke out. SARS did in fact spread rapidly – to 29 countries and territories, infecting about 8 000 people and causing an estimated 774 deaths. But it was soon contained, and effectively lasted only one season.

Ten years later, when MERS emerged, I was again concerned, but perhaps a little less so, given the successful containment of SARS a decade earlier.

The fact that SARS and MERS did not become full-blown pandemics was to a large extent the result of effective global public health and containment measures taken at the time. But there was also something about the viruses themselves that suggested, at least to me, that they were unlikely to pose a large-scale threat to humans. To understand my view on this, it is necessary to say a little about the molecular biology of coronaviruses.

Coronaviruses are large, enveloped RNA (ribonucleic acid) viruses. Their name comes from their distinctive protein spikes visible under an electron microscope, which create the effect of a crown or halo at the edges of its spherical mass. All of the coronavirus strains that we know about have undergone recent animal-to-human transition: either a virus mutates directly to humans, or it goes through an intermediary species, which facilitates its further mutation into a human pathogen – something that can cause disease in humans. In the case of SARS, MERS and SARS-CoV-2, the species of origin is believed to have been bats, specifically horseshoe bats, which are natural reservoir hosts for many coronaviruses. The intermediate species for SARS-CoV and MERS-CoV are thought to be palm civets and dromedary camels respectively.

The intermediary host for Covid-19 was from the start suspected to be the Malayan or Javan pangolin, live specimens of which were being sold in southern China at the Huanan Seafood Market in Wuhan in the province of Hubei. Wuhan is widely believed to have been the physical origin of the Covid-19 outbreak, as the earliest cases were in the vicinity of the seafood market. In China, the meat of the pangolin is considered a delicacy and the scales are believed to have medicinal value. As a result, these animals are traded, alongside bats and other animals, in so-called wet markets throughout the country. Initially, the evidence pointed to pangolins as the intermediate host for the SARS-CoV-2, but subsequent data indicate otherwise. There is also a school of thought that the virus originated from the Wuhan Institute of Virology laboratory. The most sinister claim of the ill-informed hypothesis is that the Wuhan Institute of Virology made the virus through gain-of-function genetic manipulation in partnership with scientists in the US and then released it intentionally or accidentally into the population of Wuhan. There is no direct evidence for this, but it is widely promoted as a conspiracy theory by right-wing groups, as well as some politicians and academics in the US and elsewhere. It is most likely that SARS-CoV-2 was created naturally as a spillover event, in the same way as SARS and MERS. Epidemiological and phylogenetic studies by the University of Arizona's Michael Worobey and others in the journal *Science* provide good evidence for the Huanan Seafood Market being the source of this event.[2] Further genetic studies from the wastewater from the Wuhan Seafood market confirmed the presence of SARS-CoV-2 with genes of various animals, most notably raccoon dogs, from one section of the market, providing further evidence of a potential intermediary host.[3] There is no comparable epidemiological or genetic evidence of the Wuhan Institute of Virology being the source of viral spread – just theories and accusations.

A report based on an investigation by the WHO into the source of the pandemic released on 30 March 2021 was still unable to conclusively identify the intermediate host.[4] It found that markets selling animals, dead and alive, in December 2019 were the 'probable source' of the pandemic and that the virus *probably* did not spread widely before December or escape from a laboratory, but this report was hampered by the lack of co-operation and transparency on the part of the Chinese government, which restricted the WHO team's access to the Wuhan Institute of Virology. China's lack of transparency in this matter has served to fuel conspiracy theories on the origins of the virus.

On their own, most bat coronaviruses are harmless to humans. They are generally not able to enter human cells and infect them. However, when a bat coronavirus enters an intermediate animal host, it can undergo recombinations of its genes and the genetically new coronavirus that emerges may then possess an ability to attach to human cells. Specifically, it develops the ability to attach to the angiotensin-converting enzyme II, or ACE2 receptor, on the host cell. This is done through the receptor-binding domain (RBD) located on the virus's protein spike. Human cells throughout the body have the ACE2 receptor in abundance. If a virus can attach to the ACE2 receptor, it is able to infiltrate and infect many different human cells.

When SARS succeeded in entering human cells in late 2002, with the help of its intermediary host, the palm civet (which looks just like a cat), it did so through the ACE2 receptor. However, the spike protein of SARS did not bind with high affinity (that is, it did not bind strongly) to the human ACE2 receptor, which meant that while the disease was serious, there were some limitations in its infectiousness. MERS was similar: the virus had a low affinity ACE2 receptor-binding protein, which, in turn, meant it was relatively less infectious and so could be contained with public health measures.

I was to some extent reassured by these limitations and anticipated them in the next coronavirus to come along, which, of course, was SARS-CoV-2. But here was something different: a significant alteration in the bat coronavirus had given the virus stronger binding (that is, higher levels of affinity) to the ACE2 receptor. This resulted in the emergence of a virus able to spread more easily than its earlier cousins. In hindsight, it is possible to see both SARS and MERS as two early warning bells heralding a third, more ominous threat to human health and well-being.

How one approaches a disease as an epidemiologist depends to a large extent on how one understands the endgame. Appreciation of the various scenarios for the endgame is important as it provides a desired endpoint that you want your interventions to steer towards. Without having a notion of what the desired endgame looks like, there is no pathway and overall direction for individual decision-making. For me, a key element in the endgame was a vaccine. In other words, is there a chance of a vaccine? Vaccines represent the most effective public health tools we have to control and even eradicate diseases, so understanding whether a vaccine is possible and when it might be available will strongly determine the trajectory of any response to a disease. But vaccines are not a silver bullet; viruses can mutate to escape vaccine immunity, thwarting the attempts to reach viral control, even with high coverage.

Of course, understanding the endgame is not simple, particularly at the onset of a new disease. It requires some understanding of the disease itself, but it also calls for an appreciation of *what is not known* about the disease. For example, in AIDS, some scientists were of the view that a vaccine could be made within a few years. Almost 40 years since the discovery of HIV, there is still no effective vaccine for HIV, either as a preventive or therapeutic measure.

As we now know all too well, one of the main reasons behind the failure to find a vaccine for HIV is the high genetic variability of the virus, owing in part to its rapid replication cycle and high mutation rate. HIV replication is highly error prone, giving rise to a number of minor variations or quasi species in a single infected individual, which then fight for dominance. It is extremely difficult, and thus far it has been impossible, to create a vaccine that can defeat so many different variations and strains of HIV. This, and some other unique features of the virus, is why we have lived with HIV for almost four decades without a vaccine.

Facing the prospect of a similar scenario in the case of Covid-19, given the rapid transmission we were witnessing around the globe, was a daunting prospect. However, there were some very significant differences between the new coronavirus and HIV that soon became evident. While both the coronavirus and HIV are single-stranded RNA viruses, a large difference between them is that HIV is a retrovirus, while coronavirus is not. In order to replicate, a retrovirus like HIV inserts a DNA copy of its genome into the host cell using the reverse transcriptase, the enzyme used to generate complementary DNA from an RNA template. Coronaviruses, on the other hand, simply replicate their RNA and cannot make DNA to insert into the human genome. Unlike HIV, coronaviruses have what is referred to as a proof-reading step in the genome replication cycle, which means the coronavirus makes few mistakes: there are relatively few mutations, and the genome remains relatively stable in copies of the virus. This is in spite of the fact that the coronaviruses have the biggest genomes (genetic material) known among the RNA virus family – around 30 000 bases long.

For someone like me, who is intimately familiar with the highly changeable nature of HIV, the degree of stability to be found in an RNA virus necessitated a 180-degree mind shift. However, like many others following developments in the field closely, I could see that it signalled promising possibilities for future vaccine development. Although, even with that knowledge, I could never have anticipated that there would be a Covid-19 vaccine in such a short time span – a feat previously unheard of.

Keeping close track of different viral strains and quasi species is now possible through genetic sequencing. In the sequencing that had been conducted in China when the novel coronavirus first made an appearance, it appeared that two different strains of the virus with separate lineages were circulating in Wuhan. The explanation for this remains unclear: either the virus mutated very quickly in the beginning, which was unlikely given what we know about its stability, or there were two separate spill-over events from animals to humans that occurred at different times. This phenomenon will be studied, and answers will arise in due course, but at that point it occurred to me that what was being perceived by scientists as two separate strains could be quasi-species of the new virus, which would present a fresh challenge with regard to development of a vaccine.

At that time, Tulio de Oliveira and I were discussing his data on the genetic sequences of circulating SARS-CoV-2 on a regular basis. De Oliveira roundly rejected the notion of a quasi-species. Based on his meticulous analyses, the novel virus was showing an average evolution of only one genome shift per month, if that. For a virus, this is extremely slow. But it was also reassuring. During the process of mutation, the more transmissible viruses tend to become dominant, muscling out the less infectious versions, which eventually wither away. This is called 'viral fitness'. The viruses that do not kill their host tend to do better than those that do, for obvious reasons, so viruses are expected to naturally evolve over the long term to become more infectious (more fit) but less deadly. In June 2020, the dominant strain of the new coronavirus in most of Europe, the UK and South Africa was D614G, and given what De Oliveira was saying, it appeared that it would be holding very comfortably to its pole position during the remainder of the year. This was an assumption that would eventually be overturned, a few months down the line.

Acutely aware of the need to stay one step ahead of the virus, De Oliveira and I continued to monitor its progression and genetic changes. It continued to show unusual stability despite the ongoing rapid global spread. On the surface, prospects for a vaccine continued to look good. However, I deliberately chose to be cautious when speaking about the issue in media interviews. Having faced my fair share of epidemics and outbreaks, I had no wish to be responsible for raising false hopes – just in case this virus still held some surprises.

The truth was that no one had ever manufactured and implemented a vaccine for a coronavirus before, so I could honestly say we really didn't know if a vaccine was possible. Because SARS and MERS – the two most dangerous coronavirus-related diseases we knew about at that point – had been contained, there had been little time to create and test a vaccine against either of these two coronaviruses, which, in any event, usually takes years. The remaining four known coronaviruses, which simply cause the common cold, do not warrant the development of a vaccine because the illness they precipitate in humans is relatively mild. Another sobering fact was that we had never been able to develop a vaccine for influenza that didn't need to be administered every year; whoever succeeds in creating a universal flu vaccine will likely win a Nobel Prize.

Given the complexity of the task and the lack of time to make a vaccine, I felt I had reason to temper my optimism. In those early months of the outbreak, though, as De Oliveira's data continued to show minor changes to the virus and vaccine trials started around the world, I became more positive in my outlook for a vaccine for this coronavirus's endgame. Other scientists had also begun to draw similar conclusions and a plan with vaccination as the goal began to form. The end of the pandemic may have been unclear, but the measures needed to get there were starting to take shape.

Understanding biology was not enough. The challenge was to instil and sustain behaviour change until medical solutions became available – a challenge that looked daunting, and perhaps beyond reach when it required tens of millions of people to act not only in their best interests, but also in the interests of others around them.

CHAPTER 13

A perfect storm

Biological science was not enough to tackle Covid-19; behaviour change
was critical. We needed to rekindle the celebrated philosophy of ubuntu,
which highlights our mutual interdependence and recognises that a
human life finds meaning through the lives of others.

In order for a virus to become dominant in a population, there needs
to be a coalescence of some critical factors. In other words: a perfect
storm. I'd seen it before, when women and girls were placed at higher risk
for HIV due to a complex intersection of behavioural patterns as well as
biomedical factors. The cycle of HIV transmission places young women at
risk of contracting the virus through a combination of behavioural choices
of having sex with older male partners and changes in the vaginal microbiome that make the genital tract biologically more susceptible to HIV
infection. Without addressing both aspects of the epidemic, the virus runs
rampant in a community. It was a balance that I had been fighting to
strike in my work for decades and so it was one I easily recognised when
Covid-19 emerged as a new viral foe ideally placed to wreak havoc. In this
perfect storm of both biology and behaviour, the virus had an advantage.

The first component of the Covid-19 storm was the infectiousness of
the virus. The original version of SARS-CoV-2 had a basic reproduction
rate, or R_0, of somewhere between 2 and 3. In other words, a person
infected with SARS-CoV-2 is likely to infect two to three other people
during their infectious period. While not as infectious as measles, which
has an R_0 of 16, SARS-CoV-2 is more infectious than SARS, MERS or
seasonal influenza. R_0 of 2 means that the virus will spread exponentially:

two infections become four, four become eight, eight become 16, and so on. At a small scale, this growth may seem manageable, but when a community reaches, say, a million infections, it becomes a deadly scenario because it can go to 2 million and then 4 million within days. Ideally, the goal is to reduce the R_0 to below 1 – the point at which it is not increasing and the rate at which new infections is occurring is effectively declining within a community.

In the early stages of the outbreak in South Africa, we were able to slow down the transmission rate through public health and social measures such as social distancing, mask-wearing and handwashing. But getting the number below 1 was turning out to be beyond our reach. One of the few countries to have succeeded in achieving this was the island nation of New Zealand, which implemented an early lockdown and closed international borders as part of that country's elimination strategy. In South Africa, as in most other countries in the world, we adopted a mitigation strategy, rather than an elimination strategy, as a more realistic target.

Another feature of SARS-CoV-2 that contributed to the 'perfect storm' was its selective impact on its victims. In older people, or in people with comorbidities, the virus meant potential illness and possible death. But for most of the young people who contracted the disease, Covid-19 presented a low risk of severe illness. Among this younger group, most of those infected were asymptomatic and entirely unaware of their condition. Because of this and by virtue of being the most mobile component of societies, younger people played the role (often inadvertently) of taking the virus out into communities and facilitating its spread to older and more vulnerable members of the population. And they did so largely unknowingly and undetected.

The ability of the virus to spread unnoticed, particularly among young people, and at the same time to cause death in others, particularly among older people or those with comorbidities, dramatically raised the stakes and generated serious implications for how it was to be managed. In the absence of a vaccine, the only means available to slow the spread of the virus was to reduce interaction and physical contact between people.

Understanding the biology of Covid-19 was not going to be enough; behaviour change would be key.

The virus demanded that we radically change our behaviour. Behaviour change, which is very difficult to achieve, as I knew well from trying to achieve behaviour change for AIDS, could be either voluntary (as in the case of recommending mask-wearing) or government-imposed (as in the case of mandatory mask-wearing) or a combination of some voluntary and some mandatory measures. The trade-off for such behaviour change, regardless of it being voluntary or government-imposed, was, of course, the economy and the curtailment of daily activities like going to school, accessing health care services, etcetera. Further, damage to mental health would be the inevitable outcome of restrictions to human movement and physical interaction. These were costs that had to be taken into account in light of the limited options on the table at the time – but it also meant restrictions of movement wouldn't be sustainable in the long term.

Getting people to change how they behaved was the priority and the best chance we had to contain Covid-19. But the nature of the disease and human behaviour made this harder to achieve. If every person was as likely as the next to contract a severe form of Covid-19, managing the response to the pandemic through behaviour change would have been a lot easier. However, the impact of the disease on individuals was not uniformly severe, which would likely make the public response to containment measures inconsistent. Each person would have a different perceived risk and, as such, would feel a varying need to adopt prevention measures. This became apparent as early as the first wave. The restrictions on movement applied to everyone equally but the benefits of containment accrued predominantly to the elderly or those with comorbidities. Meanwhile, younger people were being required to make major sacrifices, which affected both their lifestyles and in some cases livelihoods, while not seeing the same rewards for their behaviour. Under these circumstances and, given the fact that it is the nature of humankind that some individuals will always adhere to rules more closely than others, it is perhaps easy to understand why support for, and compliance with, lockdown restrictions was always likely to have a limited lifespan.

Nonetheless, it remains true that in this storm, the actions of only a handful of people who chose not to make sacrifices in their own lives were enough to put countless others at risk of infection, sickness, and possible death. In a super-spreading event, just one person can cause untold harm by passing on the infection to more people than is typical of the virus (in the case of Covid-19 this would be an instance where one person infected more than three people). To illustrate the super-spreader problem, I would recount how just one person in South Korea, referred to as patient 31 (because she was the 31st patient to be diagnosed with Covid-19 in that country), led to hundreds of infections when she went to church and to a buffet lunch just before she was diagnosed with Covid-19.

At this critical juncture, where behaviour could curb the spread of Covid-19, we had the opportunity to either recognise or reject our mutual interdependence. In some cases, rejection seemed to be on the ascendancy in the world – or at the very least in the US, where President Trump was taking every opportunity to applaud his own swift recovery from Covid-19 and downplay the seriousness of the disease for individuals who contracted it. This same flaw is to be found in the reasoning of those individuals who protested their right not to be restricted by government-imposed regulations; those who would argue that it was their choice to run the gauntlet of infection if they so wished, and to carry on with their normal lives, especially if they were healthy and knew that picking up infection would likely be inconsequential for them. By focusing so entirely on their own freedoms, this cohort ignored the risk they were imposing upon others by exercising and, in turn, robbing others of the chance to exercise their own rights. In the midst of a pandemic, weighing up the different rights presents many challenges. I tended to look at it as curtailing a person's rights was justified when their actions placed others in harm's way, that is, no one had the right to knowingly harm others. But this required continual assessment of the nature of the harm posed to others and the nature of the impact of curtailing an individual's rights.

I found no simple answers, just a continuum of possible answers that fluctuated as the risks and benefits varied. It wasn't as simple as letting people do what they wanted, when considering the potential harm to society as a whole. The fact that many people had lost friends and loved ones to the virus was a painful reminder that science still had its limitations in the face of a novel, highly infectious and potentially deadly virus. In the absence of a vaccine or treatment, I was painfully aware in 2020 that the main weapon we had to contain the virus was prosocial human behaviour. Prosocial behaviour is where people behave in ways that promotes the common good rather than focusing only on individual benefit. But convincing people of this came with its own challenge.

Every Sunday, Quarraisha and I walk along the Durban beachfront promenade. This weekly routine was placed on hold during those early months of the pandemic, as the city beaches had been closed to swimmers since the March lockdown in 2020. In mid-October, after the restrictions had eased to allow the beaches to reopen, we resumed our usual Sunday outing, albeit with the addition of our masks. We arrived to see hundreds of people, crowding not only on the sand, but the promenade and in the parking areas. These masses of people at the beach were commonplace during the Christmas holidays at the end of the year. But this time it was a celebration of a different kind – people were appreciating the relief from the Covid-19 restrictions, revelling in their ability to go outside and be around others. But, while others enjoyed the return of their freedom, I worried about the implications of such mass crowds with few, if any, preventative measures. I worried that large gatherings could lead to an increase in the risk of infection.

The following morning, Health Minister Mkhize and his wife were diagnosed with Covid-19. I was interviewed on SAFM radio by the astute and highly experienced journalist Stephen Grootes about a possible impending rise in the tide of infections. I was still rattled by the scenes I had witnessed the previous day on the beachfront, and I spoke of my concerns about people abandoning the Covid-19 public health prevention measures. And, of course, while it's true that being outdoors reduces the risk of infection, there are a number of other factors in any beach trip – including the use of overcrowded public transport to get there – that place people at risk of getting or transmitting infection, where masks could make a difference. It was about more than a simple trip to the beach. The scenes that I had witnessed foreshadowed a much larger problem at hand.

A second wave would be 'inevitable', given the challenges in getting people to change their behaviour and continue with a few simple public health measures. This was the warning I issued during my SAFM interview and subsequent news reports picked up on it. With the end-of-year holiday period (which traditionally starts on 16 December) of 2020 looming, I was genuinely concerned about what that meant for the movement of people across the country – and in turn what it meant for South Africa's next wave. During the first wave, it is estimated that between 10% and 20% of the population became infected; a far cry from the 66% that would be needed for herd immunity. So, a second wave would occur in the midst of little protective immunity. The gains made during that first lockdown and wave could easily be undone if people continued to revert to risky behaviour.

Fuelling my concerns at that point in time were reports of super-spreader events involving students at universities. One such instance involved University of Fort Hare students who had an all-night party at a tavern in early October 2020 and another party a week later. Some of the students who had contracted the virus during these two events, possibly without them even being aware of it, were then sent home from the university, which is based in the Eastern Cape, taking the virus with them to their families and to people in other provinces.

The Fort Hare case was by no means isolated. In Cape Town, an event at a Claremont nightclub, saw 63 people contracting Covid-19 in early October, the majority of them in their final year of high school. This was a precursor to a similar, but even bigger problem at the end of November when the week-long Ballito Rage Festival, held in the north coast village of Ballito in KwaZulu-Natal, went ahead as usual. The event traditionally attracts thousands of high school leavers from around the country. In this case, it was estimated that more than 1 000 infections in students and their families could be linked to the Ballito Rage event.

Compliance and support for government interventions was high at the start of the stay-at-home lockdown in March 2020. A Human Sciences Research Council survey at the time indicated that 78% or four out of five of 12 300 respondents said they were willing to make sacrifices to their individual freedoms in order to be safe.[1] Interestingly, the lowest willingness was among high-earning white men over 55. However, as time passed, and even after some restrictions were eased, fatigue and complacency had set in. With time making the first wave seem remote and with infection rates in the post-wave ebb, people were becoming more reluctant to continually sacrifice their freedoms for a virus that did not seem to be a serious risk to them.

Everyone was growing impatient for the day when they could go back to 'normal', to the point where the government was met with increasing resistance for reintroducing measures after they had been eased. As someone who was perceived as having control over these regulations, I also faced a growing backlash for continuing to stand behind the use of masks. So, while I was trying to promote an approach of using public health measures to reduce risks in certain settings, I was coming under increasing pressure to abandon them. The arrival of the Beta variant in November 2020 made my position on continued precautions even more important. Not only was the Beta variant easily infecting those who had been infected in the first wave, it was also causing more serious disease. Caution was needed again!

Amid pressure to abandon Covid-19 restrictions, I had an opportunity to reflect on the challenge and to draw upon some of the lessons from AIDS that were beneficial to our Covid-19 response when I was asked to deliver the 57th Cartwright Lecture, which is part of the Dean's Lecture series at Columbia University, in November 2020. The Cartwright Lecture is a prestigious annual lecture dating back to 1881. Past lectures have been delivered by Nobel Prize winners, including Sydney Brenner and Paul Nurse. The invitation had come before the advent of Covid-19, and I had planned to talk about HIV. When it came closer to the time, however, I realised the bigger issue was the complex biological and behavioural challenges produced by Covid-19, and so I pivoted my lecture accordingly. That year the event was online and because it was to be delivered in New York time, it took place in the middle of the South African night.

Part of my lecture examined the lessons that we had learned from the HIV epidemic that might be helpful in the context of combatting the current Covid-19 pandemic. The confluence of factors – the perfect storm – needed to be tackled to break the chains of transmission. In the HIV response, the dictum 'Know your epidemic' was critical to guiding the response – and so it proved to be in Covid-19. First, it was important to know where the problems were. Identifying hotspots would help us figure out what was driving the epidemic. We went the same route with Covid-19, using geographical locations of the homes of infected individuals to identify potential hotspots, which could be sites for high transmission of infections, and to determine the source of spread in these hotspots. The key lesson I drew out was that when it is difficult to get everyone in the population to maintain safe behaviours, whether in HIV or Covid-19, one option is to focus on areas at highest risk. Making people aware of their risk is key to this approach since behaviour change has a stronger motivation in a situation of perceived risk.

Second, we also understood the value of HIV testing and being able to test quickly. When I first started working in HIV, the testing was new, and we lacked confidence in its accuracy. So every routine antibody test had to be confirmed through a second test, which was a time-consuming, expensive and tedious laboratory procedure called the western blot method. Within a few years, however, everything changed in testing. New rapid on-site tests became available, meaning patients could have results in minutes rather than days. Shorter testing time meant a shorter wait for treatment, which in those days could mean the difference between life and death. The same was true of Covid-19: the shift from PCR to rapid antigen point-of-care testing made a big difference. Instead of waiting for two to three days for a result, we could have results in 15 minutes. This was key to enabling us to institute isolation, contact tracing and quarantine – all key components in our response strategy and driven entirely by the capacity to test quickly. Importantly, behaviour change could be facilitated by knowledge of infection status through routine rapid testing. So, I have repeatedly promoted home testing but even three years later it is not available in South Africa – perhaps because of a misplaced concern that people would not do the test properly at home.

Third, we understood through our work in HIV the importance of community health workers. These were trusted health education providers who could engage with people on the ground in places they knew. In response to Covid-19, South Africa had quickly mobilised the nation's network of community health workers. From past experience with HIV, we increasingly understood the value of working 'with' people, rather than 'on' people and this kind of community-based response proved to be far more effective in changing behaviour and increased testing. The recognition that communities need to be part of any successful process was also behind the minister's decision to include representatives of a range of community-based and faith-based organisations in the second Ministerial Advisory Committee so that their insights could also be part of guiding our country's response.

Fourth, the value of leadership was another lesson from HIV, to recognise how important it is to have consistent role models. At a critical time in the national response to HIV, we had a powerful leader in the form of President Nelson Mandela, who actively embodied the philosophy of ubuntu. During Covid-19, we had a wise and empathetic leader in Cyril Ramaphosa – a man who understood the need to be open to scientific advice, but also the need for decisive action in responding early to the pandemic. It was important for our leaders to take the lead in showing people the desired risk-reducing behaviours. As part of this effort, Ramaphosa demonstrated on national television how to put on a mask. Though it made him look a bit awkward because the mask covered his eyes initially, his actions showed that he was leading the way with masks, even if he had not yet perfected putting it on yet.

Fifth, our HIV response taught us the importance of a prevention toolbox – the collection of measures that can be used, according to the particular setting, to fight the virus. Just as we had experienced in the HIV epidemic, we knew that looking for a single silver bullet approach was not going to be the answer to Covid-19. We rejected measures such as natural-infection-induced herd immunity very early on, choosing instead to work with a full prevention toolbox. This meant the toolbox we adopted aimed to counter the danger of the five Ps: People in Prolonged, Poorly-ventilated, Protection-free Proximity. In other words, we promoted prevention measures, from the toolbox as the situation demanded it, like opting for outdoor spaces where possible or masking indoors.

Finally, for me, one of the biggest lessons from the HIV pandemic was the recognition of humankind's mutual interdependence and the need for global solidarity. The global AIDS movement demonstrated how a shared vision, responsive leadership and individual actions could change the course of history. AIDS had changed from a fatal disease to one where antiretroviral treatment was made available even in the most remote villages in Africa. To make this possible, the US President's Emergency Plan for Aids Relief (PEPFAR), the largest commitment by any country towards a single disease, contributed resources and funds to expanding access to HIV-prevention interventions and treatment and supporting HIV-related services in Africa. This was a shining example of how global co-operation enabled the continent of Africa to prevail against HIV, realising mutual benefits in collaboratively fighting a disease. This global solidarity and shared vision provided the fundamental pillars that enabled society to respond effectively to the pandemic threat of HIV.

In South Africa and parts of southern Africa, ubuntu is the celebrated philosophy that guides the way in which human life and interactions are perceived and indeed lived from day to day. Roughly translated as 'I am a person because you are a person', it foregrounds the interconnectedness and mutual dependence of human beings. It recognises that a human life finds meaning through the lives of others. Implied in this philosophy is the importance of the collective, even when it requires some individual sacrifices along the way. Ubuntu was our best antidote to the perfect storm driving the spread of the virus.

I have often said that our country, which saw the successful overthrow of the apartheid regime largely through the efforts of a mass democratic movement, was in fact built on the principle of short-term sacrifice for collective rather than individual benefit. Countless people put their lives at risk, and in fact lost their lives in the struggle against apartheid. It was not an easy path to take – in fact it was deadly for some – but people chose that path because it held the prospect of a higher goal with collective benefits: a new democratic order, a new society in which the rights of all people would be recognised.

I also observed the culture of short-term sacrifice in the widespread 'stokvel' system in South Africa, an informal community-based savings system, which sees members of communities and families voluntarily pooling their money in a collective fund so they can enjoy the benefits once or twice a year when it is their turn to receive the lump-sum payout. Old Mutual, one of the South Africa's largest insurance companies, which has a long history in the country, was initially built on the stokvel principle.

Towards the end of November 2020, Pope Francis wrote an article published in *The New York Times* that moved me deeply and resonated with my own thinking about people's interdependence and captured the message I might have written to the world if I had a fraction of his eloquence and audience.[2] In his plea that people resist the 'virus of indifference', the Pope argued that if we were to come out of the pandemic better than we went in, we needed to recognise our common humanity. To me, he was talking about ubuntu – even if it had some other name in his vocabulary.

His words were as follows: 'To come out of this crisis better, we have to recover the knowledge that as a people we have a shared destination. The pandemic has reminded us that no one is saved alone. What ties us to one another is what we commonly call solidarity. Solidarity is more than acts of generosity, important as they are; it is the call to embrace the reality that we are bound by bonds of reciprocity. On this solid foundation, we can build a better, different, human future.'

The Pope's words and sentiments resonated with me. Partly as a result of our experiences when we joined the anti-apartheid movement in South Africa, both Quarraisha and I developed a strong sense of social justice and solidarity with those less fortunate. In our case, that translates into our shared commitment to improving the lives of others – and an enduring belief in the power of excellent science to achieve it.

As a scientist, I had multiple challenges maintaining scientific excellence and keeping abreast of scientific developments, conducting research, providing scientific advice and educating the public on the science of Covid-19. My focus was on 'big picture' questions in science, drawing in part on the network of global expertise I had links with, in an effort to further a collective response to the pandemic. In conducting research, I am fortunate to be part of a big team that involves researchers in CAPRISA and beyond. Through the research conducted by CAPRISA with our many partner organisations, we were able to generate scientific knowledge rapidly and we published over 100 journal articles on Covid-19 – both original contributions and editorials – in the first two years of the pandemic as a small contribution to understanding the perfect storm driving SARS-CoV-2 infections and developing effective ways to counter it.

CHAPTER 14

Covid-19 scientific contributions

*It was a time when science moved quickly. It had to. My scientific
contributions, besides my advisory roles and media engagements,
included publishing a peer-reviewed Covid-19 article about once a
month in leading science journals.*

Writing scientific journal articles is a time-consuming and challenging task. It needs large blocks of time to think carefully about the
data, to review the literature and to explain what the analysis is pointing
to. When I was appointed to chair the MAC, I already had nine jobs
– four senior academic positions at Columbia, Harvard, Cornell and
KwaZulu-Natal universities and five overlapping research unit leadership
positions – that kept me busy. The research units that I am director of
are the UNAIDS Collaborating Centre for AIDS Research and Policy,
the DSI-NRF Centre of Excellence in HIV Prevention, the MRC unit
on HIV-TB pathogenesis and treatment, and a Global Virus Network
Centre of Excellence. All four of these research units are embedded within
CAPRISA, and so their workload overlaps with my workload as director
of CAPRISA. On top of these existing responsibilities, I was now adding
the MAC responsibilities as a 10th job, leaving very little time for me to
contribute to the scientific literature. Despite this, I had to make time to
ensure I was also an active scientist in Covid-19.

One of the most well-known scientific contributions I made was not
in a scientific journal but in the media. It was my prediction on when
South Africa would experience its fourth wave of Covid-19 infections. On
17 August 2021, I gave an interview to a journalist working for Bloomberg.[1]

By then, media interviews were commonplace and were regularly fitted into my schedule, so I didn't think much of it. I don't get briefed on the questions before I do interviews. I prefer not to go in feeling rehearsed, so that I can answer any questions spontaneously as they arise. In that particular interview, the journalist kept asking me when South Africa would see its next wave of infections. My initial few answers were non-committal, but she was quite persistent in trying to nail me down on when we could expect to see a spike in Covid-19 cases again. So, in an attempt to settle the question and move on, I explained to her that I was expecting South Africa to experience a fourth wave of infections and that the wave would start on 2 December 2021. And it did!

In March 2022, I was asked by the Minister of Health to brief the senior team in the department on what the epidemic trajectory would look like and what they should be planning for. In that presentation, I added the 99-day inter-wave period to the date on which the fourth wave had ended to explain that I expected the fifth wave to start on 8 May 2022. I provided a lot of detail on the caveats in this prediction, the principal one being that the prediction was predicated on the past Covid-19 temporal trends continuing into the future. It turned out that I was off in my estimation by one day. South Africa passed the threshold of cases for the fifth wave on 7 May 2022. The fifth wave, which was due to Omicron BA.4 and BA.5, was fortunately a small wave as Omicron BA.1 and BA.2 had left behind substantial cross-immunity to these new Omicron variants. Given that no completely new variant emerged in 2022 (just sub-lineages of Omicron), as they had in the first two years of the pandemic, I stopped providing estimations for the next wave after the fifth wave.

As a scientist, predictions on waves were of little academic interest to me; this is the rightful domain of mathematical modellers. I had other important scientific contributions to ponder. Of the 25 journal articles I published in the first two years of the Covid-19 pandemic – at an average of one article each month – a few stand out as worthy of mention here. My first Covid-19 article was a detailed description of 'The South African response to the pandemic', which was published in the *New*

England Journal of Medicine in June 2020.[2] It drew heavily on the eight-stage response described previously. I learned later that several others had found it helpful in their own planning and had even used stages similar to the ones I outlined.

In May 2020, out of the blue I received a query from one of the editors of *Science* about the intersecting AIDS and Covid-19 epidemics and how Covid-19 was disrupting AIDS programmes. Many of the opportunities afforded to me in Covid-19 are rooted in the decades of time spent toiling away at the much slower-moving, but still serious HIV pandemic. Quarraisha and I jointly took on this interesting task and published a perspective on how 'Covid-19 affects HIV and tuberculosis care' in *Science* in July 2020.[3] In this article, we outlined how South Africa's long history of fighting the twin epidemics of HIV and TB helped provide the infrastructure and resources that enabled such a rapid response to Covid-19. This highlighted why building research and clinical infrastructure for the long term was more important than focusing on short-term gains. The day after this paper appeared in the journal, I received an email from Dr Thomas Quinn, who is one of the world's leading HIV researchers based at Johns Hopkins University and the NIH, commenting on how important he felt the HIV–Covid-19 interplay was and letting me know that he was citing it in an article he was writing on this issue. This is exactly what we hope to achieve in our journal publications – that other scientists find the information useful and use it in their research and writings.

What followed in the next several months were several articles published in the top medical and scientific journals, each tackling new aspects of the pandemic as they emerged (see Appendix 1). Among the most relevant and significant of these articles related to the variants, as South African scientists were often the first to gain insight into some variants of concern, due to our cutting-edge surveillance collecting data, from testing and sequencing to hospital admissions and deaths.

One of my highly cited Covid-19 papers was written with De Oliveira in March 2021. In the midst of substantial uncertainty regarding variants of concern at the time (Alpha, Beta and Gamma), the editor of the *New*

England Journal of Medicine asked me to do a podcast on variants for the journal. Coincidentally, one of the editors of *The Lancet* also contacted me to do a *Lancet* podcast on the Beta variant, which ended up being their most listened to podcast for the year. This showed me that people wanted to know more; they were looking for information about these new versions of SARS-CoV-2 and they wanted to understand variants.

That was exactly what I set about doing, with De Oliveira's assistance. In the March article titled 'New SARS-CoV-2 variants – clinical, public health, and vaccine implications' in the *New England Journal of Medicine*, we spelled out what we knew about these variants.[4] It showed the importance of learning and adapting. Variants had presented a curveball during a time when the world thought the virus had struck out. When a curveball comes at you, you can't keep ducking; you have to hit it at some point. And that's what we had to do with variants. We had to use the information available to get better at understanding and predicting them and re-evaluate what this meant for the future of the pandemic.

In late 2020, I had been working on potential Covid-19 endgame scenarios when I was contacted by the International Science Council to attend a meeting to discuss the potential contribution that the council could make in Covid-19. I shared some of my thoughts around the Covid-19 endgame options and they struck a chord. The council launched a major initiative drawing upon hundreds of scientists across the world from varying disciplines to work on this problem. I served with Sir Peter Gluckman, President of the International Science Council, Sir David Skegg, New Zealand's Chief Covid-19 Science Adviser and Peter Piot, who was by then appointed as Special Adviser to the President of the European Union, on the committee overseeing this project. We encapsulated our approach to this conundrum in a short article in *The Lancet* in 2021 titled, 'Future scenarios for the COVID-19 pandemic'.[5]

The concerns about what the variants would mean for the future of the pandemic were growing and led to a collaboration with colleagues from the Pasteur Institute in Paris, and the article focusing on 'SARS-CoV-2 variants and ending the COVID-19 pandemic' was published in

The Lancet.[6] I was particularly concerned that we needed some way of quickly determining whether our Covid-19 vaccines would remain effective against new variants. But we did not know which immunological marker indicated protection against Covid-19. I felt this was now urgent and needed to be spelled out. I published a letter in *The Lancet* outlining a priority in vaccine immunology titled 'Vaccines and SARS-CoV-2 variants: The urgent need for a correlate of protection'.[7]

South African scientists were at the forefront of producing several important articles on vaccines, variants, immune responses and clinical impact of variants, among others. I felt so proud when I opened a new issue of a top medical journal to see articles in the journal from South African scientists. There was no question that South African researchers from across the country were producing groundbreaking research on Covid-19. At the forefront of the variant research was also a growing crop of young scientists who represented new talent entering the scientific field. On the laboratory end were Dr Khadija Khan and Dr Sandile Cele, both of whom I hold in high regard. These are two highly talented young researchers in the African Health Research Institute, being mentored by Dr Alex Sigal. Sigal had established the cell-lines in his laboratory to grow SARS-CoV-2 under stringent Biosafety Level Three (BSL-3) conditions. As a result, he was able to grow and study each new variant as it emerged. A major benefit was the work that Cele was doing in the lab, testing the blood of vaccinated people to see if the antibodies in their blood killed the new variant. Cele's work was being lauded across the world and he published several of his findings in top journals. In his article in *Nature,* he showed how 'Omicron extensively but incompletely escapes Pfizer BNT162b2 neutralization',[8] a finding that raised concerns among many of us that the Pfizer vaccine would not protect against Omicron. Khan, on the other hand, showed in her *Nature Communications* article that 'Omicron BA.4/BA.5 escape neutralizing immunity elicited by BA.1 infection'.[9] We were seeing this in the fifth wave in South Africa – that people who had Omicron infection previously were getting infected again with BA.5 and Khan had provided us with the reason for this observation.

On the more clinical side was a young up-and-coming star, Dr Waasila Jassat. She is a public health specialist, who worked with Dr Lucille Bloomberg at the NICD to set up active surveillance of South Africa's hospitals through the DATCOV system, and she was also someone I played a small role in mentoring. Her analysis on the impact of Omicron variants on hospitalisation and death was among the top 10 most downloaded from the *Lancet* pre-print server. Titled 'Clinical severity of COVID-19 patients admitted to hospital during the Omicron wave in South Africa', she showed how Omicron led to more clinical cases of Covid-19 but fewer hospitalisations and deaths compared to Delta and Beta variants.[10] It was an impressive contribution deservedly published in *The Lancet Global Health*. It has been incredibly gratifying to see so many upcoming young people emerging with new ideas and doing really good scientific research.

The research community is small and it needs to keep growing with young people with fresh ideas. Science thrives on innovation. We need young talent to continue elevating the research being done in South Africa by pushing the boundaries of knowledge. Mentoring the next generation of research leaders is necessary to keep South Africa at the forefront of medical science and to ensure that the country is replenishing its scientists and its science communicators.

Science communication, for me, is not limited just to media or my advisory role. In my article published in the journal *Public Understanding of Science*, I tried to capture the complexity of 'Communicating in the midst of a pandemic'.[11] Pre-Covid-19, my main means of communication was through scientific publications and that is a trend that not only continued but increased during the pandemic. It was a time when science moved quickly; it had to in order for the world to stay on top of this new virus. As research and breakthroughs happened at lightning speed, the world of scientific publishing also had to keep up. Journals had to accelerate their timeline to get studies out to the public as quickly as possible, while the rise of pre-print servers opened the floodgates for information to be shared, even before peer review.

Now, during Covid-19, we were faced with a scientific community that wanted new information rapidly and where journals were being pressured to meet this demand by providing fast turnaround times for review and approval. As someone who viewed peer review as the gold standard and served on the board of several journals, it was a period of adjustment for me as well.

Typically, an article would take months to craft. It would mean sitting down for hours, going through the data and parsing it down to the most relevant points. Then would come the writing process itself, which of course meant drafts and rewrites before new drafts and more rewrites followed. All of this before it went off to the journal for editing and then we would get comments and feedback to be incorporated from other experts who would review the paper. After all of that, once the revisions were finalised, that's when the study would be ready for publication, and we would see it in an issue of the journal months later.

In 2010, a decade before Covid-19, I had my first foray into a different way of publishing. When the CAPRISA 004 trial was nearly complete, we began discussing where we wanted to publish the results. There were several contenders – all top journals – and we needed to make a decision about who to approach. In the end, we decided to split the three papers across three journals, with the first one going to *Science*. I called up Dr Barbara Jasny, who was then an associate editor at the journal, to ask her if *Science* would be interested in publishing the results, once they were available. Her response was cautiously positive. Yes, she would be keen to publish the results, depending on what they showed.

Two months later, the study was unblinded (where it was revealed which participants got a real drug and which received a placebo). We now knew that the results were positive and that tenofovir gel could prevent HIV infection. Upon seeing the unblinded results, I left the room to call Jasny straight away and she replied: 'Yes, it's a go.' *Science* was keen to publish the article with the trial results, provided it passed peer review. But I also laid out our conditions for publishing the article in *Science*. First, we wanted the article to go live online at the same time as we were publicly announcing the results at the AIDS conference in Vienna, and the second was that the article be made open access so anyone could read it without paying a fee. Neither of these represented what *Science* did as a journal, particularly providing the article without the paywall. I had to submit a written motivation for making the article free access and by the end, they agreed to our conditions, and we were ready to go.

It was a really tight timeline. The deadline was a mere month away, just two weeks of which were for us to actually write the article. It was far less time than I was accustomed to and was the fastest I have ever written such a technical article. But we made it. After two weeks of writing, we made the submission and waited a week for the reviews to come back. The edits took another week and then finally it was done. By mid-July, as we walked up onto that stage at the conference in Vienna, the paper went live on the *Science* website.

Nobody knew what had gone into getting it there – outside of those of us who had been working to make it happen behind the scenes. Months later, Jasny and I met up while I was in Washington, D.C. for a trip. She brought me some Oolong tea and we celebrated the feat it was to get that paper ready in time and have it be published in *Science*. Everything we had done to get it there was well worth the effort and I would undoubtedly do it again. Back then, I thought that would probably be the most stressful circumstances under which I submitted an article and had it published within one month.

Fast-forward to November 2021. De Oliveira's team announced that a new variant called Omicron had been discovered in South Africa. The next day, the Department of Health called me in and asked me to participate in a press briefing to explain what the highly mutated form of the virus meant for the pandemic. I gave the presentation on 25 November and, as was becoming my new routine, the days that followed were filled with several interviews. I was being asked by news outlets around the world to talk about the new concerning variant. Shortly thereafter, a different request came through.

In my inbox, while checking my emails, I saw a message from Dr Richard Horton, editor-in-chief of *The Lancet*. I had first met Horton back in 2000 when I had approached him to serve on a panel at the AIDS conference in Durban. We'd stayed in touch after that, and we had served on a few *Lancet* commissions together. I'm also a member of the board of *The Lancet HIV* and *The Lancet Global Health*. *The Lancet* is among the world's leading medical journals and is a highly reputable publication. Covid-19 upped the ante for the journal and saw them entering a whole new league.

When it comes to journal rankings, the unit of measure used is called an impact factor. Impact factors are calculated as the average number of citations an article published in the journal in the last two years has received. Although not without its controversy, the number serves, rightly or wrongly, as a proxy for the stature of the journal and a higher number indicates more prestige for the publication. The *New England Journal of Medicine* has held the top spot in the medical field since impact factors were introduced in 1975. That is, until now. In 2022, *The Lancet* clinched its new standing as the world's leading medical journal with an impact factor of 202 – a significant rise from its pre-pandemic factor of 79.

A large part of how they achieved this newly earned status was due to how the journal approached pandemic publishing. Horton attributed this to the speed at which they covered things. Like most of the top-tier medical journals, *The Lancet* puts resources into fast-tracking its processes, so peer-reviewed papers on Covid-19 could be released within days instead of months. *The Lancet* was the first to report on the outbreak in Wuhan at the start of 2020. They wanted to be ahead of the curve when it came to sharing the science of Covid-19, and Omicron was no different.

In his email, Horton said he'd seen me on Sky News and BBC News in the UK and wanted me to write an article for *The Lancet* on the new variant. I wrote back informing him that De Oliveira would be best placed to share data on the new variant, copying Tulio on my reply to Horton. The next day, De Oliveira wrote back explaining that there was still significant work to finalise the article on the Omicron mutations. Horton wrote back to me, inviting me to submit what we knew about the epidemiology of Omicron. The deadline: the same day! In essence, it meant that we had about eight hours to write this article. I had never analysed the data and written a paper in that little time before, but I also knew I couldn't pass on this request as the world needed access to this information. The announcement of Omicron had created panic waves in the public and South Africa had the additional challenge of being subjected to multiple travel bans. This variant looked like it was going to spread quickly, and the world needed to prepare. So Quarraisha and I sat down and got to work on writing the article for *The Lancet*. Quarraisha is someone who can always keep me on task. It was no surprise that we partnered up to tackle the submission. As spouses who work together, our thoughts and approach are often in sync, which makes the writing process go much faster. And she frequently knows what I'm trying to say before I can get there myself (although that particular skill set of hers is not limited just to work).

We started by going through the available data we had on Omicron to see if we could decipher a trend. Yes, the doubling times were much higher than Delta and Beta and the epidemic curve was rising much faster. Omicron was much more infectious and was spreading more rapidly than any of the previous variants. We tried to rope in De Oliveira and his colleague Lessells but could not reach them at short notice. In any case, our focus was on the epidemiology of the new wave of infections, not on the mutations in the virus. We did not yet have a clear picture of the clinical severity of Omicron as we only had anecdotal accounts of it being less severe. We chose not to include anything on severity – this would be more appropriate when the data were clearer on this issue.

As we neared the eight-hour mark, Quarraisha and I finished off the article and emailed it through to Horton. Being able to produce a paper that held relevance in such a short time span was possible partly because I had been closely monitoring developments in Covid-19 and had the epidemiological data readily available. A few hours later, we got the review back with an email accepting the article provided the edits required were addressed. The article appeared online on *The Lancet* website that very evening! The whole experience was a whirlwind and was the antithesis of what I had grown accustomed to over the years. While I understood the need to expedite publishing and keep up with the dynamic nature of the pandemic, I don't believe that speed should ever compromise the quality of the work being done. Keeping in mind that the environment now dictated shorter time frames, my mission remained to provide high-quality research, but just in less time. The article in *The Lancet* was a good example of that.[12] I gathered later that it was the first article with data on Omicron published by any scientific journal. The article was profiled on the cover of the following week's paper issue of *The Lancet*. Very quickly, it has garnered over a thousand citations, a rare feat when it comes to journal articles.

During Covid-19, science contributions had two other particularly important roles to fulfil. One was an advocacy role where injustices needed to be highlighted and confronted. The second was its role in conveying the truth, thereby unmasking and challenging lies and misinformation.

Coming from a history of anti-apartheid and AIDS treatment activism, advocating against injustice in Covid-19 came naturally for me; almost a muscle memory reaction. Injustices abounded in Covid-19, but I focused on a few issues where I felt that I could make an impact. One of these issues was the way in which the world was stigmatising South Africa for reporting the discovery of the Beta variant, just as China had been stigmatised for the original variant when President Trump referred to it as the 'Chinese virus'. Instead of referring to it by the interim name based on its key mutation, 501Y.v2, the new variant that we had announced was being called the 'South African variant'. I took every opportunity to rectify this and continually made the point that it was not even known if this new variant did indeed emanate from South Africa. It could have come into the country from anywhere and the country's good surveillance system just happened to be the first to identify and report it. When I respectfully corrected a CNN reporter for unknowingly saying 'South African variant', the clip of this went viral on Twitter with my image being doctored to show me in dark sunglasses. I felt it was important to avoid creating new opportunities for stigma to grow in Covid-19. This problem was eventually solved when the WHO created a naming system based on the Greek alphabet and 501Y.v2 was replaced with an easier name, Beta, which avoided any reference to South Africa.

In Omicron the discrimination was even worse, South Africa was punished for bringing this new variant to the world's attention and was being penalised with travel bans that interrupted critical supply chains to South Africa. Even worse, the UK, the US and several others extended their travel bans to several other African countries as well, even though most of them had not even reported a single case of Omicron infection. I could not help but see the racist element to this, as Hong Kong, which had uploaded an Omicron genetic sequence onto GISAID even before South Africa had done so, and the Netherlands, which reported Omicron shortly after South Africa, did not get travel bans. I was vocal on this issue in the media, especially in the international media like BBC, PBS and CNN. The first country to impose an Omicron-related travel ban on African countries was the UK. My daughter Safura and I wrote a no-nonsense stinging op-ed in a prominent UK newspaper, *The Times*, in which we commented that '… the world needed to build bridges to work together in dealing with this mutating foe but instead some choose to build barriers and punish southern African countries with travel bans'.

My most visceral reaction as a scientist who stood for human rights was against global vaccine inequity. Besides the numerous media comments, podcasts and written viewpoints I contributed in support of global vaccine equity, I joined the infectious disease-focused editors and editorial board members in penning an editorial in the *New England Journal of Medicine* titled 'Addressing vaccine inequity – Covid-19 vaccines as a global public good'. But I became even angrier when I learned how wealthy countries were wasting vaccine doses at a time when most African countries had not yet received their first supplies of Covid-19 vaccines. I joined Professor Jeffrey Lazarus, who is head of health systems at the Barcelona Institute of Global Health and academically affiliated with the University of Barcelona, to capture my outrage at the way in which vaccine doses were being wasted. The article titled 'COVID-19 vaccine wastage in the midst of vaccine inequity: Causes, types and practical steps' was published in *British Medical Journal Global Health*.[13]

My efforts to challenge injustice extended to several other issues, but I was generally careful to include proposed solutions or preferred actions in my writings and comments on Covid-19 injustices. Put simply, I prefer to be constructively critical rather than to just convey put-downs. But my tolerance in being constructively critical was being tested by the quack doctors who kept promoting and prescribing unproven treatments like ivermectin.

The pandemic became the ideal breeding ground for fear, panic and desperation to take hold of people. An environment like that makes it easy to peddle harmful and potentially dangerous treatments, with these medical cures even being touted by doctors.

What may have started with good intentions was now putting people's lives at risk. In the first few months of the pandemic, when the case numbers were still relatively low and there was a dearth of research into possible treatments, the door had opened for the off-label use of drugs used for other conditions to be repurposed for Covid-19. In some cases, medical professionals had good intentions, merely wanting to offer hope to their patients and provide comfort through the perceived protection of medications like hydroxychloroquine and interferon, or more homoeopathic solutions like drinking hot water with garlic and lemon. But times had changed by 2021. There were viable treatment options for Covid-19 and effective vaccines available. Yet, still some doctors remained insistent on choosing treatments for their patients that had no evidence behind them.

One of the most commonly used ineffective medicines was ivermectin as a treatment for Covid-19. At one point, when accessing the drug was illegal in South Africa, people were even resorting to using an animal formulation that was used on farms to treat animals for parasites. The use of ivermectin as a treatment is rooted in bad science and ideology. In early 2020, when people wanted to generate information on possible treatments quickly, some early trials were rushed. This meant the studies were poorly designed, badly conducted or had too few people enrolled to test the drug, rendering the results flawed and, in some instances, misleading. One such misleading study was from Egypt by Ahmed Elgazzar and others.[14] The study showed about 90% efficacy with ivermectin treatment, but the study showed evidence of fraudulent conduct and was withdrawn from its pre-print website (it had never been published in a peer-reviewed journal). But that misleading study led some doctors to prescribe ivermectin for Covid-19.

But by the time ivermectin was disproven, it was too late. The (false) information was out there and the medication had been popularised around the world. Doctors continued to prescribe ivermectin almost with religious fervour long after mountains of evidence had accumulated showing that it had no benefits in Covid-19 treatment. Even though several meta-analyses (studies that combined all the available data) showed that ivermectin provided no clinical benefit in Covid-19 treatment, some doctors stubbornly refused to switch the treatments they prescribed to their patients. This choice actively placed their patients in harm's way. It robbed patients of proven treatments that do work, while ivermectin can cause serious side effects with little benefit.

The evidence is clear that medications like ivermectin (and fluvoxamine) do not work as Covid-19 treatments. The WHO has recommended *against* the use of ivermectin and fluvoxamine for Covid-19. Doctors who disregard this WHO advice should be held accountable for their decision to ignore the evidence available to them and continuing down this anti-science path. This is an ongoing battle. I have been involved in several lawsuits by providing expert affidavits against doctors who continue to prescribe these nonsensical ineffective treatments. In one instance, a doctor from Cape Town claimed to have treated 3 000 patients with ivermectin!

It was also a fight I took up in top medical journals. One of my 2022 Covid-19 publications was an editorial with Dr Nikita Devnarain, a talented young scientist at CAPRISA, which was published in the *New England Journal of Medicine* and titled 'Time to stop using ineffective Covid-19 drugs'; in it we argued that '… there aren't always right answers, but some answers are clearly wrong. With respect to clinical decisions about Covid-19 treatment, some drug choices, especially those that have negative WHO recommendations, are clearly wrong. In keeping with evidence-based medical practice, patients with Covid-19 must be treated with efficacious medications; they deserve nothing less.'[15]

As we repeatedly stand up for the truth as scientists, we know that we are not alone. In reading his book titled *Spike: The Virus vs. The People – the Inside Story*, I got to learn how Sir Jeremy Farrar FRS was dealing with the Covid-19 science-to-policy challenges in the UK. It was reassuring that we were not alone in dealing with this. Farrar was someone I could count on to bounce off ideas on the viral origins and other aspects of Covid-19. Scientists generally read widely to understand the latest studies and see what new information is being shared by our colleagues. We also rely on the expertise of people who are leaders in their fields, some of whom happen to be friends and colleagues. High on that list was Dr John Nkengasong, a leading virologist and colleague, whose expertise and collaboration I valued immensely. His leadership of the African Covid-19 response, as Director of the Africa CDC, was laudable. His warm personality and outstanding leadership made him the go-to person in Africa. My extensive network with scientists across the globe was helped by my participation in a number of high-level Covid-19 committees, including the Lancet COVID-19 Commission; the Africa CDC Consortium for COVID-19 Vaccine Clinical Trials (CONCVACT), which involved 20 clinical trial sites to rapidly launch vaccine trials across the continent; the African Task Force on Coronavirus; and the International Science Council, the global voice of science.

Science epitomises our mutual interdependence as a global community of scientists. We depend on each other, and we use the research findings of others to help define what our findings mean. It is by sharing new pieces of information that we have individually learned along the way that we can continue to build our collective knowledge and prepare for the next scientific advance to benefit us all. And as I undertook my research on Covid-19, I knew that I could count on several colleagues from around the world when I needed some assistance. The network of scientists I had across the world proved to be critical at a time when I most needed the support of global collaborators.

CHAPTER 15

Global pandemic collaboration

Global collaboration in science provides enormous benefits, avoiding parochialism and enabling scientists to focus on their 'big thinking' approach to disease control.

Building expertise to deal with infectious diseases is not something that can be done overnight. Luckily, South Africa had ample options on hand to call on for assistance. Similarly, around the world, in 2020 scientists and researchers were putting their heads together on how to combat this new disease: Covid-19. The pandemic served as an equaliser, with everyone, regardless of their background, starting on a blank page for how to address this new virus. With so little known, it was greatly beneficial to have multiple perspectives and opinions informed by different backgrounds. Locally, in South Africa, the MAC served this role – bringing together over 50 experts across disciplines to brainstorm what the country's response should look like. But at the same time, there was also a much larger network at play, where the world's leading scientists were coming together to share their thoughts on possible solutions.

Just as with the knowledge itself, these networks and connections did not happen overnight. Through my decades-long history with viral infections and epidemiology, I had been forming relationships over many years with many scientific peers across the globe. The foundation for many of these went back to the early days of HIV when we were similarly faced with a new, unknown virus and trying to learn as much as possible. We were, in a manner of speaking, novices then, in our field of HIV research. Regardless of where we lived or worked, we were all confronted with and learning about this new virus together – very much in the same way that we were beginning to learn about SARS-CoV-2 and Covid-19 (except that communication back then was less immediate).

Faced once again with a similar problem of how to fight off a pandemic during a time when there was little evidence-based research, I knew that it was vital to take advantage of the collective scientific expertise available, both locally and internationally. Canvassing different views and sharing information is important for building knowledge and testing assumptions. Furthermore, ongoing communication and networking were critical in ensuring that I was familiar with the views and thinking of other leading scientists, even if I might not agree with them.

It meant I could better fulfil my role in leading the MAC, providing advice to the government and passing on accurate information to the public during television, radio or newspaper interviews. To ensure I was getting a diverse range of views in order to have the best chance of effectively dealing with the new coronavirus, I began reaching out around the world to the senior Covid-19 scientists who were leading their countries' responses.

Among the first people I contacted was Dr Anthony Fauci, the then lead government Covid-19 adviser in the US and Director of the National Institute for Allergy and Infectious Diseases at the NIH. This was not the first time we would work together. Fauci and I have collaborated over several years on HIV-prevention research.

In addition to my personal communications with Fauci, our paths crossed publicly several times during that tumultuous year of 2020. This included the First International Covid-19 Conference, hosted by the International AIDS Society as part of the AIDS conference in July, when we both shared a platform with then White House Coronavirus Response Coordinator Dr Deborah Birx as the three speakers of the opening session. Our paths crossed again when we were selected as joint winners of the John Maddox Prize for standing up for science in December. On that occasion, the president of the Academy of Science of South Africa, Professor Jonathan Jansen, described Fauci and me as 'a powerful example

of research collaboration between the Global North and Global South …
here is a hopeful and inspiring example of what is possible when research
partners and partnerships bridge this dangerous divide then (HIV/AIDS
pandemic) and now (the Covid-19 pandemic)'.[1] Jansen's comments
revealed an insight into the 'big picture' nature of scientific research, a
view of science that understands the reality that no virus in our inter-
connected and globalised world can be defeated by individuals or even
teams of individuals without extensive international collaboration. Our
paths crossed again in 2021 when we met to review progress on our HIV
antibody studies. And it was particularly pleasing to see Fauci and his
wife, Dr Christine Grady, at the 2022 National Academy of Medicine
Annual Meeting, after which they both joined Quarraisha and I for lunch
in Washington, D.C. a few weeks after Fauci's retirement announcement.

Fauci is someone I knew I could count on if I needed scientific
information or advice, as were his colleagues at the NIH, and those were
the kind of people I was seeking out for input on the global Covid-19
response. Two others I reached out to were Dr John Mascola, head of the
Vaccine Research Center (VRC) of the NIH, and Dr Barney Graham,
who has spent many years working on coronavirus vaccines at the VRC.
Graham and I know each other from more than two decades ago when
we both served on an NIH committee that reviewed the US Centers for
AIDS Research. I hold him in high regard as an expert on coronaviruses as
he had developed a coronavirus vaccine following the first SARS outbreak
and was working in early 2020 with Moderna on the SARS-CoV-2 vaccine.
At the end of a long day after an AIDS meeting in Tanzania several years
ago, we walked together along the beach and there he introduced me to
an amusing rubber skin-tight water-shoe that he wore to protect his feet.
It had a skeleton of the foot painted on it.

To better tackle this virus, we needed global input from leading experts
around the world; the more people willing to share insights from their
own experiences, the better. Each country's response and outbreak could
help paint a fuller picture of what this virus was doing on the ground –
and in turn inform how we could best contain it. So, I connected with

my counterparts and scientific colleagues in other parts of the world. As part of an International Science Council initiative, I linked up with Sir David Skegg, an epidemiologist who was New Zealand's chief Covid-19 scientist. Skegg and I had served together on the WHO Scientific Advisory Committee on Reproductive Health and, like me, he held a university leadership position. Among the many others were Dr Jeffrey Lazarus of the Barcelona Institute of Global Health in Spain; leading behavioural scientist Dr Susan Michie, who was on the UK Covid-19 advisory committee and Dr Jong-Koo Lee, public health expert in South Korea, who also served with me on the Lancet COVID-19 Commission Task Force for Public Health Measures to Suppress the Pandemic. Dr Eric Goosby, who had previously led PEPFAR and was on President Biden's transition Covid-19 task force, had been in touch with me for, inter alia, a contribution to a special journal issue on Covid-19. Goosby is a long-standing friend and colleague who has visited CAPRISA many times. Some of the others were Dr Arnaud Fontanet, an epidemiologist at the Pasteur Institute, who served on France's Covid-19 scientific advisory committee, and Dr Anders Tegnell, state epidemiologist and adviser to the Swedish government, with whom I delivered the Nobel Inspired Public Lecture on the 'The meaning of science in the age of Covid-19' in October 2020.

The colleagues I had been in touch with included dozens of African scientists, some of whom were Dr Alash'le Amibiku from Nigeria, Dr Miriam Were from Kenya, Dr Pontiano Kaleebu from Uganda, Dr Francine Ntoumi from the Democratic Republic of the Congo, Dr Souleymane M'boup of Senegal and Dr Emelyn Shroff of the Seychelles; many of them through the weekly Africa CDC Covid-19 consortium meetings I chaired. Dr Shroff, Dr Agnes Chetty and their colleagues in the Department of Health in the Seychelles had regular Zoom meetings with me when their second wave hit, as they were among the countries I had been asked by the Africa CDC to assist with epidemiological and scientific advice. The whole team in the Seychelles were great to work with as they undertook various epidemiological analyses to understand their breakthrough infection problem. I arranged for 20 samples from the Seychelles to be sent to De Oliveira at KRISP for sequencing, so that we could establish which variant was responsible. I would often tease Shroff about the Zoom background she had, which looked idyllic, and she invited me, in response, to visit the Seychelles. I still have to take up that open invitation.

I also have another open invitation resulting from the scientific advice I provided; this to Disney World in Orlando, Florida. I had been contacted by Disney World in early 2021 to do a webinar on Covid-19 for their team and to provide some scientific advice on the Covid-19 response at Disney World. Their challenges were fascinating and required some out-of-the-box approaches, given the number of indoor activities and large restaurants in these parks. Since I do not charge for my education and advisory services, they gave me a standing invitation to Disney World as a VIP visitor – not sure what this entails but I hope to get the opportunity to take up this invitation one day.

Working with so many impressive international scientists and organisations helped keep the focus on the 'big thinking' approach to disease control. Comparing notes and sharing information with these experts, who were often guiding their own countries' and organisations' responses, helped me to better appreciate what it would take to provide advice on the South African Covid-19 response in a more informed way. In many instances, the early national response to the pandemic in South Africa also served as a positive case study for other countries. Several of my colleagues would refer to what we were doing in South Africa in the advice they were providing in their own countries.

I was also communicating with Chinese scientists who, given the ostensible origins of the coronavirus in Wuhan, were literally ahead of the curve when it came to responding to the pandemic. I was in contact with Dr George Gao FRS, Director of the China CDC, Dr Yiming Shao, Chief Expert on AIDS at the China CDC, who was involved in their Covid-19 vaccine development, and Dr Zunyou Wu, the chief epidemiologist at the China CDC's Division of HIV prevention. Gao was an author on one of the first articles written on Covid-19, a highly cited publication in *The*

Lancet.[2] I had reached out to Wu when we were trying to source rapid Covid-19 test kits for use in South Africa to get his feedback about the Chinese experience of rapid testing and reputable suppliers. Regardless of what politicians say, scientific information between China and the rest of the world is relatively free-flowing. As scientists, we communicate not just when we need to – but because we have to.

I found working at this global level to be a critical adjunct to the thinking and views I was encountering at home in South Africa. Sometimes we become constrained by being inward-looking; being part of a global community helps maintain perspective about what the priorities are.

I was therefore honoured when Dr Tedros asked me to serve as Special Adviser to the Director-General of the WHO. In December 2022, I was formally appointed to this new role as special adviser on pandemics, a role where I had the opportunity to be of greater service on a wider landscape. One of my tasks in this role was to support epidemic intelligence and especially the WHO's Hub for Pandemic and Epidemic Intelligence in Berlin.

Working with some of the world's greatest infectious disease scientists helped to give me a useful dose of perspective and humility and taught me the wisdom of the 'big picture view' of science. In this way, I could see beyond the petty differences and concentrate on what we could learn in a high-stakes war against Covid-19 from the discussions being held and the choices being made by scientists around the world.

Reinforcing the importance of global collaboration and learning from others, I worked with the Department of Health to host a series of MAC webinars with several countries to learn about their responses to Covid-19. The MAC hosted individual sessions with the leading Covid-19 scientists from China, Russia and the US, among others. The webinars were organised officially through diplomatic channels, where the Department of Health made the arrangements through each country's embassy in South Africa. For example, the webinar with the US had presentations by Fauci, Dr Jeffrey Sachs, an economist from Columbia University, and Dr Eric Rubin, editor of the *New England Journal of Medicine*, and was hosted jointly by the US Ambassador to South Africa and the South African Minister of Health.

But I also saw how politics overtook matters in international relations. The Cuba–South Africa relationship was an example that was brought home to me during the pandemic. We learned from the media about a Cuban medical contingent coming to South Africa – none of us on the MAC was aware of it – and it soon became public knowledge. The matter was subsequently raised at the MAC. We wanted to know what skills and human personnel shortfalls required Cubans to assist. Specifically, we were trying to understand what plan of activities the government had that could not be done by South Africans and required Cuban assistance. When we enquired, we learned that there were actually no specifics as to what the Cubans were coming to South Africa for, except that they were either trained doctors, public health practitioners or epidemiologists and that they would be deployed to work with provincial governments. I was surprised to learn of this, as we hadn't seen any health personnel plans that showed local shortcomings or called for external assistance. I saw it as simply a political act on the part of Cuba to make its personnel available to South Africa and our country accepting this, even if it was not really needed, because of its relations with Cuba.

When the issue of Cuban assistance for Covid-19 emerged, I cast my mind back to other forms of unnecessary Cuban assistance that South Africa has either sought or accepted when offered. The one that came to mind immediately is South Africa's deal with Cuba on the training of medical students. This initiative had purely political motives as far as I could see – there was no needs assessment as to what the shortfall in doctors was, why the country's medical schools could not meet it, and why students should train in Cuba as opposed to any other country, especially since medical schools in South Africa have specially allocated seats for students from other countries in Africa such as Botswana. Why then send our students to Cuba? The more important question is: who are the students going to Cuba and who is selecting them? The reason this question is important is because there is no transparency in the process of selection, even though those selected received a taxpayer-funded all-expenses-paid education. It turns out, from the information I gleaned, that it is mostly a political process, and that provincial politicians and high-level government officials have direct influence in the selection process and send in names of their preferred candidates, sometimes even family members or friends. The Cuba medical student training programme has become a mechanism to use provincial government money (each province funds its selected students) to create a new kind of gravy train, with some genuinely deserving students studying medicine in Cuba interspersed among them.

The South African medical students who train in Cuba have to undertake part of their training in South African medical schools, so that they can qualify with a South African medical degree, even though they had not completed their entire degrees with the rigours of the local training. This meant that they obtained a South African medical degree when most of their medical studies were in Cuba, and they did not need to meet HPCSA rules for foreign-trained doctors.

In essence, this Cuban programme became a mechanism for some provincial officials to select the students, whose matric grades failed to meet local medical school admission requirements, to then get into a South African medical school anyway through a back door opened by initial training in Cuba. Perhaps there will be an inquiry into this programme some day that will reveal the full extent of these problems.

The arrival of Cuban doctors to help with Covid-19 provided me with some idea of the extent to which the South African government might go just to use the opportunities of joint activities with Cuba. So I should not have been surprised when the government committed hundreds of millions of rands on a deal for unneeded Cuban medical personnel to come to South Africa's aid. South Africa seems to have deep pockets when it comes to Cuba – deep enough for the South African National Defence Force to purchase millions of rands worth of interferon from Cuba to treat Covid-19 when this was not a safe or effective treatment for the disease. The MAC responded to this news with an advisory stipulating that interferon was not a recommended treatment for Covid-19. Despite this, thousands of doses of this drug were purchased and delivered to South Africa. Fortunately, it seems that military personnel were not, in the end, treated with this Cuban medication, though I think the military may have lost the money it had already paid Cuba for it.

Notwithstanding this dalliance with Cuba, the international interactions that the Department of Health facilitated in the form of MAC webinars were welcome and an important part of ensuring that we were keeping abreast of international developments. It is all too easy to fall into the trap of thinking that we know best and that those who do not know our local situation have little to offer us. Fortunately, most of the MAC members recognised the value of nurturing and maintaining global connections in science and many had well-established global scientific networks.

One of the benefits of this global collaboration is the worldwide recognition of science conducted in South Africa. Our research contributions on HIV and, more recently, Covid-19 are well known internationally. And the consequence of raising the stature of South African science in the world is that it shines a spotlight on the important contributions our remarkable scientists make.

CHAPTER 16

Science in the spotlight

As scientists, we try to promote the use of evidence in policy development by shining a light on the important policy contributions of science through awards and in our everyday activities.

The media spotlight was never far from science during the first two years of the Covid-19 pandemic. I was called upon to do a steady stream of media interviews and the media coverage that followed these often shone a light on the importance of science. Further, each time local scientists received an award or prize for research contributions, the media portrayed this as an example of how science was contributing to health, particularly highlighting the role of South African science in improving health.

In December 2020, I shared the annual John Maddox Award with Anthony Fauci, who was the US government's chief pandemic adviser at the time. The award, a joint initiative of the charity Sense about Science and the international scientific journal *Nature* is named after John Maddox, former editor of *Nature*. It recognises the work of individuals anywhere in the world who promote sound science and evidence on a matter of public interest, facing difficulty or hostility in doing so. This award garnered substantial media attention, both in South Africa and internationally. As Fauci said when he accepted the Maddox Award, if you can't explain something simply, you probably don't understand it yourself. I myself find inherent joy when engaging with the public and talking about science. Communicating complex concepts to a lay audience is both enjoyable and rewarding! And it keeps me on my toes.

That year, the Maddox Award recognised our efforts to assist our respective governments in their Covid-19 responses. At that point, I had been chair (and later co-chair) of the MAC for about eight months. In a written motivation, the Academy of Science of South Africa, which took the initiative on their own accord to nominate me, noted that my public television broadcasts in particular had produced a 'tangible shift' in public opinion around Covid-19 measures. The 'shift' emanated from the pandemic information I had shared with the public, the scientific information they needed to understand the pandemic, and how public health prevention measures reduced the spread of the virus.

I was honoured but also humbled by the award; among the hundreds of nominations that year were two Chinese scientists, Ai Fenn and the late Li Wenliang, both of whom worked in the Central Hospital of Wuhan and were involved in sharing information that raised awareness about the infections they were seeing in their hospital in December 2019. Ai was questioned by her hospital superiors while Li was accused by the Chinese police of spreading rumours about the new virus. In a sad twist of fate, Li paid the ultimate price for his work, succumbing to Covid-19 in February 2020. As the Maddox Award organisers noted, these two doctors had gone above and beyond their duty in raising the alarm on the virus, considering their positions within the public health system, and probably being highly aware of the consequences they could face.

My Chinese colleagues had faced the contempt of the state for merely sharing scientific information. Fauci, too, had to swim against the tide that was former President Trump – at least until the November 2020 presidential elections. He was required on several occasions to contradict comments made by President Trump, for example on the benefits of hydroxychloroquine and other 'remedies' such as disinfectant injections and exposure to light. Because of this opposition, Fauci became the target of harassment and death threats, as did his family.

I know what it feels like to be in the unenviable position of being on the opposing side to one's own president – I had been directly involved in challenging President Thabo Mbeki and his administration on the issue of HIV/AIDS denialism and its impediment to treatment, which my Maddox Award citation specifically mentioned. But with the advent of Covid-19, I found myself working in a largely supportive political environment – at least as far as the government was concerned. Advice from mainstream scientists was actively solicited rather than shunned by the Health ministry. This is not to say that I was entirely spared the political fray. Representatives of political parties ranging from the Democratic Alliance to the Inkatha Freedom Party, the ANC and Economic Freedom Fighters (EFF) sought to use my public comments on Covid-19 to bolster and defend their political positions. This was particularly pronounced on the issue of the initial stay-at-home hard lockdown – and its subsequent lifting. The EFF, which is a radical populist party in South Africa, went so far as to label me 'Dr Death' for my support of the reopening of schools after the lockdown. When I stepped down after a full year at the helm of the MAC to refocus on my academic work, the party issued a statement welcoming the move, describing me as a 'failed adviser' who consistently protected the interests of capitalism over human life.[1] It seems, according to EFF logic, that encouraging children to go back to school equated to protecting the interests of capitalism.

Many media articles in early 2020 sought to compare the South African government's response to HIV to its handling of Covid-19. That was a useful exercise – a reminder of a stony path of denialism that we should not be tempted to stumble down again, especially as former President Mbeki still propounds his ill-advised AIDS denialism up to this day. Having been personally involved in challenging that path, it is with relief that I acknowledged the Ramaphosa administration for its more transparent approach to Covid-19 and its proactive overture to scientists, which put science centre stage in its response, even if the government did not always act on the scientific advice it received. Daily press statements and regular live television broadcasts by the minister, and periodic live broadcasts (affectionately referred to as family meetings) led by the president were unheard of in South Africa before Covid-19. Yet, during the pandemic, they became routine. In my view this approach had the positive effect of raising expectations from a public that was thirsty for information. To me this was a signal of a maturing democracy, a citizenry that demanded more accountability and transparency from its government, which is a good thing.

I took some pride in the fact that my comments and advice rendered during my term as MAC chair had been used not only by one or two political parties but by almost all of them, and at various times, in order to bolster their respective political arguments and ideological positions. It meant that I was doing something right: *sticking to the science.*

It was therefore ironic that I was handed the University of South Africa (UNISA) Chancellor's Calabash Award in 2021 by past President Mbeki at a glittering function held in Johannesburg. The award ceremony took place the day after the Minister of Health announced at a press conference that South African scientists had discovered a new concerning variant, named Omicron. I was juggling media interviews in between preparations to attend the UNISA ceremony. Mbeki was the Chancellor of UNISA at the time and the award he handed me was in recognition of my scientific contributions to the Covid-19 pandemic response. The irony in this case is particularly profound. The award recognised the central role of science in the Covid-19 response, while he had himself attacked science in the AIDS epidemic. He has steadfastly maintained an illogical contention that 'a virus cannot cause a syndrome'. But it must have floated above him that the award he gave me was for my work on SARS-CoV-2; which also causes a syndrome with diverse conditions ranging from neurological effects such as loss of smell or taste to pneumonia and stroke. In fact, SARS-CoV-2 stands for 'Severe Acquired Respiratory Syndrome CoronaVirus-2'. The fact that SARS-CoV-2 causes a syndrome is even etched in its name! And the person who deprived thousands of South Africans of life-saving treatment because he did not believe a virus causes a syndrome was now handing out an award for contributions related to a virus that clearly causes a syndrome.

Later that month, I received the Conference on Public Health in Africa (CPHIA) 2021 Lifetime Achievement in Public Health award. Two such awards were made by the African Union and Africa CDC; the other was to Professor Jean-Jacques Muyembe-Tamfum from the Democratic Republic of the Congo, who is one of the doyens of African science and is the recipient of the Third Hideyo Noguchi Africa Prize. My CPHIA award led to substantial social media traffic from across the continent, recognising my contributions to building science in Africa.

For scientific prestige, the Hideyo Noguchi Africa Prize is right up there. It is a highly competitive award and is only given every five years. Unlike most other prizes, the Noguchi prize is an official award made by the government of Japan and the winner is selected by the prime minister of Japan, based on a shortlist of candidates made by a selection committee of top scientists. The Noguchi prize has two categories, one for 'medical research', which is awarded for scientific contributions, and one for 'medical services' awarded for providing health care. Quarraisha and I were honoured to have been selected for the Fouth Hideyo Noguchi 'medical research' prize in early 2022, especially since we were in very good company – our good friend Professor Peter Piot was the recipient of the 1st, and Professor Brian Greenwood, who ran the UK MRC Gambia Research unit for many years, received the Second Hideyo Noguchi prize. Quarraisha and I travelled to Tunisia to receive the prize at the joint Japan– Africa meeting, which was attended by 38 African state delegations. In 2023, we visited Japan for a week as guests of the Prime Minister's office. During this week, we met with the Prime Minister in his office and with the Emperor and Empress in the Royal Palace. We gave lectures at Nippon Medical School and visited the birthplace of Dr Noguchi. He is an icon in Japan, with his portrait featuring on the 1 000 yen note.

For recognition of scientific contributions, the Gairdner awards are up there with the prestigious best as these are Canada's highest science awards. In 2020, Quarraisha and I were jointly honoured to be awarded the John Dirks Canada Gairdner Global Health Award for our research contributions in HIV, but by the time we actually received the awards, we were also being acknowledged for our contributions to Covid-19. The award specifically recognises individuals making an impact on global health research. While all five annual Gairdner awards celebrate the pinnacle of excellence in medical science, the Global Health Award that Quarraisha and I received also acknowledged efforts in 'improving the health and wellbeing of those facing health inequities worldwide'. In our joint Gairdner laureate lecture on 23 October 2020, Quarraisha and I traced our 30-year scientific search for workable and effective technologies that could make a difference in the lives of girls and young women, technologies that were alive to the power imbalances that tend to characterise a high proportion of male and female sexual relationships in Africa. In the face of these realities, the need was for technologies that gave agency and control over infection risk to women without them having to negotiate compliance with their partners – as is the case with condoms.

For pomp and ceremony, few can rival Vietnam's VinFuture Prize. There are four VinFuture prizes that are awarded annually by the VinFuture Foundation. Quarraisha and I won the 2022 prize for scientific contributions in developing countries in both HIV and Covid-19. We were particularly pleased to learn that The World Academy of Sciences had nominated us. While we were excited about going to Vietnam to collect the award, getting there proved to be a major challenge because the country had closed its borders and were allowing almost no flights in, as it had a zero-Covid policy in January 2022. It took us four days to get to Hanoi – we flew from Durban to Johannesburg to Frankfurt to New York and then to San Francisco, where we waited for two days to catch a specially chartered Vietnam Airlines flight out of San Francisco with the other prize winners and selection committee members. On arrival, we were tested for Covid-19 and taken to a hotel for our three-day quarantine requirement.

The day after we completed quarantine, the VinFuture Prize ceremony was held in the Hanoi Opera House, which is modelled on the oldest opera house in Paris. We had to get to the Opera House two hours early as all 500 attendees were required to have an on-site Covid-19 test so that the event could proceed mask-free. The ceremony was attended by the Prime Minister of Vietnam and several members of his cabinet. We were handed our awards on stage by the Ministers of Finance and Defence. The highlight of the evening was the surprise appearance of John Legend, who sang three songs before we were called up to the stage to collect our awards. The award included a medal, certificate, trophy and a hand-painted portrait of each of us. The award also included a short holiday in Vietnam – we chose to visit Ho Chi Minh City, which was an amazing experience given its central role in the history of the US war in Vietnam. While we were in Vietnam, we gave lectures at the university and established an exchange programme for Vietnamese medical students to visit CAPRISA in Durban. The first group of four students from Vietnam had a fruitful visit and we plan to continue the programme for the next few years.

A surprise award in 2020 was an honorary leadership award bestowed by South Africa's national weekend newspaper, the *Sunday Times*, which hosts an annual 'Top 100 Companies' awards ceremony. The award ceremony included a congratulatory message from Martin Kingston, CEO of Rothschild, who said, I was a 'voice of reason and reassurance in highly uncertain and challenging circumstances', able to 'allay initial levels of panic and concern' and that I took time to patiently explain things. In my own comments on receipt of this award, I explained that my contribution was a small part of what several scientists are contributing in educating the public and demystifying the science from the start of the pandemic.

Quarraisha and/or I have now received pinnacle science awards from several countries, including Canada, Japan, France, Kuwait, and from the African Union, but our scientific contributions have not been deemed worthy of a similar recognition in South Africa. I learnt that I was deemed not worthy when I was nominated by colleagues for the Order of Mapungubwe, which is bestowed by the South African President.

Importantly, in receiving our many awards, Quarraisha and I spoke proudly of how South Africa's many great scientists and their scientific talents were on full display during Covid-19 and that countless South African scientists made major contributions to the pandemic response and to elucidating the science for the public. I viewed each award as recognition of the wider importance of science and science communication, particularly as it was becoming clearer to everyone that we were likely to face more pandemics caused by new zoonoses in the future. In the face of a viral enemy too tiny to see with the naked eye, South Africans and all the world's people could draw hope from science as a powerful weapon at their disposal. Not only could a growing body of science inform the behavioural changes needed to mitigate the risk of infection, it could also, as the science evolved, provide them with longer-term hope in the form of diagnostics, treatments, vaccines and an understanding of the conditions for immunity. But that would take time. Until then, we were guided by our collective experience and knowledge of other diseases.

I was also at pains to point out the high degree of uncertainty in which we were working. Uncertainty is not an unfamiliar quality to people working with science; after all, scientific conclusions are, by their nature, *interpretations* of data. This means that differences in interpretation can and should occur between individual scientists all the time as part of the scientific process. These differences have the effect of producing more robust scientific outcomes.

In the context of Covid-19, however, the levels of uncertainty were extremely high. At a time when science was seen to be assuming new importance in decision-making and in the demystification of the novel coronavirus and the disease it caused, we were facing major limitations in our knowledge. Particularly at the start of the pandemic, there was a lot we did not know about Covid-19. We were required to make recommendations, in the absence of Covid-19-specific research and evidence, based on the way we understood the behaviour of other more familiar diseases, such as influenza. Under these conditions, following the science was not as straightforward as it sounds. In the midst of that uncertainty, providing science advice and undertaking public education are quite challenging.

But, despite all of that complexity, science is still the best weapon we have to deal with what Albert Einstein called the 'bewildering chaos of perceptions'. We can deal with those competing pressures and interests better, and more objectively, if we follow the best available scientific evidence, despite its shortcomings. In that way, we arrive at the best possible solution – a solution that might not be perfect, but it is much better than any of the alternatives.

One key element in the test of time of scientific contributions is the number of times a research publication has been cited, that is, specifically mentioned or referenced by other scientists in their scientific writings. Each time a journal publication is referred to by other scientists, it is recorded in various databases. Thomson Reuters manage the Web of Science, which is one of the largest databases on citations. This database keeps track of the number of times each scientist is being cited by other scientists.

In 2020, for the fifth year in a row, I was ranked by the Web of Science among the world's most highly cited researchers. While the concept of citations may be obscure to most, for a scientist, a high citation rate is the gold standard of success. It is a marker of scientific contributions that puts one in a position of academic and intellectual leadership, as it indicates research that is being widely used by other scientists over the past decade. The annual Web of Science list of the most highly cited researchers includes about 6 000 scientists from all disciplines of science. Among all my achievements, to feature on the Web of Science list of the world's highly cited researchers – which includes a number of highly accomplished scientists – is a major achievement of my career, one that I regard very highly.

Being on this list goes well beyond an acknowledgement of the quality of the research itself. It means that one's work is having an impact; it is influencing the work of other scientists around the world; it is pushing the boundaries of human knowledge; and it has the potential to produce positive outcomes for society. These factors were all part of the reasons I pursued a research career in the first place.

While the excitement and kudos over citation rankings remain confined to the halls of academia and research institutes, the spotlight on science was most sharply focused in the mainstream media and social media. In a paper published in 2017, science communication researchers

Dr Marina Joubert and Dr Lars Guenther placed me among 211 South African scientists – less than 1% of the scientific workforce of the country – who were then considered 'visible' in the public sphere.[2] When Joubert was conducting research for her PhD about the public communication behaviour of publicly visible scientists, I was among her interviewees. Citing 2016 statistics, she noted that I had appeared in about 455 articles and news items and had been on eTV about 20 times and on SABC 16 times (the number of media appearances and mentions were monitored by a commercial media monitoring service).

Because of my pre-existing visibility and past experience of dealing with epidemics, journalists started approaching me for comment about the impending Covid-19 pandemic, even before the first case in South Africa. Media houses were realising the reality of an enormous, internationally significant story. So even before the first case was reported, and before I was appointed to chair the MAC, I had a regular TV slot on Newzroom Afrika, which I would sometimes share with my daughter Aisha, as she was a regular on this channel. I appeared frequently on eNCA. Later, I had a regular daily 5.30pm live slot with Stephen Grootes and Cathy Mohlahlana on the *Pulse* show, also on Newzroom Afrika.

However, it was the live television broadcast on 13 April 2020 that unexpectedly took my media profile to a higher level: in the first five months of 2020, between January and June, I featured in 583 print media articles, 381 broadcasts (TV and radio), 2 609 online articles, and 16 000 social media posts. In the following year, 2021, I featured in 1 063 print media articles (~3 per day), 1 217 broadcasts (TV and radio) (~4 per day) and 5 810 online articles (~16 per day). In summary, I was on TV, radio, print articles or online articles on average every hour in 2021 (that is ~23 per day, every day of that year). In terms of geographical distribution, 36% of the articles/broadcasts were within South Africa, while the remainder were in several other countries across the world, with the US, UK and India as the top three countries.

Engaging with the media is an educational responsibility for me, as I care not for the publicity itself. On occasion, I would come away from an interview with a sense of deep satisfaction in having addressed some important issue – in these instances, there was mutual benefit. I benefited from having to explain a scientific concept while the reader/listener benefited from gaining a new insight into Covid-19. I found that constructive engagement between scientists and the media creates a space for science education and the promotion of science – with benefits that accrue to the collective in the form of a more empowered and informed citizenry. In return, the occasional warm fuzzy internal feeling from having done something useful and good is my deeply appreciated reward.

The media in South Africa plays a role in driving public opinion and government policy – I witnessed this influence at close range in the push for HIV/AIDS treatment in the early 2000s. I have, over the years, served on national and international platforms to champion science, emphasising its indispensable role in dealing with global challenges such as climate change, food insecurity, disease and epidemics. In 2017, Quarraisha was the convenor of the Durban chapter of the March for Science, the global movement that had its genesis in the US. Initially targeting the Trump administration's perceived anti-science stance on human-caused climate change, the campaign proved to have resonance throughout the world. In May 2019, marches were held in 150 locations around the globe. For each of those participant countries or cities, the motives for defending science may reflect a slightly different texture or emphasis, given prevailing circumstances. For example, concern about a government reduction in use of scientific evidence in decision- and policy-making was a big motivator for participants in the West, as were fears of cuts in government funding for research and reductions in access to government data for scientific research. For most African countries, including South Africa, the need for more state-level investment in science and scientific research, seen as critical to protecting and growing the status of science in society, is another important aspect of the marches.

We scientists have a privileged position in society. As scientists, we try to promote the use of evidence in policy development by illuminating the importance of policy contributions of science. We need to remain vigilant that those in positions of authority are acting rationally in the public's best interests, not just through marches and protests but also through shining a light on science through the media, awards and in our everyday activities. But I had also come to realise that we needed to go beyond *defending* science to *building trust* in science.

CHAPTER 17

Building trust in science

A key factor in building trust is honesty. People want honest evidence-based explanations that can help them understand the situation, make up their own minds on what to do and give them a sense of control over their own lives.

I have long held the view that we need some scientists who are not only *practitioners* of science, but *educators* of science too. This applies to communicating the outcome of scientific research as well as enhancing scientific literacy more broadly. In addition to science education, scientists can play a role in building people's confidence and trust in science. Science literacy – which includes an understanding of scientific concepts and the way in which science is produced – gives people tools to make better decisions in their lives and bestows upon them greater agency in social, political and economic processes. As my 40-year career in research testifies, I am committed to using the power of science to improve people's lives and to help societies advance.

By carefully engaging with the public, especially through the media, it becomes possible to build public trust in science. Public trust in science does not mean that every person necessarily understands the nuts and bolts of the science; it means they broadly trust the scientific method and peer-review system; they trust the country's scientific institutions; and they have some confidence in the scientific consensus around a particular issue – such as the wisdom of vaccinating one's children against diseases such as polio or measles. Public trust in science also means that people are able to see the benefits of science to society, especially when the science is conducted for the public interest, rather than for corporate or political interests.

Generally speaking, science is seen as too complicated or boring by mainstream media, which prefers dramatic headlines and pithy soundbites. In addition, a scientist's day-to-day work is not glamorous: much of the slog happens behind the scenes and it is only when there is a major discovery, with clear implications for people's daily lives or well-being, that the work tends to become publicly visible and, even then, it may reach only a select audience.

Covid-19 changed the landscape for scientists dramatically. In fact, among the positive spin-offs of the global pandemic – if one is forced to look for such a thing – has been a fuller understanding and appreciation of scientists and the way they work. In the pre-Covid era, when I told people I was an epidemiologist, I was often mistaken for a skin doctor. Now, many more people are aware of the discipline of epidemiology and what epidemiologists actually do. The intense public interest in Covid-19 and the media coverage of it has meant that many more scientists have been flushed out of their laboratories and into the media spotlight. As a result, people also now better understand that the world's scientists and researchers can and do play a role in shaping decision-making and government policy.

Anecdotal evidence from around the world suggests that as a result of Covid-19, more young people are now considering scientific research as a career path. I hope this is true and that the greater interest in science, facilitated in large part through the media's coverage of Covid-19, bodes well for future investment in science education and training at all levels, particularly in Africa.

Hopefully, people also understand a little more about scientific method, the painstaking process through which science happens: methodical and rigorous processes that build evidence, piece by piece, often in the context of high levels of uncertainty rather than via the stereotypical 'Eureka!' moment. Perhaps it is more obvious now that scientific research is often not a linear process. When we embarked upon a national response to

Covid-19, for example, the world was using our past experience of influenza as a model for disease control. But Covid-19 soon took a different path to influenza, as was evident in the speed of its spread, mortality rates and clinical features – to name just some of the divergences. But based on rapidly accumulating evidence, a new Covid-19 model was forged. This pivoting is part and parcel of the frequently messy process of growing science and the global body of knowledge.

Closely allied to the responsibility to improve science literacy is the duty to inform. Throughout the Covid-19 pandemic, the point of my media engagements was not just the sharing or explication of new scientific information and discoveries. My job, as far as I was concerned, was to keep people properly informed, help them understand the complex pandemic world they found themselves in and to help them navigate the tsunami of information – and misinformation – coming their way on a daily basis.

Having a public profile facilitates public communication, but it comes with some strings attached. In her article in the *South African Journal of Science* published in July 2020, in which my function as a 'media star' is dissected, Dr Marina Joubert, a leading science communication researcher from Stellenbosch University, wrote that a sign of high public visibility is when the media start to take an interest in a scientist's personal life, and when such visibility is 'sustained by controversy'.[1] In my case, she was able to tick both check boxes. Several journalists started to take more of an interest in my personal background. Some took an interest in my family, which was fine – all of them, as I indicated earlier, were making valuable contributions in their own right to the Covid-19 response and they had something to contribute.

When I became involved in a lawsuit against the local city government in Durban, where I live, over the illegal construction of a building in my neighbourhood, despite the fact that the issue had nothing to do with epidemiology or the pandemic, the media coverage was extensive and was heavily angled on my personal involvement in the case rather than the case itself. This is despite the case itself being an interesting example of how a developer demolishes a protected heritage building to construct an apartment block called 'the Currie Road monstrosity', breaking several building regulations in the process. Six municipal officials were identified by the city's own internal investigation for having bypassed proper procedures in approving plans that did not comply with the law – none were fired. As a result, this court-declared illegal development continues, with lawyers actively ensuring the construction proceeds, while the city turns a blind eye to incompetence or corruption in its own midst by choosing to side with the developer in the latest court case.

So much for the first check box. As for the second, the answer is less clear cut. I would like to believe that my visibility was sustained less through controversy than the need for accurate scientific information and comment. As a general rule, I do not actively court controversy, although I do not shy away from it either. Generally, in life, my approach is not a combative one – I see more value in winning people over and I find a respectful approach is far more productive as a rule. In media engagement, my approach is as follows: a) explain the situation, the reasons for the current situation, the available evidence and its implications, b) note any advances or changes in views expressed previously, c) avoid attacking or defending individuals or institutions, d) acknowledge uncertainty where it exists and e) be forward-looking, explaining what may be expected next. In other words, I focus on the science.

That is not to say that I was not a lightning rod for people trying to create controversy and capitalise on my visibility. In May 2020, I found myself personally accused by a lobby group based in Durban of benefiting from substantial funding – over R944 million – from Bill Gates, who was at that time the subject of all manner of bizarre conspiracy theories about Covid-19. The sum alone was astronomical and beyond any prospect of being true. But the accusation gained momentum on social media. The allegations against me were vague, but they insinuated something underhanded on my part. I initially felt that they were not deserving of a response, but on the advice of a colleague, I put together a message in response and sent it to a WhatsApp group that had been circulating the accusations. I refuted the allegations, arguing, inter alia, that as adviser to the Gates Foundation, I did not personally receive grant funding from the foundation as that would constitute a conflict of interest. My response went viral and was then, predictably, picked up by the mainstream media. When I was contacted by a journalist who asked whether I had received any funding from the Gates Foundation, I refused to comment any further as I felt that I had made my point. In fact, it later turned out that two CAPRISA researchers had received funding from their US collaborators who were in turn being funded for the research by the Gates Foundation. I was not aware that the source of those two grants was the Gates Foundation. It is almost impossible for me to keep track of the various grants that scientists in CAPRISA secure and to determine if it is indirect funding from the foundation. Both these grants were completely unrelated to my work and I was not involved in either project. The story purporting to 'expose' me as a recipient of research grants from the Gates Foundation made the front page of a local Durban newspaper. It was an example of not letting the facts get in the way of sensationalism. The newspaper article is no longer available online[2] – a sign that it probably should never have been published in the first place and a lesson in how easily one can become the target of disinformation peddlers.

The controversy about differences between scientists on the MAC was another, much larger, source of distraction. I lost count of how many times I told a journalist that dissent among scientists was normal, to be expected and, to some extent, desirable, given the way that science is produced. Among top senior scientists – people who run research institutes, units or university departments, facilitating and managing differences of opinion and interpretation of evidence is not just common – in fact it is par for the course.

When she wants to embarrass me, Smita Maharaj will recount quotes from journalists telling her how much they appreciate my honest and tell-it-like-it-is responses. This comes from my commitment to science – but it also comes from the enjoyment I get personally from sharing my knowledge, and the satisfaction I experience when I help people understand the underlying reasons for a situation, in language they can understand. I do this best in real time. In an interview situation, I am rarely ruffled. I prefer not to know the questions beforehand as I prefer to 'think on my feet' as I can readily order my points, quickly recall facts and figures (admittedly, not quite as promptly as I could when I was younger), and convey evidence-based facts in a calm and reasoned way, without hype that may provoke alarm, particularly given the high levels of anxiety experienced during the pandemic, especially in the early months. I also try to be as inclusive and personal as possible, speaking in the first person – partly to convey what I regard as a collective responsibility and, to some extent at least, a collective destiny.

At a content level, I prefer to respond off the cuff to almost any relevant question that is thrown my way. I found out long ago that preparing answers is time-consuming and leads to me giving unnecessarily long-winded and detailed answers. Also, my answers then look staged and lose some of the spontaneity and immediacy of my messaging. My preparation for interviews is really simple: *stay informed*. And I do this anyway as part of my daily routine, reading copiously, devouring journal articles as well as mainstream media reports. When Covid-19 broke out, I certainly had much more to read, but the pattern essentially remained the same.

Experience has taught me that, after credentials and expertise, the most important quality of a public communicator is his or her ability to engender a sense of trust in an audience. The pandemic brought with it an insatiable need for information on the part of the public, but not just any information; more than ever, it became clear that people needed reliable and accurate information and explanation from a trustworthy source.

Earning public trust is not as straightforward as it seems. As Joubert argued in her *South African Journal of Science* paper, an expert is able to garner *respect* on the basis of their expertise and academic credentials, but not necessarily *trust*. Trust goes beyond respect and is predicated on a range of factors that include accuracy, clarity, consistency of messaging, as well as less tangible, more personal qualities such as intention, sincerity and empathy.

I would say a key factor in building trust is honesty, particularly about what is not yet known by science and therefore remains uncertain. As Bertrand Russell said, 'The trouble with the world is that the stupid are cocksure and the intelligent full of doubt.'[3] Sticking to the evidence and avoiding speculation as far as possible is essential. During stressful times, what people do not need is someone using their status to make dramatic headline-attracting claims or telling them what to do or how to think about the pandemic. They need honest information and evidence-based explanations that can help them make up their own minds; and give them a sense of control over their own lives.

Challenges at the advice-to-policy interface

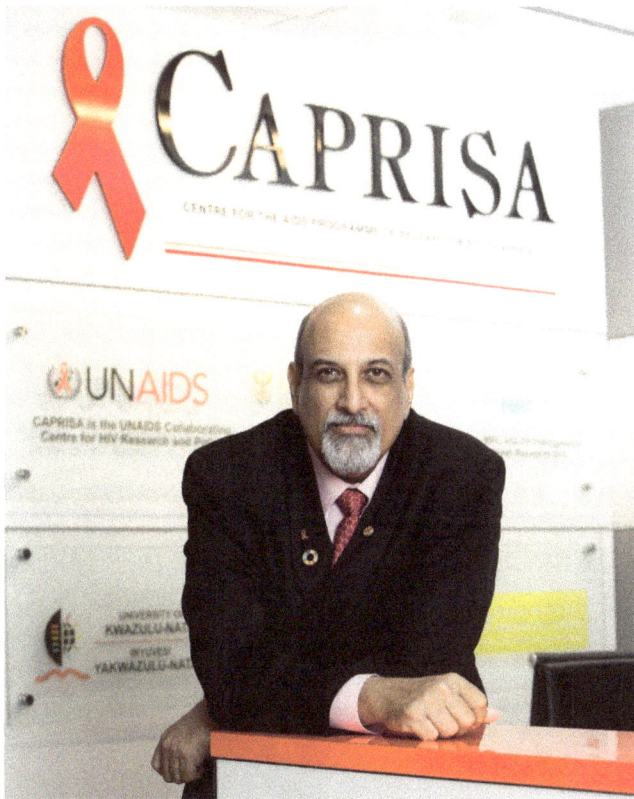

Salim Abdool Karim in the foyer of the CAPRISA headquarters at the Nelson Mandela Medical School campus of the University of KwaZulu-Natal in Durban.

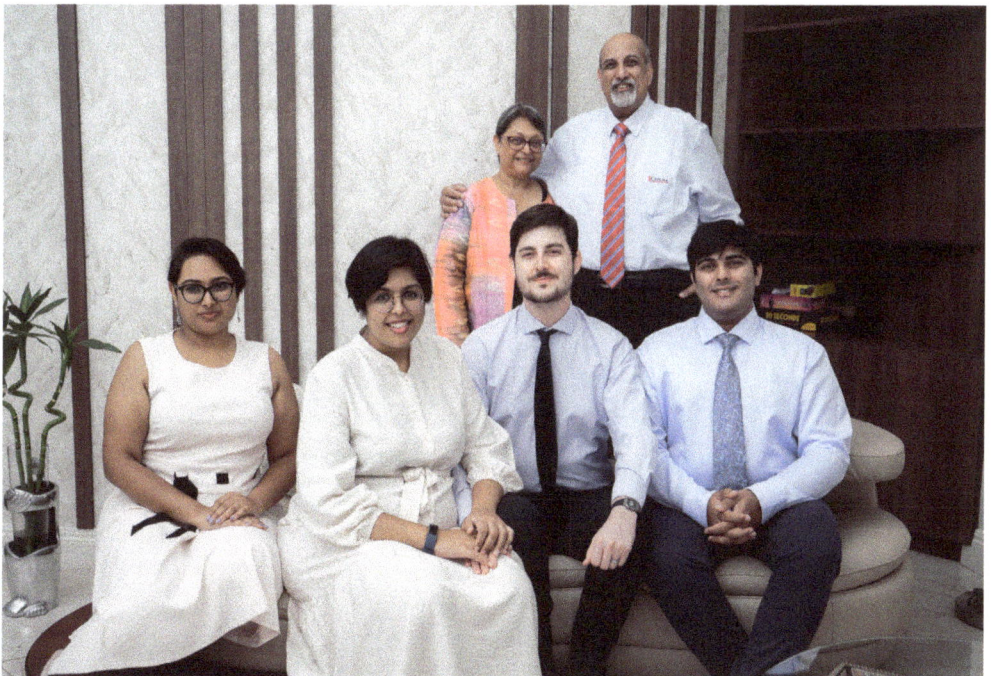

Abdool Karim family portrait: Salim and Quarraisha are standing, while daughters Aisha (left) and Safura are seated with son-in-law Ivo Peres and son Wasim.

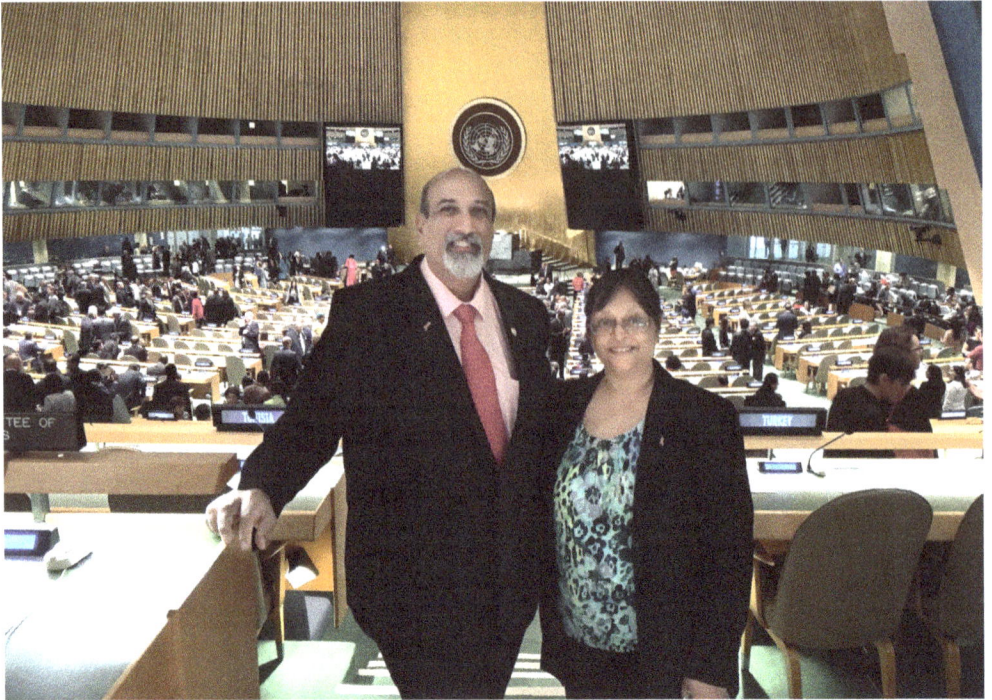

Salim and Quarraisha Abdool Karim at the UN High-Level Meeting on AIDS in the plenary hall at the United Nations in New York.

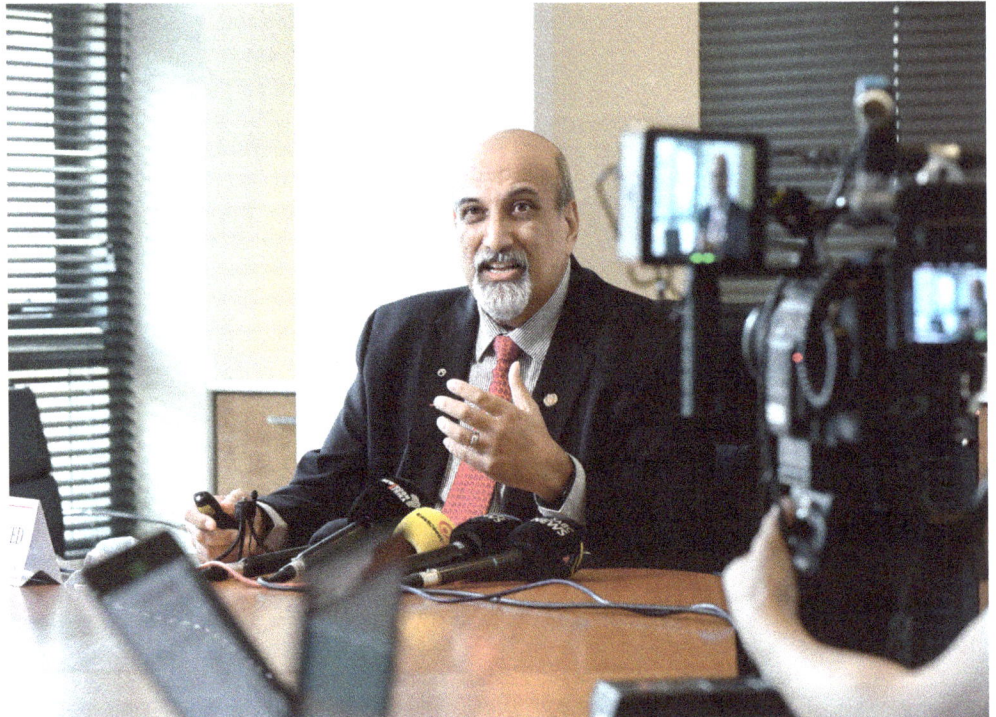

A televised media briefing on Covid-19 shortly after the second wave of infections.

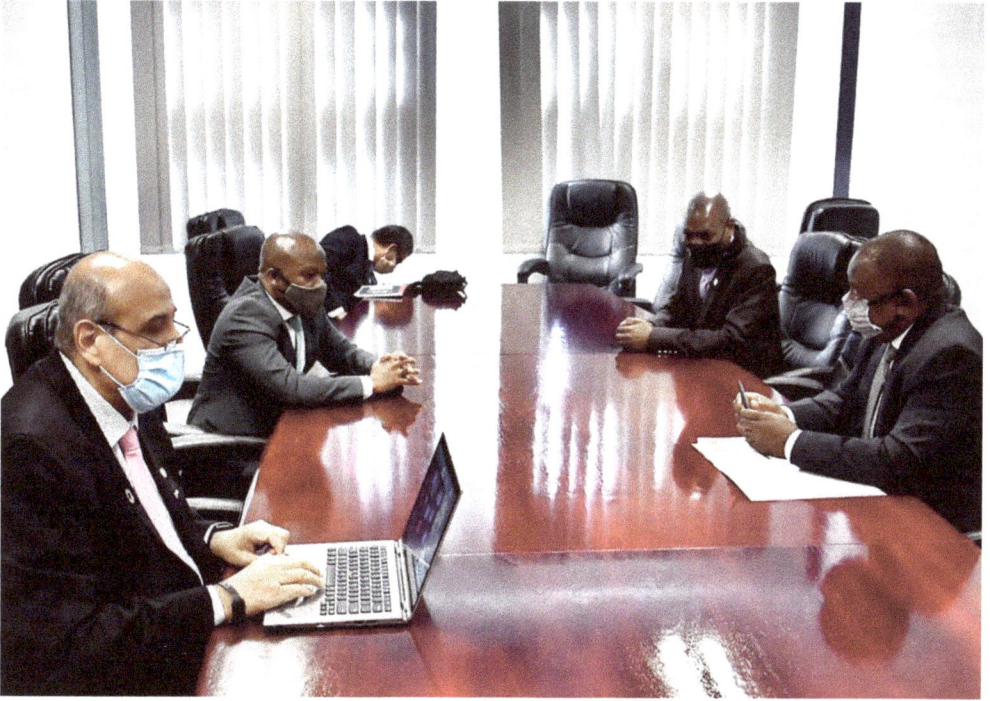

Preparing to do a Covid-19 presentation in a meeting with KwaZulu-Natal Premier Sihle Zikalala, Health Minister Zweli Mkhize and President Cyril Ramaphosa at the command centre in Durban.

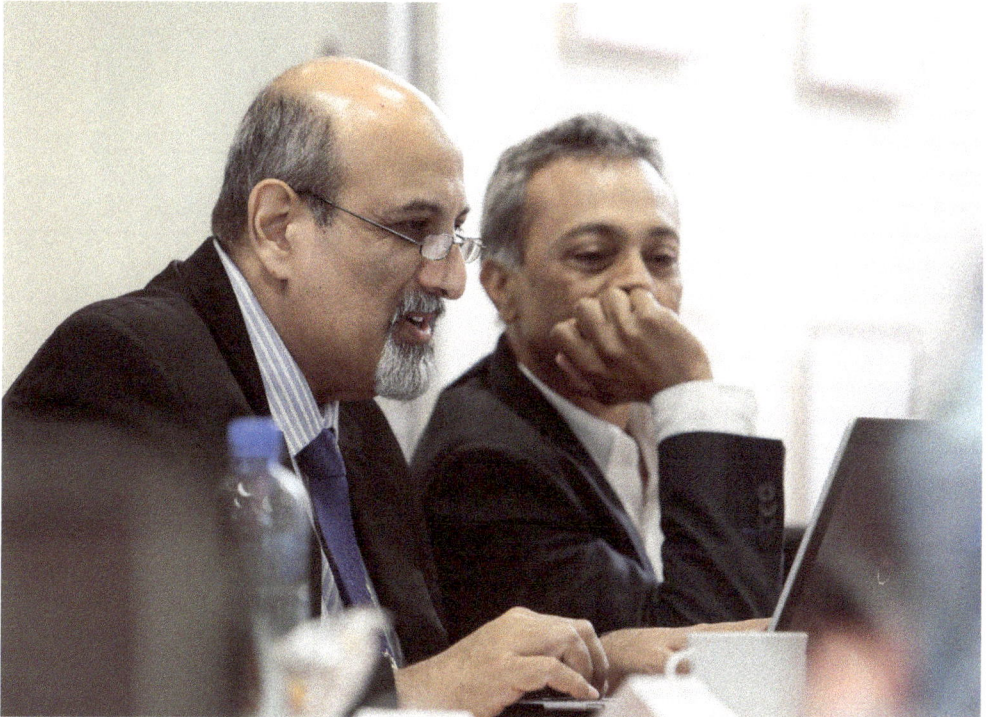

Working on a policy document with Yogan Pillay, Deputy Director-General in the Department of Health.

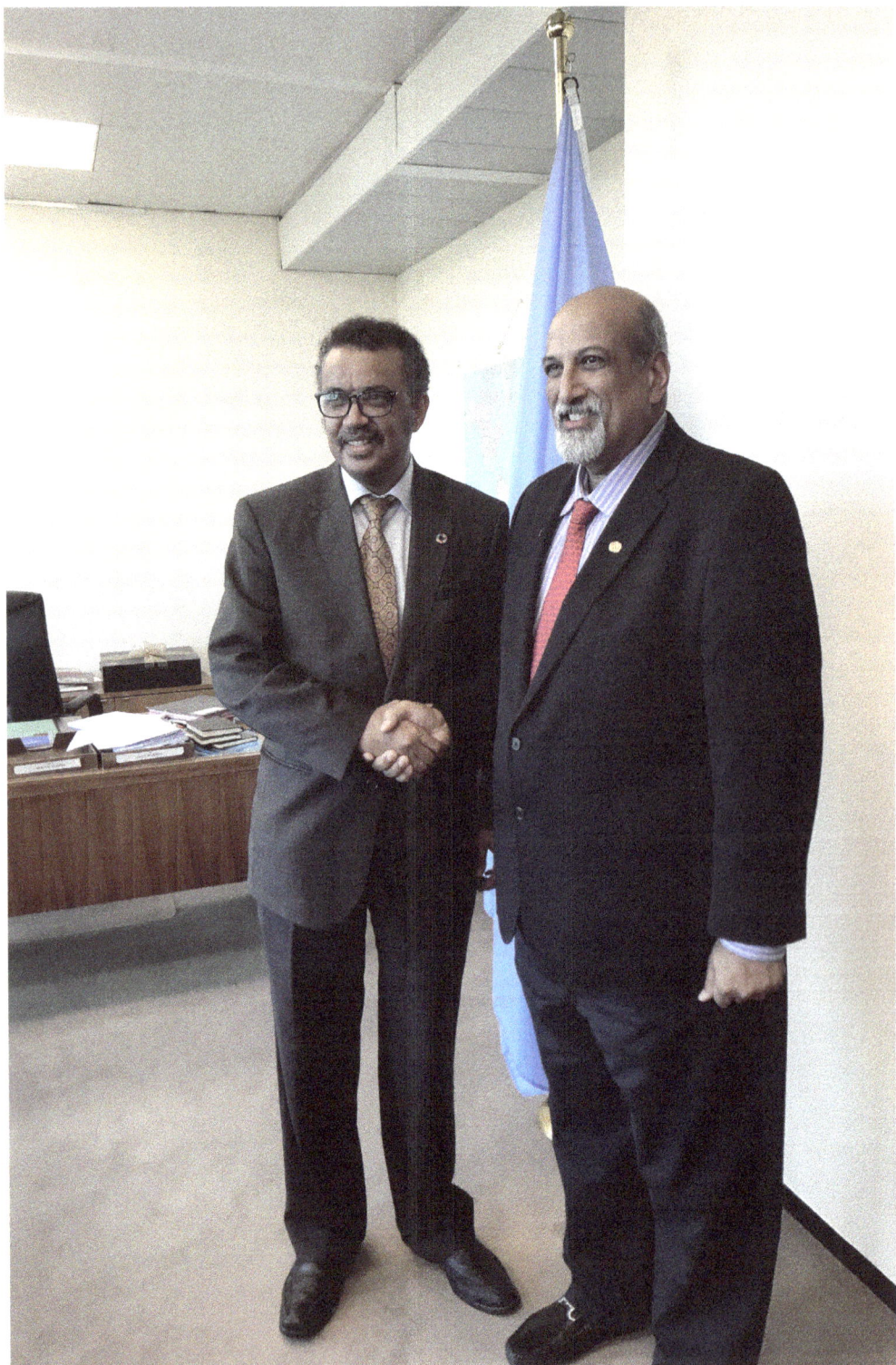

Meeting with WHO Director-General Tedros Ghebreyesus at the WHO Headquarters in Geneva.

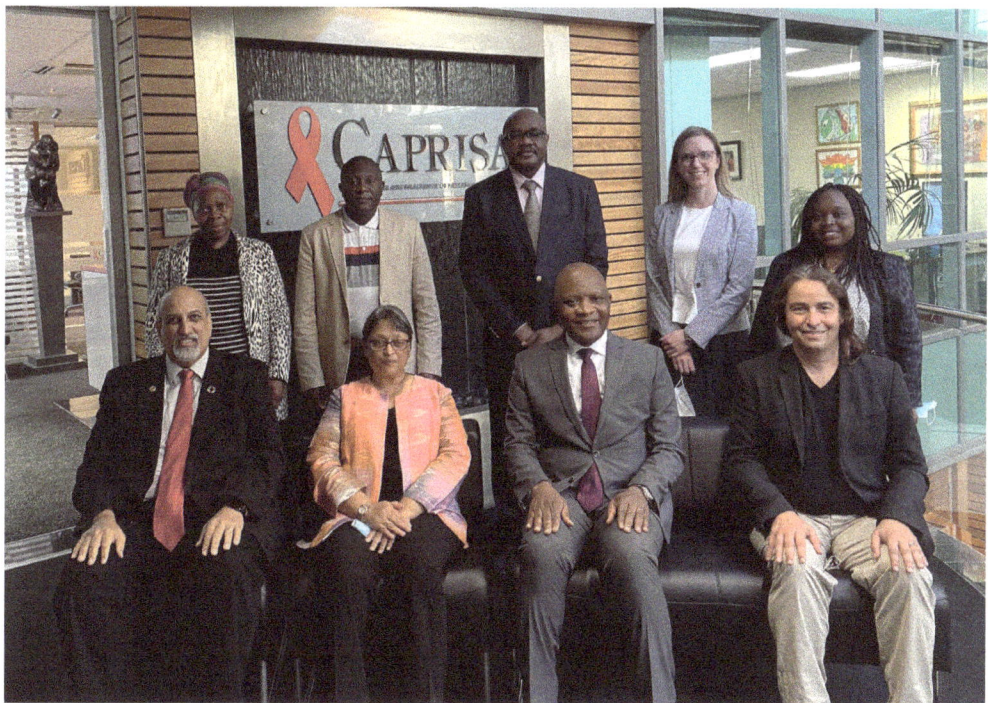

Africa CDC delegation visit to CAPRISA and KRISP in Durban. Standing (from left): Hlekani Liesbeth Mangate (NDoH), Edward Matlaila (NDoH), Nicaise Ndembi (Africa CDC), Andrea Thiel (Africa CDC) and Laura Ambe (Africa CDC). Seated: Salim Abdool Karim (CAPRISA), Quarraisha Abdool Karim (CAPRISA), John Nkengasong (Africa CDC) and Tulio de Oliveira (KRISP).

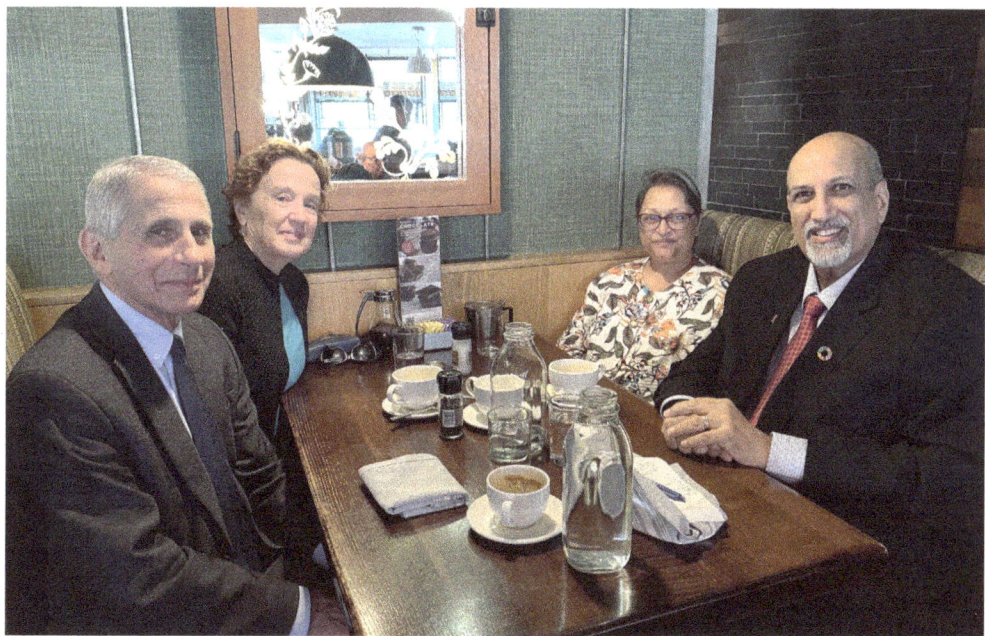

Clockwise: Anthony Fauci and Christine Grady at lunch with Quarraisha and Salim Abdool Karim during the 2022 Annual National Academy of Medicine meeting in Washington, D.C.

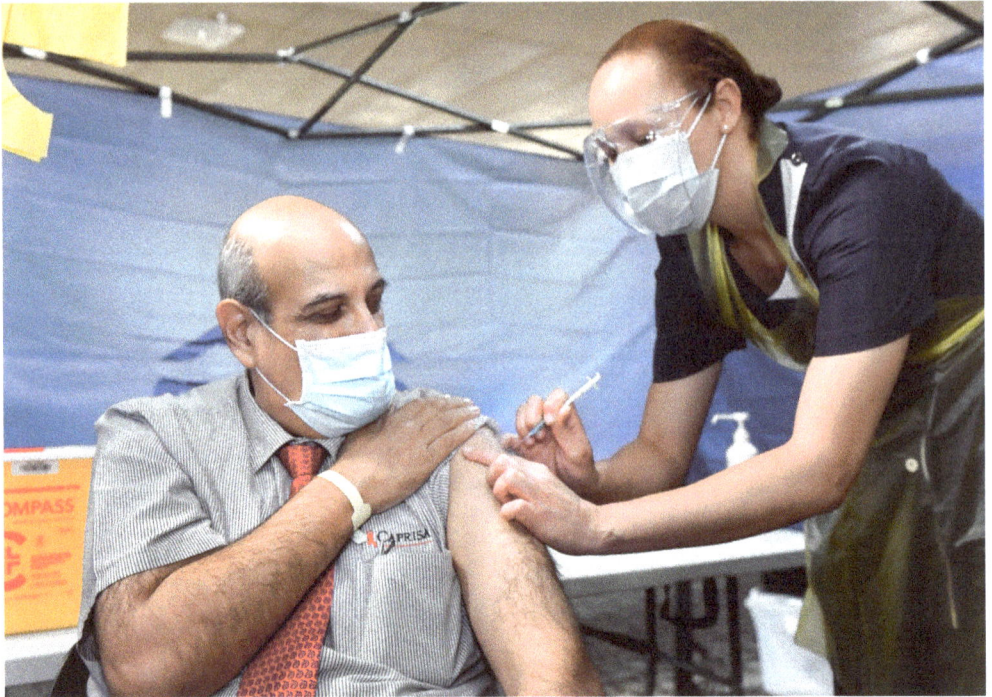

Receiving a Covid-19 vaccination at the St Augustines Hospital vaccine site.

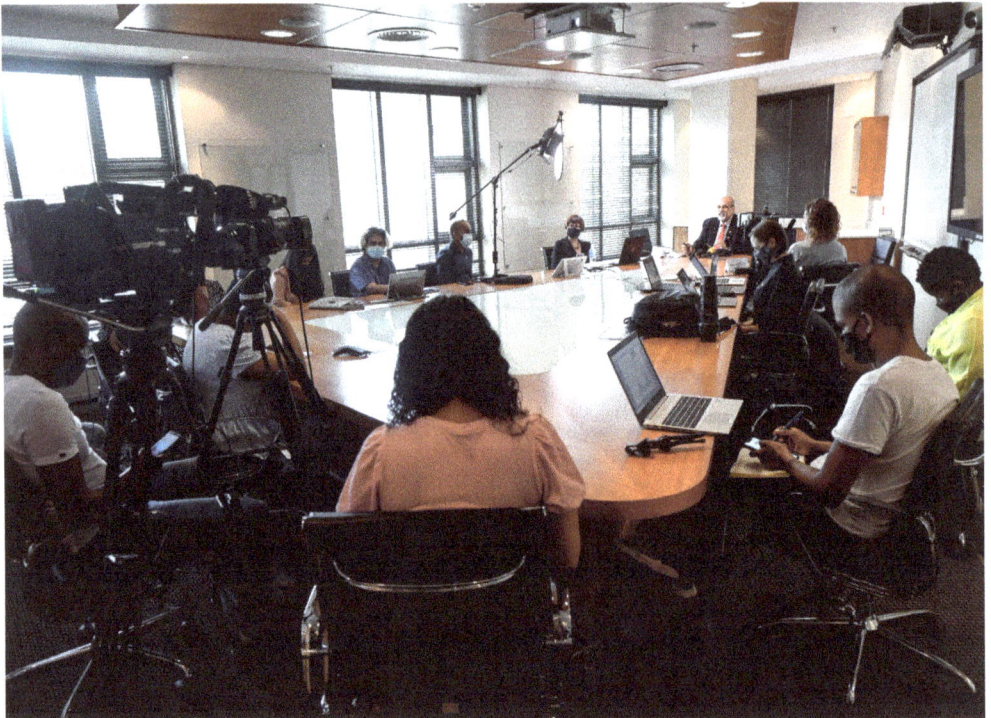

Briefing the media in the CAPRISA boardroom on the Covid-19 situation on the one-year anniversary of the first case of Covid-19 in South Africa.

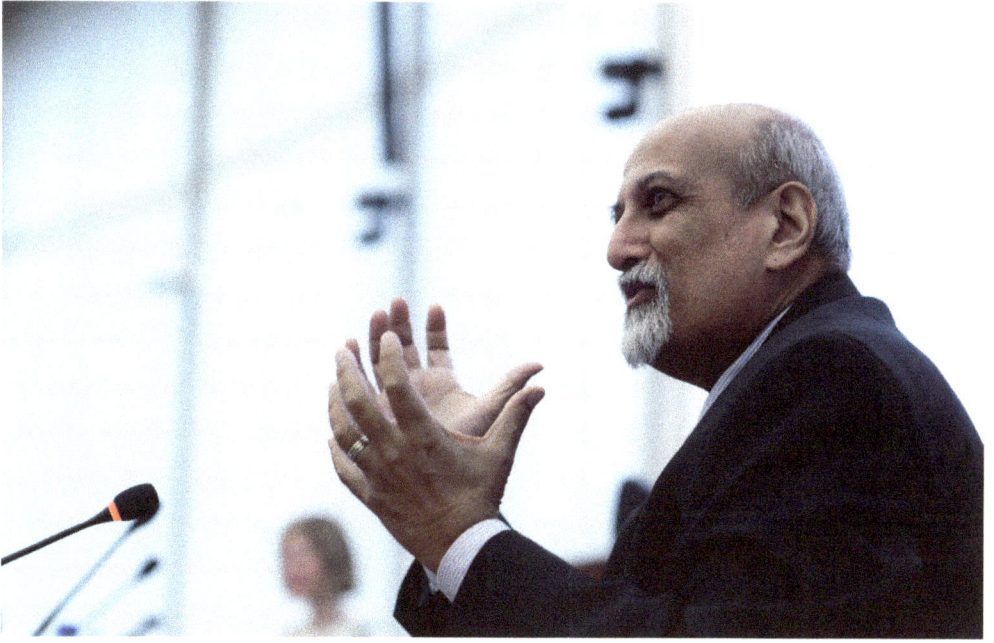

Salim Abdool Karim delivering the keynote address at the World Health Organization, World Intellectual Property Organization and the World Trade Organization Joint Technical Symposium held in Geneva on 16 December 2022.

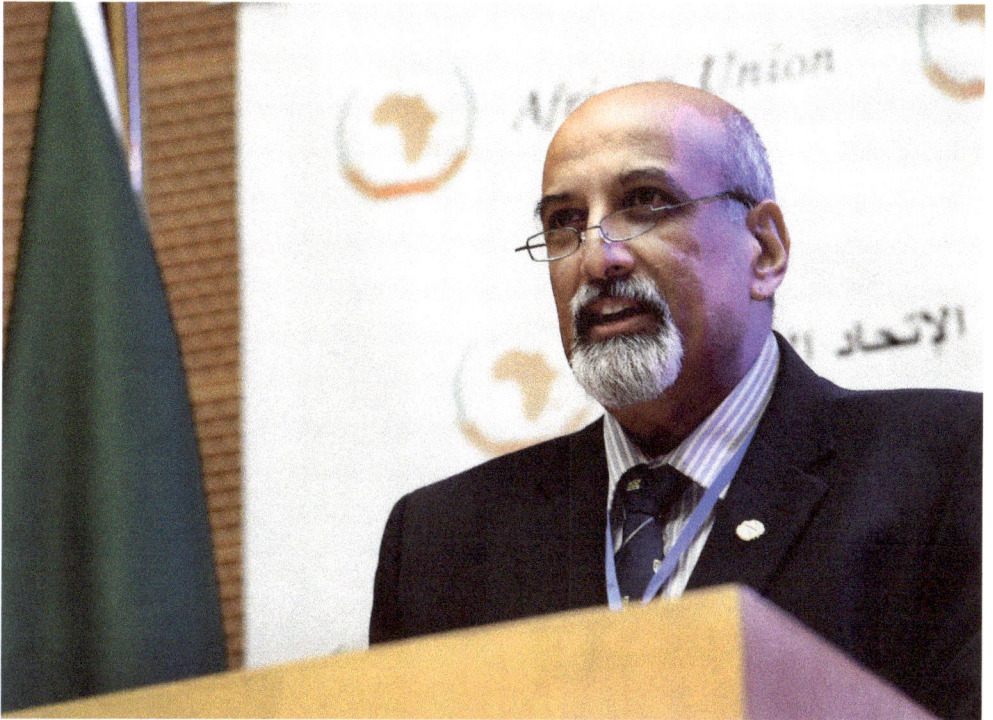

Salim Abdool Karim addressing the African Union General Assembly on receiving the Kwame Nkrumah Scientific Award.

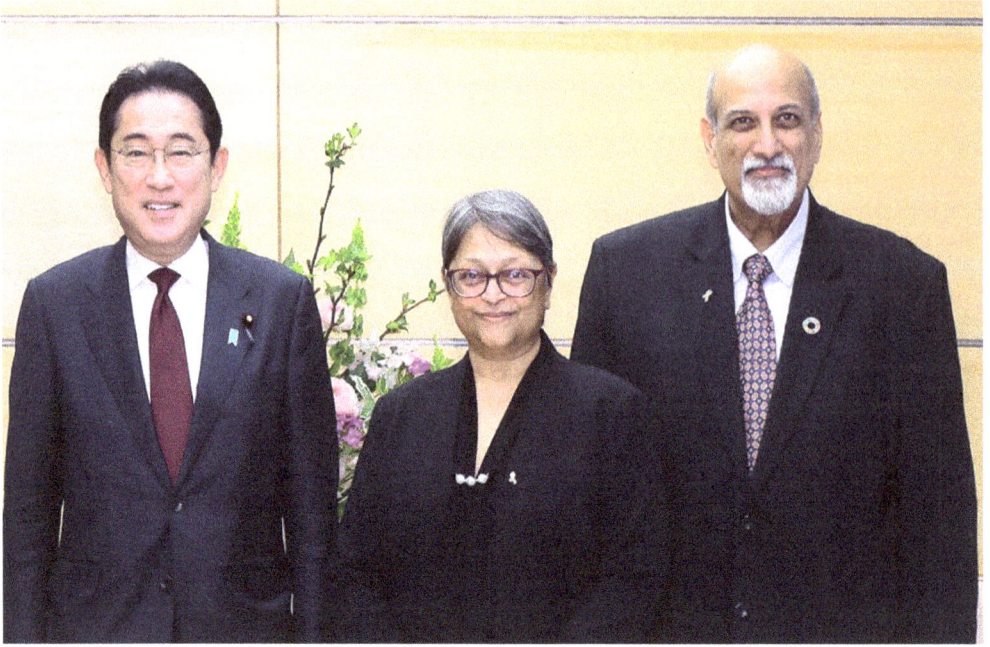

Prime Minister of Japan, Mr Fumio Kishida (left), meets with Quarraisha and Salim Abdool Karim, laureates of the Fourth Hideyo Noguchi Africa Prize (Medical Research category) during their visit as guests of the government of Japan.

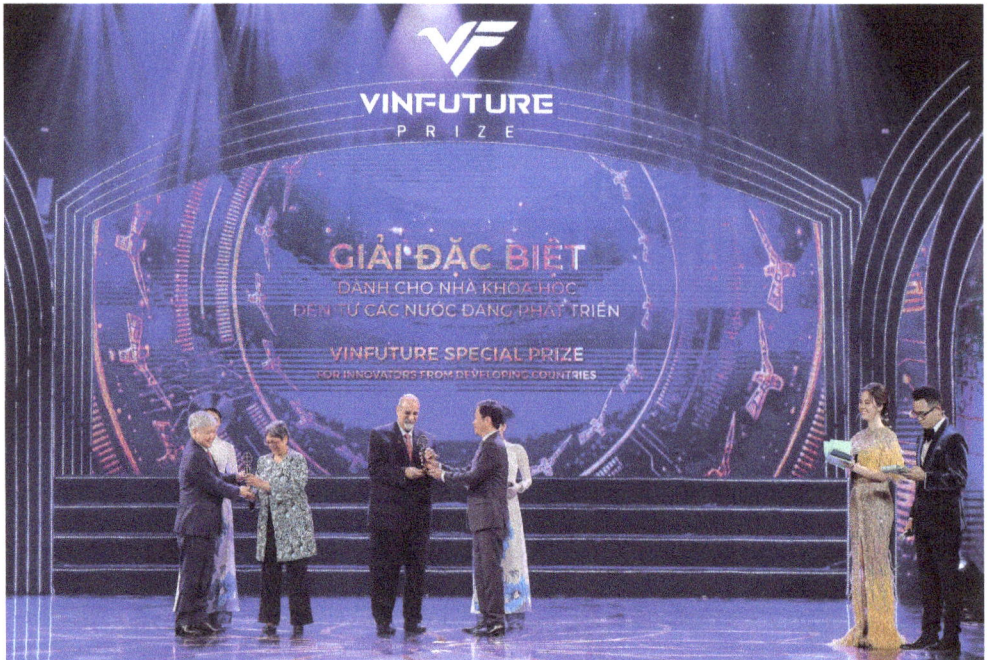

At the VinFuture Awards Ceremony at the Hanoi Opera House, Mr Do Van Chien, Chairman of the Central Committee of the Vietnam Fatherland Front, presents the VinFuture Special Prize to Quarraisha Abdool Karim, while Salim Abdool Karim receives it from Dr Tran Tuan Anh, Head of the Central Economic Commission of Vietnam.

Leading the MAC –
attaining sufficient consensus

*Following vigorous debate, the MAC had to come up with a decision
– we had to agree on what the best advice would be in response to each
question. That was our task and responsibility – and we did that for
every one of the first year's 119 advisories.*

Throughout my career, I have been thrust into leadership roles.
Although I can't say whether that is a direct result of my personality
type, I do feel that there are certain traits or qualities that help someone
become a successful leader. While I am not one to put a lot of stock into
personality types, as most people are a blend of characteristics, I regard
my younger self as a Type A personality: goal-oriented, ambitious and
competitive. I thrived under pressure and was constantly pushing myself
to achieve new milestones. But now, in my sixties, I like to think that I
have mellowed a bit and have begun to embrace my more Type B traits.
I am focused on the bigger picture, as opposed to short-term goals. My
relentless drive is now focused towards the greater good and building up
others to collectively reach this dream.

Type A and Type B are two personality categories, a typology for the
pattern of emotions, thoughts and behaviours that make each individual
who they are. Not everyone fits neatly into these two personality types.
Some people may have traits of each personality type to varying degrees
or may demonstrate different traits in different situations. Very generally
speaking, people with Type A personalities are usually ambitious, competitive and aggressive. They are those drivers waiting at traffic lights who

shift their car into first gear more than once and keep half an eye on the opposite light so as to be the first one to take off when the lights change. They just want to go. They are impatient and they do not like to be held back. They are quite simply *driven*, mostly by personal ambition. People with Type B personalities are usually patient, flexible and laid-back. They are, by contrast, more measured and their pace is more even. People with Type B personalities are described as those who take the time to stop and smell the roses. They are willing to play the long game. They are able to glimpse the bigger picture and are seemingly not distracted by the less important minutiae. I oversimplify, but you get the picture …

To climb the ladder in an organisation, Type A personality traits need to come to the fore. The more entrepreneurial and risk-taking qualities enable a person to progress and advance. Passion and a strong work ethic pave the way to becoming a leader – but once you achieve that, level-headedness and patience become more important. The job of a leader then becomes working with and supporting people, many with Type A personalities who focus on getting things done. It falls to the leader to take their views on board, facilitate their personal progress and map out a path they can follow for the organisation's overall goals.

While a manager explains the rules that should be followed in order to complete a task, a leader is more preoccupied with ensuring the vision is being reached, without holding on too tightly to a rigid set of rules. A leader facilitates and decides on the collective vision and an appropriate way forward, ready for eventualities where the conventional path ends in a brick wall.

Beyond my research activities, I run a regular eight-part interactive programme on leadership and mentorship for academic leaders, specifically aimed at the University of KwaZulu-Natal Medical School deans and department heads. The course aims to provide those in academic leadership positions with the tools to become effective leaders. As part of this leadership programme, I encourage the participants to place their trust in their substantive achievements; to let their academic stature convey their leadership standing rather than the title on the door of their office. I emphasise the importance of getting things done through others, the value of servant leadership in the programme and argue that academic leaders have to put other people's needs and careers ahead of their own, facilitating their subordinates' academic growth and development; in other words, to facilitate other people's success as a reflection of a leader's success.

I apply this concept in my own life with the people I am fortunate enough to lead. It simply translates into putting others first. On a practical level, it involves actively canvassing and engaging with all ideas and views.

Listening to and engaging with others' views and opinions was particularly important in the Ministerial Advisory Committee, where I was dealing with a number of expert scientists. Effective leadership required diplomatically dealing with strong opinions, especially when — occasionally – they are intertwined with big egos.

Many of the scientists on the MAC were at important growth stages in their careers, still climbing up the academic ladder, aiming to become deans or heads of university departments. My task as the chair and leader was to draw out the best in each of the members and tap into their knowledge, experience and talent. At the same time, we needed to build a common vision of what we were trying to achieve as the MAC so that we could all pull in the same direction. To achieve this, I would have to use an inclusive approach; we would be stronger as a collective. Being a collective also meant appreciating diverse views and having a multiplicity of minds giving their attention to common issues, but producing views and opinions that may be divergent. This does not mean you never reach a consensus – that would be counter-productive. It means that, working with evidence and rationale, you develop a collective position that most people agree is the best or close-to-best option. Having said that, I also believe in picking one's issues and battles: don't waste time fighting all the small issues because they will tire you out before you get to the more important ones.

After the first few meetings of the MAC during the early days of the pandemic, it became apparent to me that the forum – at 51 people with full attendance – was too large to allow everyone a reasonable chance to be heard, particularly given that we had some Type A personalities. The MAC discussions tended to be dominated by a small group of people who had a lot to say, and mostly they were valuable comments. But I became increasingly concerned that this small group also happened to be, with a few exceptions, white. While their race was not the problem *per se* in this case, I was concerned that the outcome of our discussions might be skewed as a result of that dominance. We were missing an opportunity to receive some alternative ideas and perspectives from a broader cross-section of medical professionals and thus failing to make use of the full range of rich expertise and talent at our disposal. It was soon apparent to me that the uneven participation was partially related to pandemic information. Not every member of the committee had access to the same level of resources and information about the pandemic. This put some of them at a disadvantage and they felt intimidated to comment in the larger group.

When I looked at this more deeply, it turned out that the more vocal members had significantly more resources and were part of or led large research teams or part of international networks, which enabled them to collect, monitor and analyse data not otherwise readily available. The others were almost entirely reliant on official publicly available information and had only their own professional experience of Covid-19 upon which to rely. While this latter expertise and insight was valuable to the committee, it was not being heard in the general MAC meetings and so was not seeing the light of day.

In an attempt to address this problem, I split the discussion on major MAC meeting agenda items into two parts. The first part was for those who voluntarily jumped in to comment or raised their hands to comment, but the second part was an opportunity for each and every MAC member, in turn, to comment. The ground rules for the second part were to be short and concise. Those who had not already spoken on the topic were invited to comment first and everyone was required to say something in the second part of the discussion, even if only to say they agreed with others or to say that they had nothing further to add. I was impressed at how many additional views we obtained in the second part of the discussion. Importantly, everyone now had a voice and was being heard in the MAC. But this still meant that we had two sets of contributors, with the small vocal group that dominated the first part of the discussion still disproportionately defining the direction of the MAC debates.

To address the imbalance, I set about creating a new way of working within the MAC in order to distribute leadership and participation opportunities, which I called technical working groups (TWGs) – smaller groups within the MAC to focus on technical aspects of our work. There were several TWGs at any one time and each existed for a few weeks until their advisory was finalised. Each TWG was chaired by a MAC member with particular expertise in that area. For these chairs I specifically selected those members whom I felt had not been able to contribute to their full potential in the large MAC meetings but whom I knew possessed valuable expertise, all the time keeping in mind the need for the leadership and membership of TWGs to preferably be demographically representative. The secretariat also kept tally on which MAC members had served as TWG chairs so that new chairing opportunities could be allocated to those who had not already had the opportunity. I encouraged the TWGs to supplement their membership, by 25% to 50%, with non-MAC members – South African or international scientists, public health practitioners and others who could bring their knowledge and experience to bear and ensure we had an inclusive approach. This helped to address another of my niggling concerns: the committee's potential insularity.

Despite the range of expertise in the MAC, it was still only made up of 51 medical scientists and health specialists and there were hundreds if not thousands more scientists and clinicians out there who could help. I felt instinctively that we could benefit from the input of a wider range of experts who were not on the committee. Several scientists, who were not MAC members, devoted substantial effort and time to help the TWGs produce high quality advisories. For example, Dr Robin Wood of UCT, who is an expert in tuberculosis transmission, provided valuable insights in the TWG that prepared the airborne and aerosol transmission advisory.

I took the view that the MAC needed to produce the best advice it could, and to do this, we needed to ensure that we drew on the knowledge of the best people available. I also felt that giving space to a diversity of views in the MAC was particularly important, given the lack of hard evidence available in the early stages of the outbreak. The irony of calls to 'Follow the science' – extremely popular in the discourse of the day – was not lost on us, considering how little science there actually was at our disposal at the beginning of the pandemic. It was in our interests to canvass different views – so as to ensure the decisions adopted were as robust as possible.

Together with the MAC secretariat, I worked on a process for drafting and finalising an advisory that would be as democratic as possible, given the time constraints we faced. After a draft prepared by the relevant TWG or MAC member had been presented and debated in the MAC, the secretariat and I would incorporate the points made during the debate to ensure it reflected the common view. This took hours and often involved contacting individual members to clarify their comments. When I felt that certain views could not be accommodated in an advisory, I would often phone the individual who had suggested the point to discuss the matter, and we would jointly discuss ways in which it might be incorporated in the advisory or somewhere else. The final version of the advisory would then be re-tabled at the next meeting so that if anyone differed with my interpretation of the discussions and the common points of view, they could make their opinions known then or within a comment window of 24 hours. Very rarely would there be problems or errors in the final version, but in the event that there were, we could issue an update.

I adopted the concept of 'sufficient consensus', which I borrowed from the 1990 CODESA (Convention for a Democratic South Africa) negotiations and applied it to our discussions to ensure that the outcomes reflected what most people were thinking and articulating.[1] Still, ensuring that everyone had an opportunity to air their views came with a downside: meetings would sometimes go well over the allotted time.

All of us were extremely busy people and the pressure on us was high, particularly when infection rates were rising, and we had to work to unrealistically tight timelines to map out actions to slow down the spread of the virus. MAC members did have sharply differing views on certain issues; especially when we were time-pressured or, perhaps, it just felt that way. I tried as hard as possible to avoid a situation in which we were split down the middle and a vote was required. In my experience, there is nothing like a partisan vote to harden positions on either side. To a large extent, we succeeded in achieving sufficient consensus. We had only one near vote – about my continuance as chair, which I will cover later – and that was not over a scientific matter. I generally tried to find the areas we could agree on and worked from there.

When a new discussion point comes up, I try to avoid polarising points to begin with. This allows everyone to start on some form of common ground and then slowly start to introduce points where they differ through the discussion. In this process, I felt that it was important to acknowledge the essence of all views and, where possible, reflect aspects of those views in the final advisory that went to the Department of Health. On the whole, this approach served us well and we always managed to find a way to move forward. While some members might have felt my approach was too accommodating, others might have felt that I should have more openly supported a position about which they felt strongly. As chair of the MAC, it was my responsibility to get us to a point where we could provide our best advice, and my credibility as fair chair had to be above reproach.

Six months after the original MAC was formed, while there was a dip in Covid-19 cases, we were faced with a different type of curveball. On 14 September 2020, Minister Mkhize changed the composition of the MAC. The new committee was more balanced in terms of expertise; while it had fewer biomedical experts, it included people with knowledge and experience in ethics, nursing and social science. I remember sitting on the couch next to Quarraisha when she got her email that evening thanking her for her service and saying that she would no longer be serving on the MAC. Naturally, the seemingly overnight shift garnered a great deal of media coverage. The media's focus was less on the composition of the new MAC and more on who was no longer on it – as well as speculating about what had led to the changes.

A popular media depiction was that some MAC members had been dropped due to their vocal criticism of government. In reality, the explanation was simple. All members whose salary came from the Department of Health – including employees of the NICD, NHLS, MRC, etcetera – were removed. It was inappropriate to have those employed directly or indirectly by the Department of Health on the committee in the first place as it meant that employees of the Department of Health were advising their own department. In some instances, departmental employees were both providers and recipients of the MAC's advice on an issue. Some of the changes in the MAC's composition aimed to reduce duplication in expertise to allow for a wide range of skills and experience on the committee. In the new configuration, the number of MAC members was cut by about half. I was to co-chair the new committee with Professor Marian Jacobs, a former dean of UCT medical school, former chair of the MRC board and someone known to be an exceptional leader in the world of medicine. Working alongside Jacobs made leading the MAC easier and the reduction in the size of the MAC enabled greater participation, though we missed the wise contributions from those who were no longer on the committee. I particularly missed having Quarraisha's wise counsel on the reconstituted MAC.

Along with our reduced membership, two other MACs were created. One was a committee to deal with Covid-19 vaccines, chaired by Barry Schoub, and the other, a multi-sectoral committee on social and behavioural change, chaired by Bishop Malusi Mpulwana. Now that the emergency of the first Covid-19 wave was over, the Department of Health needed a lot more guidance on Covid-19 vaccines and on longer term behavioural and social change in anticipation of future waves.

By the time the MAC was reconstituted in September 2020, the first epidemic wave had passed and science was, for the most part, holding its own against the array of competing real-world interests. But there were rougher seas ahead: a second surge, fiercer than the first, would see us reaching infection rates of over 10 000 per day, necessitating the introduction of new national restrictions. Initially predicted to happen after Christmas 2020 and New Year festivities, the resurgence came earlier, starting its climb in late November. At the time, it was believed to be driven by pandemic fatigue in general but also by teens and young adults who were celebrating en masse the end of a disjointed and frustrating academic year. That earlier-than-expected spike was bad enough, but in mid-December we received worse news, which partially explained our predicament: a new highly transmissible variant, then known as N501Y.v2 (later called Beta), had been detected in South Africa and was making its way steadily across the country.

It was up to the MAC to come up with guidance in the uncharted territory of new Covid-19 challenges, including variants. That was our job – and we managed to do that. Every advisory – all 119 of them produced by the MAC during my time as MAC chair or co-chair – was supported by the members of the MAC. As far as I can recall, no one had ever rejected an advisory, even if they held strong opposing views during the discussions. This reflected on the maturity of the MAC members and their willingness to find a path forward, even if it was not exactly what they wanted. This willingness to compromise on less important issues in order to make progress on the critically important issues enabled the MAC to generate, on average, two advisories a week during my tenure. My task as its leader was to steer the process that enabled the MAC to achieve this. But the steering was not always being done in calm waters ...

CHAPTER 19

From advisory to policy and implementation

In its first year, the MAC produced 119 advisories, out of which 96 were fully implemented, 19 partially implemented and four were not implemented at all. The 81% (96/119) implementation rate of its advisories confirmed the valuable contribution of the MAC.

When the MAC was established, it was very clear that scientific advice was not just desired but actively sought by the Department of Health in order to feed into its decision-making process. Initially in March 2020, Health Minister Mkhize would phone me almost daily at the end of his day, usually at around 11pm, and would raise the pandemic issues with which he had grappled during that day. Occasionally they were simple issues requiring straightforward answers that I could respond to immediately over the phone. Most of the issues, however, were complicated and required broader consideration. I would take those issues back to the MAC, which, in those early stages, was meeting almost every day or every second day. After discussion at the MAC, I would relay the gist of our debates and the guidance we agreed on verbally to either the minister or Acting DG Anban Pillay.

Very quickly, it became clear that we needed a more formal mechanism for the advice, one that reflected the scientific rationale and evidence for the advice the MAC was providing. Together with the MAC secretariat, I devised the concept of a written advisory as an appropriate vehicle through which to convey the reasoning and advice of the MAC. The advisory format consisted of three parts: a problem statement, evidence and recommendations.

By early April 2020, written advisories had become the standard way for the MAC to provide advice in response to requests from the minister or Acting DG. But the feedback loop to learn what eventual decisions were made based on our advice was tenuous, as it relied on the minister providing verbal feedback to the MAC when he was available to attend. Given his active involvement in the Covid-19 response on the ground in the provinces, he could only attend MAC meetings occasionally. As a result, there were breaks in between when we did not know whether our advice was being followed. But when he did attend, Mkhize's feedback usually described how the MAC advice had been adopted, sometimes with practical modifications to match capabilities on the ground or to incorporate other advice, such as that from the WHO. We were generally confident in the first few weeks that the Department of Health was finding our advice useful and was following it. At least in its early stages, the pandemic response was following the science.

The contention that the government was not listening to the scientists proved to be a concern among some in the MAC and more broadly. There was an assumption that because the government said it was 'following the science', the MAC was the *only* place where this scientific advice should be sourced. This meant that the MAC should be regarded as the advisory committee to the whole of government, should be *the* final authority on all matters scientific and, further still, that the government was obliged to follow the MAC's advice.

During the lockdown, I had repeatedly heard the question – what's the point of having scientists to advise you [referring to the government], if you are not going to listen to them? The question reflected the view that the government should not be allowed to determine what advice it would follow. It also reflected the view that when science advice is sought by the government, it should simply follow the science advice received and not seek other advice or consult more broadly to get alternate views, in case this leads to decisions differing from the MAC's advice. Worryingly, it conveyed a lack of trust in government to seek advice, consult multiple bodies (not just scientists) and weigh up the diverse sources of advice and information to make the best decision.

If the sentiments in the question were followed, then the government's task would be simply to rubber-stamp the MAC's views, making the MAC all-powerful in defining the national Covid-19 response. This view was akin to a power grab, and it did not have my support. I encouraged the Minister of Health to seek many views. In my opinion, the MAC had a voluntary role to provide non-binding advice. 'It is not a board of directors,' I said on more than one occasion. The MAC had no decision-making powers, could issue no instructions, and could not insist its advice be heeded. Neither the minister nor the Department of Health was accountable to the MAC on each item of advice – but they were accountable to the electorate and the people of South Africa more broadly. Furthermore, while the MAC comprised some of the country's top scientists, it was not the only source of scientific advice. The government received advice from the WHO, Africa CDC and a number of current and former scientists in its employ. The job of the MAC was not to make policy decisions. Nor was it involved in planning, implementation or execution; that was the responsibility of the Department of Health and the government.

Our job was to plough through the rapidly growing mountain of journal articles and other material to provide the best available evidence to support the Department of Health personnel to do their jobs to the best of their ability. Put simply, our role was to provide the best scientific advice for the Department of Health to consider when making Covid-19 policy decisions. I took the view that it was the MAC's job to start with a question, to collect evidence and produce a set of recommendations that constituted advice to the minister and Department of Health that was non-binding. At first, we collected information based on questions posed by the Department of Health. After a few weeks, we began to take the initiative to identify a gap or problem in the national response that war-ranted a MAC advisory. But, as our terms of reference stipulated, at no stage were we responsible for policy-making or delivery or co-ordination of services related to the Covid-19 response.

For a large part of my career, particularly in the latter stages, I have served as an adviser to many different national and international organisations. I do not expect them to take all the advice I offer. In fact, if my advice or that of other advisers were to be uniformly accepted, in my mind that would signal a lack of discernment on the part of those asking for the advice. The role of adviser is typically a behind-the-scenes, backroom role. However, the exigencies of the pandemic elevated the public status of science and scientists, drawing them out of their laboratories and conference halls into the media limelight – not just at home, but around the world – and that created its own set of dynamics.

In South Africa, individual appointments to the MAC naturally came with a sense of national importance and prestige. The profile of the MAC and its scientists rose sharply after the first live television briefing on 13 April 2020, in which some of the key MAC figures, including myself, were introduced to a wider South African public and we were able to offer the reassurance of science being made available to policy-makers in what were choppy, uncharted seas. For some in the MAC, it may have been difficult to reconcile their sudden public profile with the role of backroom mentor. After all, there was a growing perception in the public that the MAC was calling the shots.

Many of the MAC members were senior leaders in their own right. They were used to being in charge, having the final say, running their own teams and organisations in the way they saw fit. When their expectations about how things should be done were thwarted, it was difficult for them to remain sanguine. At a MAC meeting in June 2020, concern over the lack of feedback from the Department of Health or the National Coronavirus Command Council (NCCC) in response to the MAC advisory on PCR testing priorities was raised – and not for the first time. Testing backlogs were growing, and results were taking too long to be meaningful for public health action. The MAC had produced a prioritisation advisory, but we did not know if this was being implemented, as the testing delays persisted. There was a feeling that issues that were being flagged by the committee as urgent were not being treated as such, and recommendations made by the MAC were not finding their way into official guidelines for testing.

I had repeatedly explained in the media and in the MAC that the MAC was not involved in implementation, but the line between offering advice and providing a service did get blurred in some instances, especially in the early days. One instance of this concerned the data management capacity of the NICD and the testing capacity of the NHLS.

In March 2020, as the pandemic gathered speed, I tried to get a handle on the tests being conducted in both the private and public sectors. Unable to make sense of the private sector data being provided by the Department of Health's data management contractor, I turned to the NICD for the data, which I thought was the logical place to find it. However, the NICD was struggling to get up to speed as a result of internal structural challenges and I pretty much took matters into my own hands, sourcing the original data from the laboratories and setting up a team at CAPRISA to crunch the numbers. Now at least, we had a system to obtain simple Covid-19 test statistics, which others were struggling to set up. This included how many tests were being done, how many of those were positive, and a profile of the patients tested and the provinces in which they were located.

Testing is a critical component in any response to a pandemic. It gives fundamental information about the size and shape of a pandemic, and, to an epidemiologist, this information constitutes the raw material for their work. In a clinical setting, delayed results present problems when it comes to making decisions about isolation and quarantine, particularly in a hospital.

To add to my frustration, in the early days of the pandemic, the NICD had come up with a highly restrictive definition concerning those permitted to test for Covid-19. It basically meant that only people who had recently travelled overseas or who had contact with a positive person who had travelled overseas could legitimately qualify for a test. It was such a restrictive definition that I found there was insufficient data available for me to get a handle on the pandemic. Fearful of not having sufficient testing capacity, all attempts by me to make the definition on who qualified for a test broader came to nought – I could not persuade them to change the definition. In addition, there was some concern about the quality of data being received from the private sector after a false positive result from a private lab in the Free State had incorrectly heralded what everyone believed was the first case of community transmission. That mistake led to a new policy where all Covid-19 positive tests in the private laboratories had to be confirmed by additional confirmatory testing at the NICD or in the NHLS. I could understand the concerns, but it was a hugely inefficient process.

By early April 2020, I had managed to persuade the Department of Health that we needed to open up the definition for those qualifying for tests, despite resistance from some quarters. Those who resisted enlarging the testing definition turned out to be right – the limitations on laboratory infrastructure proved to be a bottleneck and limited our early response to the pandemic. I am not blaming anyone; everyone was trying to do things for good reason. But the net effect was that we hamstrung ourselves. Test kits were difficult to obtain, and the testing process was long. Put simply, we did not have the capacity to undertake the level of Covid-19 testing needed to identify the initial chains of transmission and try to slow or stop transmission while the pandemic was still in its infancy. Also, the data we needed on the spatial distribution of Covid-19 could not be generated and so was not available when it was needed initially.

It took a few weeks before the NICD's data management systems became functional and started to produce the necessary information. It was great to see the NICD taking up its rightful role of lead agency for surveillance during an epidemic or pandemic. But there were ongoing concerns about inadequate testing capacity (see advisory on 2 June 2020 – 'Advisory on the urgent need to address the current challenges in testing through prioritisation for the SARS-CoV-2 daily test targets'). I had previously worked with Barry Schoub, who was the founding director of the NICD, in preparing the country's pandemic response. In my view, the principal source of scientific advice to guide the Covid-19 response should be the NICD. I had discussed with the minister that we needed to be careful that the MAC did not usurp the legally mandated role of the

NICD. The situation was made even more complicated by the fact that there were over a dozen scientists from the NICD who were members of the MAC. In essence, they were working in the MAC on matters that the NICD should have been dealing with; in some instances, they were effectively advising the Department of Health about what to tell the NICD to do. One option was for the MAC to assist and support the NICD in its science advice to the Department of Health. This would enable the NICD to play its rightful leadership role in the pandemic response and relegate the MAC to an appropriate backroom support role. But time was of the essence, and this would just have added a layer of complexity when we needed to be fleet-footed. And so, the MAC continued providing advice directly to the Department of Health.

I was clear that our job was to provide advice and to let the Department of Health decide if it wanted to accept or reject our advice in its policy-making and implementation. Overall, we had a pretty good conversion rate from advice into policy and implementation though. The MAC secretariat had developed a tracking system, which showed the implementation status of each completed advisory. When I stepped down from the MAC at the end of March 2021, we had produced a total of 119 advisories, out of which only four were not implemented at all, and 19 were partially implemented. The four that were not implemented at all were the recommendations to scrap Covid-19 tests for travellers coming into South Africa by land from neighbouring countries (issued in December 2020); the recommendations of tighter restrictions for an 11-day period over Easter 2021 (issued in March 2021); the recommendation to scrap thermal scanning at airports (17 March 2020); and a recommendation that taxi capacity be limited to 70% (version 1, 3 July 2020). It was not a perfect score, but the 81% advisory implementation rate (94/119) was certainly high enough to confirm the value of the MAC.

After repeated calls from the public, the media and even the MAC, in August 2020, the Minister of Health agreed that the MAC advisories should be published online, including those that had been produced thus far. Initial resistance from the ministry to the idea had been based on concerns that they would be construed by the public as government policy rather than what they were – advice – and that this might create confusion in the minds of the public about outcomes. This was something that I, too, was concerned about. I worried about creating more confusion around the government's policies, especially where MAC advice had not gone into the policy-making process – a phenomenon that did transpire on some occasions. For example, when the MAC recommended that the isolation period be reduced to eight days instead of the 14 days recommended by the Department of Health, the public was confused as to whether isolation was eight or 14 days. When I was asked in the media about it, I had to explain that the policy was 14 days but that the MAC had recommended, in response to a query from the Department of Health, that it be changed to eight days. The confusion was around whether to follow the current government policy or the advice of the MAC, which had not yet been considered by the Department of Health. I felt that the advisories should be made public a few weeks after they had been submitted to give the Department of Health time to consider the MAC's advice so that policy could be aligned with the advice to avoid confusion when there were differences. But these problems emanating from the advice to policy delay paled in comparison to the benefits of transparency that emanated from the publication of advisories.

While I preferred that the advisories only be made public after a short delay, I was very pleased to see that once the advisories were in the public domain, it helped address the concerns that the government was not being sufficiently transparent, that the government was not heeding the advice of scientists and that the government was dragging its feet on implementation. Now the public could judge for themselves whether or not that was true. Still, nothing in this space was ever straightforward and our advisories sometimes had to traverse a complicated political path – whether in government or in the public sphere.

CHAPTER 20

Following the science?

*In the midst of deep frustration with government-imposed Covid-19
restrictions on freedoms, the Covid-19 response was badly damaged
when inappropriate, unjustifiable and unnecessarily intrusive
regulations on the purchasing of clothes provided glaring evidence
that science had not been followed.*

Since we were building the ship as we were sailing it, a challenge
emerged in relation to whether the government was consistently following the science. The expectation that the government would always
seek and follow the advice of the MAC – from both within the committee
and among members of the public – stood out as a significant challenge
to its smooth sailing. Perhaps this was a product of its origins as a lashed-
together raft, rather than an elegant schooner with a sleek hull.

As I have explained, the MAC was an advisory committee of the
Department of Health – it was *not* an advisory committee of the
government more broadly. While it was clear that the Department of
Health was generally following the MAC's advice, there was concern
related to the occasions when other departments of the government
did not seek the advice of the MAC. There was no obligation on any
government department to seek the MAC's advice, and it may not even
have been appropriate or practical to seek it for every Covid-19 response
policy decision. Regardless, the concerns about government policy not
following the science mostly occurred when the Department of Health
was not consulted, and the advice of the MAC was not sought. This
problem came to the fore during the extension of Alert Level 5 (stringent

stay-at-home lockdown) and, thereafter, the transition from Level 5 to Level 4 (less stringent, partial stay-at-home lockdown).

The initial decision to impose a three-week stringent lockdown from 26 March to 16 April 2020 did not involve the MAC (the committee was only established on the day of this announcement). I subsequently learned that this lockdown had been labelled Alert Level 5. On 15 April, the National Coronavirus Command Council (NCCC) extended the Alert Level 5 for another two weeks up to 30 April. No advice was sought from the MAC on this decision. I later learned that the NCCC had based their decision to extend Level 5 on a mathematical modelling presentation. I did not personally support the extension of Alert Level 5 and had suggested a systematic easing of Level 5 over the course of a week, starting on 16 April. Even though I was annoyed by their decision on the extension and let my annoyance slip in some media interviews, I gave the NCCC the benefit of the doubt since an evidence-based decision could not be made on an issue where little or no data were available. While there was no obligation on the NCCC to consult the MAC, there was some frustration within the MAC that our advice was not sought on such an important issue, particularly as we had not been privy to the modelling evidence provided to the NCCC. I subsequently met with the Acting DG Anban Pillay and DDG Yogan Pillay to convey my displeasure at this NCCC decision and made sure that they were aware that the MAC was available to advise on such matters in future.

The concept of lockdown alert levels was new to me – as it was to almost everyone, including those in the MAC and in government. I gathered that the government had developed the alert levels by taking its cue from other countries around the world that had developed similar grading systems to define the level of stringency in the restrictions in response to the pandemic during any period. The South African alert level system, for example, was similar to that used in Australia. In essence, the system of 'levels' in South Africa embodied the desire on the part of government for a phased and controlled approach to imposing or lifting restrictions – referred to as a 'risk-adjusted strategy'. When asked by the media about the defining features of each level, I could offer no insights. The MAC had provided no advice on the alert levels at that stage and was not party to those decisions.

The problem got worse when on 1 May 2020, the NCCC lowered the alert status to Level 4. At that point, infection rates were still low, but the threat of the first wave was looming. There was keen anticipation that South Africa would ease some of the restrictions on personal freedoms that had been in place for the past five weeks, so as to allow a partial recommencement of economic and social activity. This optimism turned out to be misplaced.

The task of defining the features of Alert Level 4 fell to another government department and did not include the Department of Health. The Department of Trade, Industry and Competition, in consultation with industry stakeholders, defined what was permitted and this was published as the Level 4 regulations in the *Government Gazette*. It listed the activities permitted during any particular level and the products that could be sold. Those activities and products not on the list were deemed by their absence to be 'not allowed'. Since this list of allowed services and goods did not fall under the purview of the Department of Health, the MAC's advice was not sought.

With these new rules, we were obviously in uncharted territory, but the regulations opened the door to a number of inconsistencies. When I visited my local retail pharmacy to pick up some medication the day after the start of Level 4, I encountered store workers wrapping many of the shelves with plastic sheets, covering up those products deemed non-essential and therefore not allowed to be sold. These 'illicit' items included perfumes and cosmetics, but not deodorant and shampoo. It made no sense at all, made no contribution to minimising the risk of transmission, and had the potential to undermine confidence in the government's approach to Covid-19 and compromise adherence to the rules.

On Tuesday, 12 May 2020, this potential was realised when the government published three sets of 'directions' in terms of the Disaster Management Act regulations, which guided the sale and emergency repairs of motor vehicles; the sale of clothing, bedding and footwear; and the operations of small businesses offering 'permitted services'. Since these regulations had been developed by the Department of Trade, Industry and Competition, I had hoped that they had their own Covid-19 advisers, as the MAC's advice was not sought and had played no role in these new regulations.

All of the directions – basically sub-regulations – imposed restrictions that appeared to any normal person to be completely arbitrary. Operating at the level of individual products rather than at sector level, they had the effect of creating a set of inappropriate, unjustifiable and unnecessarily intrusive regulations. For example, in the case of car sales, no children were allowed to be in car dealerships or used car outlets under Level 4. This meant that any prospective car owner who was also a parent could not take their children to help choose a new family vehicle. It was odd, to say the least. The same was true of the 'permitted businesses' listed in the regulations governing the operation of micro and small entities – those with the smallest profit margins and arguably the hardest hit by the lockdown.

The guidance relating to the sale of clothing, bedding and footwear was most concerning and later attracted the most public interest. Not unusually, my attention was first drawn to these regulations by my daughter, Aisha, as soon as they were made public. 'Did you know you can only buy closed-toe shoes, not open-toe shoes?' she announced incredulously at the breakfast table. There was more: 'Did you know you can buy a short-sleeved T-shirt only if it is "promoted and displayed as undergarments for warmth"!' It did sound bizarre, and when I looked at the full list of clothing that was permitted to be bought and sold, I realised that her indignation was not misplaced and that the list had enormous repercussions for the government in relation to perceptions of the public on whether these were justifiable.

In their attempt to limit the number of people taking trips to retail stores, the Ministry of Trade, Industry and Competition had come up with a list of individual clothing items they believed South Africans might need over the next few weeks as the country headed into winter. But the 'directions', as they were known, came across as arbitrary, petty, unworkable and, frankly, ridiculous. The importance of public health interventions as the means to keep people safe was being lost in the emphasis on what products were being made available.

As soon as breakfast was over, I sat down at my work desk at home and called Ms Jane Ridden, head of the MAC secretariat, and asked her to convene a meeting of the MAC sub-committee chairs for later that day. 'What's on the agenda?' she asked. 'Only today's regulations from the government,' I replied.

If you take a big picture view, the problem with the regulations was part of the fallout that comes from building a ship while sailing it. Usually, government regulations undergo a long and finely calibrated process before their publication. But in the case of regulations for the Covid-19 response, time was of the essence. The regulations needed to be produced rapidly because the levels were constantly changing. In this instance, broader consultation might have resulted in a more sensible and practicable outcome, but this had been sacrificed on the altar of urgency. There was another factor contributing to the propensity for nonsense: there was no precedent for this specific sort of regulation.

Deputy DG of the Treasury Mr Ismail Momoniat, who I knew as 'Momo' from our days as student activists and whom I held in high regard for his steadfast anti-corruption stance, was invited sometime later to attend a MAC meeting to speak on the issue. He drew our attention to the advantages of a regulation *blacklist* (what he called a negative list) – listing items or activities that were not permissible – versus a regulation *whitelist* – a list of activities or items that were permitted. After he had made this distinction, I was convinced that a blacklist, if needed at all, was a better approach in regulations. There were only a few things that posed a problem in relation to viral transmission and super-spreader opportunities, and these could be captured as a short blacklist. It would be more meaningful to identify the riskiest activities and list them with a clear rationale for each item on the list of what you *cannot* do rather than what you *can* do.

I raised the issue with the minister and at the NCCC in one of my presentations later but was disappointed to see that the next sets of regulations published were also made up of whitelists. The resulting problem was that the regulations were seen as unjustified government intrusion aimed at curbing personal freedoms. I also felt this way at times when I could see no reason why warm chicken was not allowed, but cold chicken was.

We were not alone in making silly decisions in an attempt to give alert levels a set of rules that distinguished each level. For example, one story I saw on the evening news was about a man who went into a store in Wales to do his shopping dressed only in his underwear because under Welsh lockdown conditions he was not permitted to buy clothes deemed non-essential. It was a protest against what he saw as arbitrary. I struggled to grasp how so many governments across the world were lurching into crises due to ludicrous lockdown rules. It was strangely comforting to know that people around the world were expressing similar outrage at unnecessarily intrusive rules. But it was also a reminder of the lack of benchmarks to guide the rule-makers. Each country that established alert levels was having to make up the rules as they went along. Few had managed to do this in a meaningful and justifiable way.

The problem for the MAC was that a large section of the general public held us responsible for this folly, when in fact we had nothing to do with those decisions and regulations. For me, it was all the more reason to critique the regulations and 'stand up for science' by highlighting the idiosyncrasies and irrationality of the rules – and this was the reason I had asked Ridden to set up the afternoon meeting.

When the four MAC sub-committee chairs met with me that Tuesday afternoon on 12 May 2020, it was unanimously agreed that the new regulations did nothing to contribute to slowing down the transmission of the virus and an advisory from the full MAC should be submitted to the Minister of Health, explaining that the regulations were ill-advised and recommending that they be withdrawn in their entirety rather than simply altered. It was felt that the regulations were detracting from our efforts in the real fight against Covid-19 and were undermining the public's confidence in the country's Covid-19 response. Glenda Gray, who was head of the research committee, one of four sub-committees within the MAC, volunteered to write the advisory within the next day or so.

On Friday, 15 May, there was still no draft advisory from Gray in my inbox. Instead, she had raised the issue in a media interview. Speaking in their personal and professional capacity as scientists, MAC members were entitled to take issue with anything at all. And they did: several criticised the actions of government on a regular basis in keeping with their own political and scientific views. Some MAC members even criticised the MAC publicly. MAC rules only proscribed members from claiming to represent the MAC (this was the prerogative of the chair) and from sharing confidential MAC information with the media. But nothing prohibited MAC members from conveying public criticism. Indeed, I had personally challenged the government on several matters, reserving my harshest criticism for human rights violations such as the Collins Khosa incident. Not only was it a member's right to express their views, but I was very keen to avoid any hint of 'group think' setting into MAC deliberations. The phenomenon of 'group think', which promotes conformity instead of debate, results in intellectual atrophy – a notion that is fatal to any organisation.

Gray's comments about some of the regulations being 'thumb-sucks' and her complaint that the phased lifting of the lockdown was 'unscientific' were justified in my view and I had already conveyed similar views at the Tuesday MAC co-chairs meeting that I convened on this matter. So, many held similar views on the regulations meant to define alert levels. But in her – unsubstantiated – claims about child malnutrition cases being seen for the first time in decades at Chris Hani Baragwanath Academic Hospital in Soweto and about the government's treatment of scientists, she went too far. That was an over-reach. And both were not true. MAC member Professor Sithembiso Velaphi, who is head of Paediatrics at Chris Hani Baragwanath Hospital, publicly provided the hospital data showing a reduction in malnutrition cases in 2020 compared with the previous four years. And the advisory implementation tracker kept by the MAC secretariat showed that there was evidence of policy or implementation of every one of the over 50 MAC advisories submitted by then.

But the damage had already been done. Gray's comments sparked a new narrative in the media: the government was deliberately ignoring the scientists and was choosing to implement a Covid-19 pandemic response to suit its own political goals. A part of me felt that the government deserved to be castigated for the mess it created with the regulations – it should not be allowed to get away with abuse-of-power actions like those regulations. But, at the same time, it was wholly inappropriate to make untrue statements. It was sad to watch this matter taint the entire Covid-19 response. The South African government had its fair share of errors in its Covid-19 response – the T-shirt and open-toed shoe regulations were glaring evidence of that.

The government's biggest error was the level of corruption within its ranks, spawned by the state of disaster allowing procurement procedures to be bypassed. I was deeply distressed to learn that employees of the state worked in cahoots with private companies to loot the public's money. The looting was on a grand scale – prices of masks were being jacked up manifold and in the absence of any of the requisite clearances, fly-by-night providers were getting multimillion-rand personal protective equipment (PPE) contracts. I gathered that there's a maxim in the world of contract corruption – that the requirements of the contract *must be met*, even if this is done at low quality, *after the corrupt get their slice of the pie*, in order to avoid an investigation for non-delivery on the contract. However, the Covid-19 corruption mongers disregarded even this elementary step, which needed to be followed to reduce their risk of being caught. They were brazen!

The Covid-19 looting was on a wide scale. It permeated multiple government departments, including Health, Police and Education. At exorbitant prices, schools were being gassed long after the MAC had advised against gassing for surface sterilisation. Even the police had widespread corruption in their PPE contracts. It was deeply distressing to learn that those responsible for upholding the law were the ones breaking it. Covid-19 PPE contracts became a looting fest.

And it did not end there. Looting of the state's money occurred with impunity. When the corrupt were occasionally caught out, the government's incapacity to bring them to book initiated long periods at home on full pay before the culprits got to an internal hearing, which often led to nothing more than a slap on the wrist. Court action, if instituted at all, may follow years later.

A communications contract between a company called Digital Vibes and the Department of Health had all the hallmarks of state looting. Politically connected individuals secured a contract with the government, allegedly with political interference by the minister, and then siphoned off large amounts, some of which seemed to make their way as payments for a vehicle and fitting out a nail salon for the minister's family members. While these findings of a Special Investigating Unit report are merely allegations, as they have not yet been tested in court, even the hint of impropriety is damaging at a time when people need to have confidence in their leadership to guide them to safety in the midst of a pandemic.

Corruption was not new, but the pandemic just created a feeding frenzy that highlighted corruption as a political crisis. Covid-19 corruption created a sense of powerlessness in the public's mind akin to watching a bank robbery from afar without being able to do anything about it. Worse, the bank's guards, who could have stopped it, were unwilling to do anything about it either and, worse still, were abetting the crime in some instances. The net effect was that public lost confidence and trust in those charged with using the public purse wisely. Trust, once broken, is very difficult to rekindle. The corruption in government had caused this breach of trust and the government was reaping deserved criticism as a consequence. Disillusionment would follow.

South Africa was not alone in this situation. The UK government announced that about half its pandemic-associated contracts were tainted for breaching procedure. Indeed, no government has had a flawless Covid-19 response, and South Africa was ranked as having among the better pandemic responses in a multi-country comparison by a Covid-19 Commission. Notwithstanding the PPE corruption, instances of military abuse and ill-considered Covid-19 regulations on clothing, reports have used our country as a global exemplar for some aspects of its pandemic response. The reality was that while there were occasions when the MAC was not consulted, the MAC's advice, when sought, was being generally followed.

While the government had its share of blame to shoulder, the work of the scientists in the MAC was now being blemished by false claims on, among others, malnutrition. At a hastily called MAC meeting on Saturday, 16 May 2020, aimed at resolving this, I had hoped that the facts would be acknowledged and the falsehoods withdrawn. But this did not happen. Instead, the MAC discussions did not make headway towards resolution; I felt that it had reached an impasse. The coronavirus pandemic was a national crisis. Any group responsible for guiding the nation in this crisis needed to be united and demonstrate a common sense of purpose. Was this failure of the MAC to guide the government's regulations a reflection of a problem with my leadership? Up until that point, I had been unaware of any unhappiness in the way I was chairing the MAC, but perhaps there was someone who could better lead the MAC out of this impasse? I decided to take a drastic step – I tabled a motion of no confidence in my own position in the MAC.

Needless to say, the motion caused quite a stir. Several members intervened to argue that there were no grounds for the motion and that I should continue as chair. When it was pointed out that it was unprocedural to consider a motion that did not have a seconder and that the committee had no authority to appoint or dismiss the chair, I had no choice but to retract it, thereby averting a vote. But my motion made it clear that I would not continue to lead the MAC if we were not going to be truthful and if the committee was going to get distracted from its mission to give the Department of Health the best advice we could on the Covid-19 response. I was also signalling that I had no interest in, or tolerance for, power plays and would not stand in the way of anyone who had ambitions to lead the MAC. While we were trying to put the issue to bed internally in the MAC, speculation about warring factions within our committee started to grace news headlines. In response to the growing media interest in this issue, Mkhize released a statement on Wednesday, 20 May 2020, challenging the four key falsehoods in Gray's media comments and stating that he considered the matter now closed.

The day after Mkhize's statement, Acting DG Pillay wrote to the MRC board recommending an investigation into Gray's actions. His bureaucratic missive seemed to take on more sinister overtones, conveying an attempt to silence critics of government. Pillay was justifiably castigated for his actions, with many attacking him for what they saw as an assault on academic freedom. His ill-considered text confirmed the very issue – that the government was suppressing scientists – that he was seeking to challenge through his letter! While the MRC board was still considering what action to take in response to Acting DG Pillay's letter, Gray's attorney reached out to me at her request, to ask if I would be willing to facilitate communication with Mkhize to resolve the matter by way of an apology. This initiative fell away shortly thereafter, however, when the indications were that the MRC board would not take further action against her on the matter.

Things might have ended there, but a few days later I received a call from a MAC member who told me that Gray had called about three weeks before the 16 May meeting, looking for support to unseat me from the position of MAC chair. I had no reason to question the veracity of this revelation, as I have been in leadership positions too long to bother about this kind of behind-the-scenes plotting. I decided that the matter was not worth a second thought – there was work to do and I was perfectly happy to continue working professionally with everyone on the MAC to get the job done.

I was struck at the time as to how this controversy grew to a crescendo so quickly, coming as it did against a backdrop of deep frustration with Covid-19 restrictions being imposed by government and concerns as to whether they were following the science.

To avoid a repetition of these disastrous regulations, I reached out to three other government departments to offer the MAC's assistance with their work on Covid-19. I was heartened when the Department of Basic Education agreed to a joint TWG with the Department of Health to develop recommendations related to schools. But I had no illusions that I could get all government departments to consult the MAC; as some explained, they preferred to consult their own scientific advisers who were knowledgeable about Covid-19 and understood the needs of their sector.

In the midst of these events, I tried my best not to get taken off track, as I had to focus on my first responsibility – to work with the MAC to do everything we could to provide advice on the Covid-19 response. Despite the slight detour of our minor internal guiles, I put my energy back into the task at hand – focusing on the science.

CHAPTER 21

Politically challenging advisories

While some MAC advisories were implemented with little, if any challenges, others had to traverse complicated political waters. The advisories on the reopening of schools, taxi occupancy and medical oxygen supplies proved to be hot political potatoes.

My work is centred around science and evidence. This is also the creed that laid the foundation for all the MAC advisories. However, a pandemic is not just about managing infections and counting case numbers. It is also about ensuring that the advice is appropriate and is feasible. Failing to do this will lead to controversy and advice that is promptly ignored. This is a lesson we had to learn with some of our advisories – a balancing act that, it turned out, came with its own set of highly contentious political viewpoints.

Advisory on the reopening of schools

At a media briefing on 18 May 2020, Basic Education Minister Angie Motshekga announced a return on 1 June 2020 for Grades 7 and 12, in line with the MAC's advice. A growing body of evidence was suggesting that children were less susceptible to severe Covid-19 than adults, although they were still likely to transmit the disease at the same rate. My concern was that we had no idea how long Covid-19 would be in our midst and we would pay too high a price if we continued to put off in-person schooling until we had defeated the pandemic. As well as the loss of school time, there was the fact that many parents were unable to return to work until their children were back at school.

We need to learn to live with the virus, was basically the point I made in media interviews. This was a growing global call in an effort to try to rationalise the ending of some restrictions, while still living in the midst of a growing pandemic. Based on what we knew scientifically about transmission, there was strong reason to believe that the controls already in place within the school environment meant it was possible to implement social distancing and masking protocols that would effectively minimise the risk to both learners and staff – a position that later proved to be correct.

Not everyone saw it the same way, however. My public comments earned me the label of 'Dr Death' from the EFF. Among a host of other claims, members of the party accused me of making decisions based on 'assumptive gut feelings' and abandoning my own scientific advice for 'economic expediency'. To this day, I have no idea what the accusations meant, but it appeared to be nonsense to me. However, it led to an onslaught of hate mail and hate comments on social media targeted at me.

Once the Education minister had made the announcement, the concern was how to minimise the infection risk of those returning children and staff. The MAC drew again on outside expertise to help draft a lengthy advisory. This was published on 26 May 2020, titled 'Getting children back to school safely', and outlined the risks and benefits of reopening schools. It was the unanimous view of the joint health-education TWG that children needed to return to school as quickly as possible with public health protocols to reduce risk to children and staff. The advisory discussed the available evidence for each of its recommendations and laid out a series of scenarios linked to measures to be taken in the event of infections within the school.

Despite the objections, fortunately sense prevailed and South African school learners started to return to at least some in-person classes from early to mid-July. Close monitoring of the situation for the remainder of that year found no evidence that schools implementing mitigation measures contributed to increased circulation of the virus in local communities. Isolated outbreaks were quickly identified and stopped in their tracks, with only some infections brought into schools from the community. Despite this, there was often panic by both parents and teachers whenever a case was identified.

This fed into the political dynamics between those who wanted schools to close and those who wanted them to remain open. The uncertainty around the risks in schools fed this polemic and it was difficult to traverse this complex arena. At one of the Africa Task Force on Coronavirus meetings, which included representatives of several African countries, I learned that this problem was much more widespread and politically even more complicated in many other African countries. In some countries, those advocating for schools reopening were politically marginalised, and they had little chance of getting their children back to school. In many ways, the issue of reopening of schools was turning out to be a predominantly political decision, with science relegated to lesser role.

Advisory on taxi occupancy

The reopening of schools was not, by any means, the only political balancing act in the Covid-19 response. The issue of taxi occupancy illustrated the limitations of 'following the science' in the face of complex political and economic exigencies and handed government critics copious quantities of cannon fodder.

During the initial stringent lockdown, taxis rarely operated. As the restrictions eased in Alert Level 4, only a fraction of taxis operated, and they were only allowed 50% occupancy. Under Alert Level 3, this was raised to 70%. On 12 July 2020, the President announced it was back up at 100% for short trips. The MAC members were understandably perplexed. In our advisory released on 3 July 2020, the MAC had recommended that taxi occupancy should not be increased above the current 70% level and that, given the risk of transmission, consideration should be given to reducing occupancy to 50% in areas where the numbers of active Covid-19 cases were high and rising.

I gained some insight into the complexity of the issue after I met with the DG of Transport, Mr Alec Moemi, and the heads of the three main taxi organisations to explain the health risks of reverting to a 100% occupancy. It was clear that the configuration of seats in a minibus taxi does not lend itself to effective social distancing, even at 50% occupancy. Skipping one seat between two commuters only left a distance of around 50cm – too small to be considered social distancing. I tried my best to explain the complex risks of infection in a taxi environment and why occupancy, window ventilation and mask-wearing were all important factors mitigating risk in a taxi environment.

The taxi owners explained that taxi operators could not operate a taxi at 70% occupancy at peak hour as this was not commercially viable for the taxi owner, particularly those not running large fleets, and to insist on this level of occupancy would effectively kill off the small guys and change the face of the industry. I learned that this had been confirmed by the Transport Department, that is, that taxis are financially viable because of their high occupancy during peak hours and that it's more cost-effective not to run the taxis at low occupancy during the off-peak hours. Moemi was in a quandary. Taxi users make up 46% of the commuter population in South Africa. Any decisions relating to taxi commuters could have substantial implications. Under the prevailing Alert Level 3 in July 2020, taxi occupancy was routinely lower than 70% anyway, given that many industries were still shut or partially operating. So, perhaps we could get away with allowing 100% occupancy knowing that taxi occupancy would generally be much lower anyway? The other option was to have the government subsidise the 30% shortfall needed to ensure the commercial viability of the taxi industry.

The Department of Transport roundly rejected the second option and so we moved from a quandary to an impasse. For their own viability, taxis would load to 100% occupancy anyway. Self-preservation would lead them to maximise occupancy regardless of any decree on lower occupancy. So, the discussion shifted to focus on how to lower the risk of transmission at 100% occupancy. Improved ventilation through open windows could be better than lowered occupancy, but it was winter and it would be difficult to keep the windows open. Masking remained the mainstay of the mitigation strategy as far as I could see, but I felt this needed more minds to chime in on the options.

I provided feedback on my taxi meeting to the MAC and the TWG on taxis was reconstituted. Six days later, we produced a new taxi risk mitigation advisory. While we adhered to our recommendation that the industry abide by the 70% occupancy mark, we also acknowledged that the decision required 'consideration of many factors besides health'. Importantly, I discovered from a journal search that two engineering students from UCT had published a study on airflow in taxis, depending on which windows were open. It was a fascinating study and provided exactly the evidence I was looking for. The study showed that maximum airflow occurred when the two front door windows were open. Opening other windows when the front windows were open did not make much difference. This provided us with good evidence for an open-window ventilation strategy. The revised advisory offered six mitigation measures, including window-jammers that would keep windows open to ensure a constant flow of air throughout the taxi, and staggered working hours for taxi drivers.

From the outside looking in, I can see how confused the regulations around occupancy appeared. And it turned out that our efforts in the MAC to mitigate risk in the taxi industry seemed to be largely without impact. As the pandemic progressed, there was little evidence to link higher numbers of infection to the use of taxis. I spent quite a lot of time thinking about why this might be the case, given what we knew about the conditions under which Covid-19 was likely to spread. I came to consider the possibility that raising levels from 70% to 100% occupancy was an insufficient increase to have any significant impact on its spread. Seventy per cent already constituted a high risk and moving to 100% made very little real difference on the ground. Therefore 70% occupancy presented roughly the same risk as 100% occupancy, and there was no real difference in neither the risk levels nor the outcome at any of these levels of occupancy – in occupancy, we had focused on the wrong issue to balance. A stronger emphasis on window-jammers would have been more important in balancing economic considerations with risk mitigation.

Advisory on medical oxygen supplies

In preparation for South Africa's first wave, we prioritised the need for steady medical oxygen supplies. Oxygen therapy was the single most effective supportive measure available for Covid-19 patients and concerns about oxygen demand and supply were constant in South Africa as they were in most other low- to middle-income countries. The MAC gave this issue substantial attention.

As 2020 progressed, evidence started to emerge that treating patients with continuous positive airway pressure (CPAP) and/or high-flow nasal cannula (HFNC) oxygen might obviate or reduce the need for invasive mechanical intervention, in other words, the use of ventilators. Early data showed that the less invasive forms of oxygen administration produced better outcomes. The evidence also suggested that the therapy was less complex and required less supervision by trained providers. It could even be used outside of intensive care units, thereby reducing some of the pressure on ICU facilities.

In December 2020, the MAC put together an internal memo to the Health minister, in which we recommended that CPAP and HFNC be promoted as alternatives to intubation and ventilation, and for use in hospital settings where ventilators were not available. It was a logical proposal, but one that depended on all health facilities having constant supplies of medical oxygen, particularly during high-demand periods.

Through his organisation Right to Care, MAC member and health systems specialist Professor Ian Sanne was part of a team that worked closely with national and provincial departments of Health to assess and bolster the oxygen supply capacity of both rural and urban health facilities. Working with commercial oxygen suppliers, Right to Care provided invaluable insights and advice, helping us to anticipate, through its modelling exercises, the potential demand for oxygen supplies from private and public hospitals during the first and second waves. It had also conducted a national audit of infrastructure and on-site storage capacity at approximately 160 health care facilities. With funding from USAID, it facilitated the installation of bulk liquid oxygen tanks at five Eastern Cape hospitals and improved the supply of oxygen cylinders to under-equipped rural hospitals.

Working closely with commercial suppliers such as Afrox, which had the contract to supply the country's public hospitals and roughly 50% of private hospitals, and Air Liquide, which supplied mostly private sector facilities, Right to Care was able to provide the MAC with daily feedback about liquid oxygen supplies and resupply across both public and private sectors during the first two waves. It provided the monitoring needed to ensure that oxygen levels were kept as high as possible – the goal was at least 50% of anticipated 24-hour need – during critical demand periods.

It was not plain sailing. In January 2021, shortages of liquid oxygen led to reserves falling below 30% at Groote Schuur and Tygerberg hospitals in the Western Cape and shortages in cylinder oxygen in district hospitals in the Eastern Cape. Afrox was forced to issue legal notices to some of its private sector customers informing them of the possibility of a diversion of all oxygen supplies to medical facilities.

Keen to avert an impending crisis and concerned by the slow pace at which upgrades to facilities that had been recommended by the Right to Care audit were taking place, given the convoluted procurement processes of government, the MAC issued an unsolicited advisory, which we called a 'Strategic review of oxygen supplies' to the minister in January 2021. Among this advisory's recommendations was a call for the departments of Health, Infrastructure Development and the Treasury jointly to engage the services of oxygen providers to help the government monitor and manage the oxygen supply chain. We also recommended that the providers be tasked with completing all procurement and implementation of infrastructure enhancements planned since July 2020.

This turned out to be much more complicated than we anticipated. The competition laws in the country did not allow the three major companies that provide oxygen in South Africa to come together to rationalise the oxygen supply between them, as this would be tantamount to collusion among competitors. Special permission was required so that this exercise did not fall foul of the law. The companies did come together and helped produce the Strategic Oxygen Supply Plan, which included working together to monitor daily quantities of oxygen available to enable expeditious redirection of oxygen away from commercial use for the benefit of medical use.

This complicated exercise, with which the MAC provided assistance, likely saved thousands of lives by ensuring continuous oxygen availability across the country. But it did not work everywhere. Despite the best efforts to assist the Eastern Cape, the dire lack of capacity in that province led to health facilities running out of oxygen. It was a stark reminder about how a person's chances of surviving Covid-19-induced hypoxia depended on which province you lived in, with those in the Eastern Cape being disadvantaged by the incapacity of the provincial health department. But this province's bungling was more systemic, as demonstrated by its now infamous modified bicycle ambulances that flouted multiple legal requirements to be regarded as ambulances.

When it came to oxygen supplies, it wasn't simply a matter of efficiency or rationality. It was very clearly a matter of saving lives.

CHAPTER 22

Alcohol and tobacco bans

While the rationale for the initial step of banning cigarettes and alcohol was unclear, alcohol bans had a major benefit for Covid-19 patient care by freeing up beds in highly pressured health facilities, but cigarette bans had no discernible benefit.

Confusion around the role of the MAC in relation to the banning of cigarettes and alcohol, to which some people are addicted, was widespread in the public mind. Many people saw the MAC, rather than the government, as being responsible for the changes in access to these from one lockdown alert level to the other and the total ban during Level 5 on alcohol and cigarettes.

On 26 March 2020, the government imposed a total ban on alcohol, which lasted until 1 June. On 2 July 2020, the ban was reinstated without warning and lifted, subject to certain restrictions, on 17 August 2020.

I learned from Professor Charles Parry, who has been researching alcohol and drug dependence at the MRC for many years, that only 31% of South Africans consume alcohol on a regular basis. So, it was surprising to me that the availability and non-availability of alcohol during the various lockdown alert levels took centre stage in 2020. Each prospective easing of lockdown levels brought with it widespread speculation about the availability of alcohol; at some point it seemed that whether or not alcohol outlets were open had become the primary way in which people distinguished one level from the next. I became quite irritated when, at times, it felt as if important health discussions about controlling the spread of the pandemic seemed to be reduced to discussions about alcohol restrictions.

However you look at it, though, the consumption of alcohol – because of its huge impact on South African society – was a significant factor in the national response to Covid-19.

The ban on both cigarettes and alcohol during the stringent Level 5 lockdown admittedly constituted an unusually severe step by the government; very few other countries had placed such severe restrictions on their populations, especially since there could be severe consequences for those people addicted to these substances. While the first cigarette ban was never repeated, the alcohol ban was lifted and reimposed with some variation a few times throughout the first year of the pandemic – and, as it turned out, with some good effect.

I was held responsible for the ban on alcohol inter alia by some misinformed Twitter users. Some implied a personal agenda – that I had implemented the ban because I was a Muslim and did not drink alcohol. The latter part is true: I do not consume alcohol; nor do I smoke. But my response as a rational person, like that of many other rational citizens, to the first bans on alcohol and tobacco was that both made little sense. I struggled to understand the rationale. Why deprive people of these indulgences when they would be enduring so many other deprivations? I wondered. A few weeks later, however, Professor Debbie Bradshaw, who heads up burden of disease and mortality research at the MRC, sent me some statistics on the impact of the alcohol ban in terms of reduced numbers of alcohol-related trauma cases, violence and road traffic accidents, and I was forced to reconsider my position. The alcohol ban was dramatically reducing pressure on ICUs and other hospital facilities, which was exactly what the country needed at that time because those health services were central to caring for Covid-19 patients.

I doubt that this outcome or its marked benefits for health services dealing with Covid-19 had been anticipated by the government when it came up with the alcohol ban, but once such clear evidence was out there, it was difficult for anyone, myself included, to deny its positive impact. The evidence was clear and compelling! And so, I became a supporter of the alcohol restrictions. Not only was the ban effective in reducing pressure on hospitals, I argued, but it also reduced the risks associated with super-spreader events, many of which involved alcohol. In the beginning, we hadn't fully grasped the central role of bars, nightclubs and taverns, both formal and informal, in spreading the virus – they accept large numbers of patrons, most of whom show little concern for social distancing and cannot mask when they are eating and drinking.

The difficulty was that the ban equally affected those people who like to have a glass of wine over dinner or a beer to relax at home at the end of the day. The real target of the ban was those who drink to excess and then drive their cars under the influence; beat up their partners or children; or go out and pick fights, that is, activities that lead to hospital ER visits for alcohol-related trauma or illness. But there was no way that an alcohol ban could be selective. And so, there were blanket restrictions that impacted on anyone consuming any type of alcohol in any setting. And the collective benefits to the health care system were substantial.

Dr Keith Cloete, the head of the Western Cape Provincial Department of Health, shared some impressive data with me. It showed how ER utilisation dropped during the alcohol ban and how it rebounded when the ban was lifted, only to drop again when the new ban was announced. The second drop was less marked because some people had stocked up with alcohol in anticipation of the alcohol ban being reimposed. What was key was that alcohol-related injuries often required operating theatres, ICU beds, ventilators and oxygen. This used up the time of anaesthetists, ICU specialists and respiratory physicians – exactly the same scarce services that Covid-19 patients needed desperately. Banning alcohol freed up the health facilities that were in big demand during the Covid-19 waves of infection.

The alcohol ban was one of the most contested restrictions – it led to several court challenges. While I was not involved in the government's policy to impose an alcohol ban and was initially a sceptic, the evidence left little room for doubt about its benefits. When the alcohol ban faced a challenge in the courts, I was confident that there was sufficient evidence to justify it and was called upon to provide the scientific rationale in defence of the alcohol ban in several court cases. The government did not lose any of these court challenges against its alcohol ban.

When it came to the cigarette ban, which lasted from 25 March 2020 to 17 August 2020, I turned again to the available evidence. When I was asked if I would prepare an affidavit supporting the government's policy on cigarettes, I declined. Research on smoking and Covid-19 was very limited at that time and I had been trying to keep up with this literature. After that call, I did another search looking for research available on the link between smoking and Covid-19. I found an informative study in the *New England Journal of Medicine* by Chinese scientist Wei-jie Guan, and others,[1] which had been published at the end of February 2020. It indicated that both current and ex-smokers tended to have higher case fatality rates on ventilators than non-smokers (smoking is definitely not good for the lungs – no surprises there). It was not clear whether giving up smoking shortly before contracting Covid-19 – which is effectively the scenario the ban would have precipitated – conferred any benefits.

Minister Nkosazana Dlamini-Zuma, who was the Minister of Cooperative Governance and Traditional Affairs at the time, also raised the risks related to marijuana: 'When people zol, they put saliva on the paper, and they share their zol.'[2] While this made for good parody on YouTube, the risks associated with this behaviour were theoretical. At the time, there was concern about spread through contaminated surfaces and so this concern was not far-fetched. But there was no actual study of risks in this setting to back up this argument.

In the end, my lack of support for the tobacco ban was inconsequential, as the government won their first case against Big Tobacco, represented by the Fair Trade Independent Tobacco Association. That came as something of a surprise to me – but I think in the absence of extensive evidence, the court took a conservative view, erring on the side of caution. Four months later, the Western Cape High Court ruled against the tobacco ban, finding that its damage to the economy and industry was disproportionately high compared with the benefits. As leave to appeal the ruling was granted, it paved the way for the government to reinstate the ban if it so wanted.

While the alcohol ban had important positive spin-offs, it is not evident if the tobacco ban produced any benefit, even as more evidence became available. What was emerging in the media was that the bans had a massive negative spin-off in the form of a boost to the illicit cigarette and alcohol markets.

With these bans, I had another concern – was this big government flexing its power? In the absence of reasoned arguments for these bans, they seemed to be particularly intrusive on individual choice. While the benefits of the alcohol ban became evident after it was imposed, these benefits would have been difficult to predict beforehand. At first impression, these bans also seemed to be unrelated to Covid-19.

The alcohol ban turned out to have many benefits; not just the glaringly obvious one of reducing trauma that keeps emergency rooms busy. For example, the alcohol ban apparently had an impact on reducing gender-based violence. GBV was a problem during the stringent lockdown but would have been much worse if alcohol had been readily available during that period. So, did these benefits warrant government intrusion into such personal matters as alcohol consumption?

My rationale was that the government already intrudes in this domain – and did so quite substantially pre-Covid. The government controls who can sell alcohol, stipulates hours of alcohol sale, where alcohol can be consumed and institutes checks on alcohol levels in drivers, to name a few. Alcohol and cigarettes are regulated quite stringently across the world, even to the extent of controlling whether you can smoke in your own home. So, the government already intrudes directly in this area – taking steps to institute temporary restrictions on alcohol access was an extension of those government controls on alcohol. The justification for implementing this additional step of controls with a temporary outright ban remains a fine line in my mind.

With these arguments in mind, I felt that, while intrusive, the alcohol ban's benefits outweighed its harms. I ended up being a strong supporter of alcohol curtailment when the country was going into a wave. But I did not support any cigarette curtailment specifically for Covid-19. However, given the dearth of information available when the bans were first imposed, would I have supported the bans then? Perhaps not.

There was little time to ponder what the advice on alcohol and tobacco may or should have been. The country was coming out of its first wave and a new question was swirling: could people get reinfected with SARS-CoV-2?

CHAPTER 23

Getting Covid-19 twice?

The issue of reinfection was important due to its implications for herd immunity and vaccine efficacy. If natural immunity cannot prevent a second infection, would vaccine immunity be able to do so?

In a media interview in May 2020 on eNCA with Sally Burdett, I was asked whether it was possible to contract Covid-19 twice. My answer was: 'I would be surprised if you can't. We should expect repeated Covid-19 infections.'

Our experience with the other four (common cold) coronaviruses suggested that reinfection was likely. Immunity to seasonal colds caused by those viruses typically lasts seven to eight months. Therefore, if SARS-CoV-2 followed the pattern of its cousins, there would be reinfections. But I also emphasised the facts: firstly, there simply wasn't sufficient evidence, and secondly, it was too early in the epidemic to make a definitive call. An early study coming out of the UK suggested that immunity to Covid-19 waned substantially after three months, but in the absence of more studies and more data, it was impossible to draw hard and fast conclusions.

However, if there were to be reinfections, I argued, we would see them first in China, followed quickly by Italy. As these countries had been the first to experience the epidemic, it stood to reason that they would also be the first to experience waning immunity from the first wave of infections. In addition, while reinfection was *likely*, I thought it would be *unlikely* that someone would experience Covid-19 twice *as a severe clinical disease*. In the case of reinfection, I expected that the symptoms of disease would probably be mild. I based this upon what we know about the way T-cells respond at first infection. T-cells are lymphocytes that are one of the white blood cells and they play a central role in the body's immune response. T-cell responses from an initial infection would likely assist in dealing with a later infection.

When the first case of reinfection was announced in August 2020 – based on a study conducted by the University of Hong Kong and published in the journal *Clinical Infectious Diseases*[1] – it fitted with my expectations on the issue. The study found that a 33-year-old man living in Hong Kong experienced a second case of Covid-19, 142 days after the first. While his first case in March 2020 had been associated with symptoms such as cough, sore throat, fever and headache for three days, his second episode was characterised by a complete lack of symptoms. He only realised he had the disease after he was required to undergo screening at the Hong Kong International Airport on his return from Spain via the UK in August. According to the study, genetic analysis suggested that the first infection was from a strain of the coronavirus most closely related to strains from the US or the UK, and the second infection was most closely related to strains from Switzerland and the UK. The fact that he was infected by two separate strains meant that the patient was definitely reinfected, rather than simply experiencing ongoing viral shedding from the first infection. In terms of vaccine development, the fact that the first infection produced an immune response that protected against disease was positive, but it was too soon to be sure.

A couple of days later, a US-based study was announced that turned the tentative optimism – and my assumptions – on its head: a 25-year-old man from Nevada was diagnosed with Covid-19 in April, exhibiting symptoms of a sore throat, cough, headache, nausea and diarrhoea. After recovering and testing negative twice, he fell ill again with Covid-19 symptoms and sought care on 31 May. A test showed he was indeed positive for Covid-19. He was hospitalised five days later, requiring oxygen support. Again, genetic analyses suggested he had two distinct viral infections.[2]

The second case seemed to contradict my thoughts and expectations of the lower severity of repeat infections, but individual cases can be misleading. In a media briefing, Dr Maria van Kerkhove, the WHO technical lead for the coronavirus response and head of the emerging diseases and zoonosis unit, eloquently echoed my thoughts when she said population-wide studies were needed on reinfection. Shortly afterwards, more confirmed reinfection cases started to emerge, with most of them showing less severe disease in the second infection. Even so, it was still too early for us to fully understand the situation.

It was around this time that a journalist called me for a response to comments made in the media by a South African scientist to the effect that Covid-19 reinfections in South Africa were 'common'. I declined to comment, noting that anything I said would be purely conjecture, given the lack of data at our disposal. Then, in mid-July, a TV news channel asked me to comment on reinfection claims made by a GP in the south of Durban. In a video clip that had gone viral, the GP said one of his patients who had been diagnosed with Covid-19 had recovered and tested negative, but three months later tested positive again.[3]

I was aware by that stage of a study from South Korea that had found that, rather than a signal of reinfection, the re-detection of the Covid-19 virus in a few cases was likely to signal the presence of persisting deactivated virus RNA.[4] It emerged that there are a small number of people who continue to shed the virus for months after initially contracting the disease, but the virus cannot be cultured and is therefore not infectious.

If natural immunity cannot prevent a second infection, would vaccine immunity be able to do so? The burning issue of immunity from Covid-19 reinfection and the lack of any reliable scientific data on the issue moved me to reach out to colleagues in the US. On 19 March 2020, I composed an email, which I sent to Dr John Mascola at the VRC of the US NIH, copying in Dr Julie Ledgerwood, who at that time headed the VRC's Clinical Trials Program. The VRC was a long-standing collaborator of CAPRISA's, having previously worked with us on HIV vaccines and antibodies, and I had a good relationship with both Mascola and Ledgerwood. I knew that they would be working on a vaccine and, as part of the National Institute of Allergy and Infectious Diseases (NIAID), their scientists would be best placed to provide answers – if there were any – to the question about immunity.

Mascola's return email came promptly and its contents showed a gratifying confluence with my own thinking around the issue: they had asked Dr Barney Graham, deputy director of the VRC and the centre's expert on coronavirus, the same question – *that very day*, he said. But Mascola's reply also confirmed the reality of what was essentially a global predicament: it was simply too soon to make a call on the issue of natural immunity. 'We don't have data to know,' wrote Mascola. 'But perhaps it is likely that, as for many respiratory viruses, there is at least partial immunity protecting against severe disease, but the durability is a question … We will know more … from animal vaccine studies soon.'

The reinfection cases and the longevity of the immune response were of critical interest because of their implications for the size of the vulnerable population and the development of a successful vaccine. If the natural response to infection could not offer long-term protection from reinfection by the new coronavirus, it meant that past infection would not contribute to herd immunity. Also, if nature cannot prevent reinfection, how likely was it that scientists could manufacture a vaccine that could do better in generating immunity that prevents reinfection? Usually, the vaccines that are manufactured in the laboratory are inferior to the natural response. For example, if a patient contracts measles, the immune response from the body provides greater protection than a medical vaccination. The SARS-CoV-2 virus, however, was proving to be wily, capable of causing changes to the human immune system that blunted the immune response. So, while traditional wisdom would dictate that a vaccine cannot do better than nature, in the case of Covid-19 this might not be true: we might actually be able to do better than nature by producing a fully fledged immune response.

By the end of the second year of the pandemic, our understanding of reinfection and immunity had grown in leaps and bounds. We knew that natural infection produced immune responses that protected against reinfection with the same strain of the virus and to a lesser extent against other viral variants. Vaccines, especially mRNA (messenger RNA) vaccines, could produce high antibody levels, equivalent to, or even higher than, those seen in patients with severe Covid-19. But both natural and vaccine immunity waned over time; by six to nine months, antibody levels were quite low. As the virus mutated over time, the newer versions of the virus needed even higher levels of antibodies to prevent clinical infection. And so, reinfection was common in SARS-CoV-2. However, subsequent infections did not lead to hospitalisations to the same extent as we had witnessed in 2020. The main reason seemed to be that waning immunity was principally a phenomenon of B-cell or antibody immunity, while T-cell immunity did not seem to wane like antibodies did. Also, T-cell immunity, which plays a major role in preventing severe disease, remained effective as the virus changed over time.

But back in mid-2020, I was flummoxed by this question. There were countless other scientists around the world assessing the data and drawing conclusions about the possibility of a vaccine and how long the immunogenicity created by the vaccine would last. When the question moved beyond 'Will we be *able* to create a vaccine?' to '*When* will a vaccine be produced?' my initial response was 'Vaccines take years', which they normally do. In my mind, I had three years as a realistic time frame. When I learned that an American biotechnology company called Moderna was already testing an mRNA vaccine in Washington State in the US (collaborating with the NIAID) literally weeks after the disease had been identified, it seemed remarkable. Pfizer and BioNTech were also developing an mRNA vaccine. mRNA technology more broadly has been a promising technology for a while but had not delivered in anything before.

Making a vaccine with mRNA was new. Unlike traditional vaccines, which rely on the insertion into the body of a dead virus (for example, rabies vaccine), a small immunogenic part of a virus (hepatitis B vaccine, for example) or a weakened live virus (for example, measles vaccine) to prompt an immune response, mRNA vaccines contain a strand of genetic code. The mRNA genetic code, which is packaged in a lipid capsule, instructs the body to manufacture a specific part of a pathogen, which then launches the body's immune response. Manufacturing mRNA vaccines is much quicker than anything we have seen before.

This was just the boost mRNA technology needed – it was at the right place and the right time. While some consider mRNA as a technology that will revolutionise all vaccines, I have kept an open mind on this question. I had been aware of work being conducted on mRNA vaccines for a long time and was alive to their promise and the challenges they had in the delivery of the vaccine into human cells. I was also familiar with the work done by Dr Thomas Cech and Dr Sidney Altman, who had jointly won the 1989 Nobel Prize in chemistry for their discovery that RNA, previously considered to be a carrier of genetic codes between parts of a cell, also actively aids chemical reactions in cells. This discovery opened the door to a new field of scientific research on a range of potential RNA therapeutic applications, including vaccines. I had the privilege of getting to know Cech when he was President of the Howard Hughes Medical Institute (HHMI). HHMI donated the funds for the institute building at the Nelson R. Mandela Medical School where CAPRISA's headquarters is located. In my interactions with Cech at HHMI, we quickly developed a rapport. Cech displayed a remarkable breadth of scientific vision and could perceive the merits of an HIV research partner in Africa. It was a privilege to sit and talk science with him. I felt like I had a whole new world of science open up to me after I spoke with him. His broad vision of science and personable style of communicating left an impression on me.

In a talk I had given a few years before the pandemic, I had spoken about the potential of mRNA. It was showing good results in animal studies but, because it was a completely new technology, there were inevitable questions about its efficacy and safety. It made good sense in theory, but the mRNA was proving to be highly immunogenic itself. I had been aware of the research conducted by Dr Katalin Kariko and Dr Drew Weissman, who had figured out a way to reduce this immunogenicity and were packaging mRNA in lipid capsules to enable the mRNA to enter cells. Their visionary research over many years served as the foundation for mRNA vaccine technology that was now being applied by Moderna and BioNTech to make a SARS-CoV-2 vaccine.

While the speed with which the Moderna vaccine – and others – was developed was certainly unprecedented, that company was already developing mRNA vaccines pre-Covid. As soon as the Chinese published the genetic sequence for the new coronavirus in January 2020, they pivoted their efforts towards the urgent development of a coronavirus vaccine.[5] The fast-tracking of this process was assisted by billions of dollars' worth of investment from the US government as part of Operation Warp Speed, a private-public partnership set up to accelerate the development, manufacture and distribution of a range of Covid-19 vaccines.

Genuinely impressed that a vaccine had gone into trial so quickly, I contacted Graham at the VRC and offered my support for international clinical trials of SARS-CoV-2 vaccine candidates. Graham put me in touch with Dr Tal Zaks, Moderna's chief medical officer at the time, to explore whether Moderna was interested in CAPRISA's participation in their clinical trial programme. Although I had a couple of teleconferences with Moderna representatives to discuss the possibility of international trials in South Africa, Moderna ultimately decided to conduct all their trials in the US owing to a more favourable regulatory environment that would reduce the time needed to produce the vaccine – an important factor, given the rapid rise in cases in the US in early 2020 and its devastating impact on health care services.

So now we could potentially have a vaccine much quicker, laying the basis for a potential endgame. But would a vaccine mean a definitive and speedy end to Covid-19? I kept my hope in this endgame scenario but deep down knew that it was unlikely. Vaccines are seldom able to offer complete protection from initial infection, which is referred to as 'sterilising immunity'. Instead, they prime the body's immune system so that when the virus comes along and tries to infect the person, there is a pre-prepared immune response ready to go into action immediately. But vaccine-induced immune responses are rarely able to prevent initial infection, and so they were unlikely to block SARS-CoV-2 transmission completely. In other words, the vaccine could prevent people becoming seriously ill or needing to be hospitalised, but they would not be able to entirely stop the spread – although they were certainly likely to reduce the likelihood of transmission and could contribute to bringing the pandemic under control.

Scientists started to contemplate the possibility that Covid-19 might become endemic, like the common colds caused by the four other coronaviruses that continue to circulate around the world. However, there was another, much greater obstacle standing in the way of our hoped-for endgame. This was the ability of the virus to mutate – and, as it did, challenging scientists and governments under increasing pressure to find solutions, the cracks in multiple firmaments began to show.

CHAPTER 24

A new variant – Beta on the rise

'I'm afraid we do not have good news ... A new variant, 501Y.v2, has been found in South Africa. The concern is that the mutations may make it more infectious, more clinically severe or enhance its ability to escape immunity.'

When De Oliveira arrived at my office for our monthly 'genomic sequencing' meeting in late November 2020, I could tell something was amiss. Usually upbeat and full of life, De Oliveira looked uncharacteristically stressed and burdened.

'Tulio! What is it?' I asked.

'Twenty-three mutations in the last month,' he replied. 'And not just any kind of mutation …'

Up until October, De Oliveira's genomic sequences showed that the virus was averaging around one or two insignificant mutations every month. Now, the number had jumped to 23 mutations in one month, with many of them in important parts of the virus.

He put his data up on my office projector screen and there it was – a gene map, which is a colour-coded ribbon showing each of the viral genes with a line below each position where a new mutation or deletion has occurred. Among the colour-coded strips in the ribbon displayed on the screen, it showed three changes in the critical receptor-binding domain (RBD) of the spike protein at positions 417, 484 and 501. While we did not know what each mutation would do, we expected that the RBD mutations would enable the virus to better attach to the cell and to escape from immune responses. When I saw those data, there was a seismic shift in my understanding of the virus. I could feel the terrain of the epidemic shifting under my feet and the vaccine-focused endgame losing its clarity.

The significance of these genetic mutations, even though we did not know exactly what they did at that time, was not lost on me, especially given my three decades of work on another shape-shifting virus. HIV was notorious for its rapid rate of mutation. The mutations in HIV were due to the faulty way in which the virus's enzyme known as 'reverse transcriptase' made mistakes in converting RNA to DNA. However, only retroviruses, like HIV, carry this enzyme. Since SARS-CoV-2 does not have this particular step in its replication cycle, the expectation was that we should not have the same problem of a rapid mutation rate. But De Oliveira's arrival in my office seemed to suggest otherwise. Still, what we were seeing was nowhere near as fast as HIV.

Were we just lucky to find this new virus? No, it stemmed from an active surveillance initiative that established good relationships between health care providers and laboratories doing the surveillance. In November, doctors in Nelson Mandela Bay in the Eastern Cape reached out to De Oliveira with their concerns about a sudden explosion in Covid-19 cases that was putting huge pressure on the hospital system in that province. For these physicians, a second wave seemed to be in progress; it had arrived much earlier than anticipated and it seemed to be moving faster than the first wave. Based on the few samples De Oliveira had collected from the doctors, he found that a new version of the virus was present in both the Eastern Cape and KwaZulu-Natal. More samples that were obtained later from the Network for Genomics Surveillance in South Africa (NGS-SA) revealed that the variant had also spread to the Western Cape. At that stage, indications were that the new variant, eventually dubbed Beta, was spreading quickly and had probably been around for weeks before being detected.

The information that De Oliveira and I had at that stage was explosive. We both recognised that we had to act on it decisively but not create panic. We put into action a plan on how best to handle this new development, starting with briefing Health Minister Mkhize. In essence, we explained that the new variant's mutations could lead to a new wave with a faster-spreading virus where everyone might be at risk, and its immune escape could create a situation where those previously infected would be at risk of a second Covid-19 infection. A more infectious version of the virus that transmitted faster would put more pressure on hospitals, I explained. But the variant's possible higher infectiousness and immune escape was conjecture on our part, as the actual effects of these mutations was not yet known. We were conveying a likely scenario.

It was not the kind of news you want to pass on to a Health minister, or anyone else for that matter. Not only would it mean a dramatic change in how we were thinking about the pandemic response, but it would also generate more questions than answers. It is a major challenge to translate science of this nature for policy-makers when there is more uncertainty than certainty. There was so much that we did not know about what these mutations could do. Would the new variant cause more severe disease? What impact would the variant have on the country's health systems? There were also implications for global public health. The discovery of a new variant – the first serious variant to be detected in the world thus far – would have a ripple effect around the globe.

Mkhize immediately understood the gravity of the situation but was typically calm and measured in his response. He asked if we were confident that this was indeed a new variant and could impact on the Covid-19 national response. His concern, which De Oliveira and I shared, was that we did not want to create panic if this variant was just a few isolated cases – we needed to be confident that this new variant was indeed spreading.

A few days later – now early December 2020 – we felt there were sufficient data to confirm that we had a problematic variant on our hands. The time taken to complete the sequencing and undertake the bioinformatics analysis meant that we got genetic sequencing information only about two to four weeks after the sample was collected. But it was becoming clear that the variant was already established in South Africa, accounting for 11% of the viruses sequenced (44 of 392) from samples taken in the first week of October 2020. We learned later that it was spreading like wildfire, comprising 60% of viruses sequenced (302 of 505) from samples taken in the first week of November 2020, and 87% of those sequenced (363 of 415) from the samples taken in the first week of December 2020.[1]

The next step was to brief President Ramaphosa. At that point, South Africa was experiencing an average of just over 8 000 new infections per day, and the number was rising rapidly, particularly in the Western Cape and in KwaZulu-Natal. Prior to the discovery of the variant, our belief was that this second wave – expected after Christmas but making an early and dramatic entrance – was being fanned by super-spreader events. In KwaZulu-Natal, Ballito had recently been the site of the annual school-leavers' Rage Festival. The event inevitably became a super-spreader, with over 1 000 people becoming infected. Combined with several other matric-related celebrations and other end-of-year student gatherings around the country, this played a role in driving the second wave, which would eventually supersede the first wave and peak at just over 19 000 cases a day.

As the evidence of the second wave was emerging, De Oliveira informed his international colleagues on the WHO SARS-CoV-2 Virus Evolution Working Group about the new variant and encouraged them to look for similar mutations in their own sequence data. British scientists on this WHO working group soon found a variant that had a mutation on the spike protein at position 501, just as we had found. But the variant they found did not have the 417 and 484 mutations.

Since they had identified large numbers of this new variant, the UK Minister of Health publicly announced this new variant with the N501Y mutation (also known as B.1.1.7 in recognition of its family – or phylogenetic – tree) on 14 December 2020. In their public announcement, the British minister explained the recent rapid spread of the disease in parts of south-east England at the time was being driven by the 501Y variant, and he acknowledged South African scientists for assistance in identifying the variant. This variant was later named Alpha by the WHO, as it was the first publicly announced variant. Our careful approach, ensuring we had more data before announcing the new variant, meant the version De

Oliveira had discovered would be called Beta, even though it was identified before the Alpha variant. The British scientists published their findings on their variant on 19 December 2020, and in an acknowledgement of the importance of global collaboration, credited De Oliveira on Twitter with alerting them about the new variant.

With the new variant now confirmed and very likely contributing to the rising infections in South Africa, President Ramaphosa was of the view that we needed to inform the nation. On the evening of Friday, 18 December, De Oliveira, Lessells and I found ourselves involved in another lengthy live television broadcast with Minister Mkhize.

We were watched not only by the South African public through all three national television channels, but by the world. The presentation was covered by international TV networks, such as Sky, the BBC and CNN, and senior representatives of the Africa CDC and the WHO were on the call. The variant had potential implications for everybody – not just South Africa. Despite the dire news we were sharing, it was an important moment for genomic surveillance in South Africa, showcasing the power of early detection and tracking in our Covid-19 public health response.

'I'm afraid we do not have good news …' That was how I started the scientific part of the presentation. Because the stakes were high, we were at pains to explain the science and its implications clearly, to give people what they needed to know to exercise control over their risk of infection. This was particularly challenging when there was so much uncertainty about how the new variant would behave.

The uncertainty even extended to what we should call the variant. The day before the press briefing, De Oliveira and I had a discussion in my office about what we should name the variant (the WHO naming system only came into existence months later). We knew the enormity of the responsibility we had, having been the first in the world to identify a variant with multiple significant mutations; the first to have discovered that SARS-CoV-2 could create new versions of itself. We chose to call it '501Y. v2'. It felt strange having to name a variant, but we opted to follow the UK's announcement of referring to the mutation's position. The variant had a phylogenetic name, B.1.351, which we used interchangeably with 501Y.v2.

Viral genetics is admittedly quite a complex area of science, and the minister took the initiative to translate the key messages of the briefing into isiZulu. We had been conscious of the danger of our presentation being perceived as overly complicated and had actively structured it so that De Oliveira could explain the technical aspects of the mutations, with me following to tease out more clearly the implications of those scientific observations. Lessells did a short presentation on the potential clinical implications, to the extent that he could. Lessells was able to emphasise the point that the new variant did not seem to necessitate any changes in clinical treatment and patient management protocols, but that these would be updated as new information emerged. I think the level of scientific discourse was quite complex for a layperson, but Covid-19 had created a new approach to communicating science – where we were trying to convey complex concepts to the public in an attempt to educate them in the midst of uncertainty.

In terms of messaging, it was very important to distinguish what we definitely knew from what still had to be confirmed. There were still many unanswered questions, but we needed to reinforce the sense of agency and personal responsibility that the new information provided to the broader public and impress upon them that our traditional lines of defence against the virus, like mask-wearing and social distancing, remained essentially unchanged by the emergence of the new variant.

President Ramaphosa had already announced, four days earlier, a raft of new measures aimed at reducing the numbers of Christmas time holidaymakers congregating at hotspots such as beaches and dams. These measures, we confirmed during the Friday broadcast, had been recommended by the MAC as they would be helpful in reducing transmission of the virus, including the new variant; we did not think that any further restrictions were necessary.

What *did we know* about the new variant? We could say that in the second wave there was evidence of more rapid and greater transmissibility, but not necessarily more deaths. We were also seeing, in the epidemiological data, some indication of higher viral load in each collected swab, which I said might also translate into greater efficiency of transmission and a higher R_0.

What we *did not know* was whether the new variant would cause a more severe form of disease. Given what is known about viruses in general, the expectation among the scientists was that the disease would be less severe, but we had insufficient data to rule out the possibility of more severe disease. 'These are not difficult questions to answer but they take time,' I said, referring to the epidemiological analyses and laboratory tests under way at the time to shed light on some of the unknowns. And, of course, there was the issue of vaccines: would the new variant be susceptible to the vaccines, which were increasingly being viewed around the world as the best chance we had of defeating Covid-19? We couldn't confidently say. Several vaccine trials, including the trials of the AstraZeneca and the Johnson & Johnson (J&J) vaccines, were being conducted in South Africa, and direct trial and laboratory evidence would be available in due course. We had no choice but to wait for more results.

What we *also did not know* was what would cause such a big change in the genome? My first thought, one shared by a host of other scientists, including some in the WHO, was that it might be the result of another species jump – similar to the recent situation in Denmark where a mutated version of the novel coronavirus had been found in minks – passed from humans into minks and then back to humans again. While South Africa did not have minks, we had other animal hosts that could get infected with SARS-CoV-2. A species jump was unlikely, but possible, I thought.

Unknown to us at the time, the *New England Journal of Medicine* was preparing to publish a contribution from a group of doctors in the US who were advancing the idea that immunosuppressed patients who were persistently infected with Covid-19 could be a source of Covid-19 variants.[2] The case was based on a 45-year-old man who suffered from antiphospholipid syndrome, an autoimmune disorder, and took heavy drugs to suppress his immune system. The man, who came to be known as the 'Boston Patient', was admitted to hospital with a fever and diagnosed with Covid-19 on admission. Regular phylogenetic analysis showed that he suffered recurrent Covid-19 infections. Gene sequencing also showed that there was accelerated viral evolution within his body – the virus was changing quickly, acquiring a cluster of 20 or more mutations at a time. When they wrote up their findings, the authors, mostly from Harvard University and Boston hospitals, noted that amino acid changes were predominantly in the spike gene and receptor-binding domain.

When we became aware of this research a week or so later, we realised that this was by far the best explanation for the development of the new variant in South Africa. But as De Oliveira and I were picking through the sequencing data in my office at the end of November, we had no evidence to establish a cause.

A week after our public announcement of the new variant, on Boxing Day 2020, I was looking forward to my annual break, after an intensive 10 months of dealing with Covid-19-related issues. My vision for that day was to try to catch some of the test cricket match between Sri Lanka and South Africa. I am an ardent sports fan, and I especially adore rugby, cricket, Formula 1 racing and soccer – in that order. You can almost always find me watching some kind of sport most evenings and well into the early morning. I like to make myself comfortable in my recliner, settle into work and keep a game or match running on the TV in the background. That means finding sports that hit the sweet spot of not needing too much focus or attention. Although I enjoy it, I have given up watching NBA basketball because I find it addictive and too fast-paced to accommodate my divided attention, as I am usually trying to do some work on my computer and watch sports on TV at the same time. Cricket, on the other hand, happens at a perfect pace. I can concentrate on my work and look up from my computer from time to time to check the score or watch an exciting replay. So, after tuning into the test match on 26 December, out of habit, I also switched on my computer to check my emails. And that was how I came across the paper by Filip Fratev on the 501 mutation, which indicated that a rotation of the spike protein significantly increased binding (affinity) to the human ACE2 receptor, making it easier to infect human cells.[3] This stronger binding of the new version of the virus to the human cell was also accompanied by a 160-fold lower binding between the spike protein and the antibody found in Covid-19 patients; that is, antibodies would now be much less effective.

There it was: actual evidence of both increased transmissibility and viral escape. *This is trouble*, I thought, and quickly forwarded the email to De Oliveira and Lessells. Boxing Day 2020 happened to fall on a Saturday, so I wasn't expecting to hear back from them soon. Almost immediately, however, their respective replies landed in my inbox. They had already seen the paper and were hard at work in their laboratories. It looked like the cricket, and our holiday break, was going to have to wait. *Let's meet first thing on Monday*, I wrote back.

Come Monday, I had given up on my leave and was back to working flat out. For about a week thereafter I devoured the steady stream of academic papers that were now being produced on the topic of Covid-19 mutations. In addition to the Fratev paper, there were two other papers I found that confirmed that the new variant was likely to be more transmissible and escape antibodies. One of these papers was a study by the company Regeneron (the same company that administered monoclonal antibodies to President Trump in an experimental treatment when he contracted Covid-19 in October 2020). The study showed that monoclonal antibodies fostered mutations at the 484 position, a key area when it comes to escaping antibodies. This study predicted that mutations would occur at position 484, but their importance was being realised now, long after their prediction.

The other paper had, in fact, been published back in July 2020 in the prestigious journal *Cell*.[4] Using theoretical modelling, it showed that changes to the amino acid at the 501 position resulted in changes to binding affinity. In a sense, the *Cell* paper had predicted the 501Y mutation before it actually happened.

The *Cell* article had been spot on! Besides 501Y.v1 and 501Y.v2, another variant with a mutation at position 501 in the spike protein was identified the following month in Japan and described by Brazilian researchers. This variant had similar characteristics to the 501Y.v2 variant and was called 501Y.v3, in addition to its phylogenetic name of B.1.1.28.1 or P.1, until the WHO named it Gamma variant.

All three of the variants had the N501Y mutation, which changed the amino acid asparagine (N) to tyrosine (Y) at position 501 in the spike protein RBD. The 501Y.v2 and 501Y.v3 variants both had two additional RBD mutations, K417N/T and E484K, which increased the binding affinity of the receptor-binding domain to the ACE2 receptor.[5]

We were right to be concerned when we first saw the mutations. Based on all the new information we gleaned from published research and discussions with colleagues, we were now quite confident that the mutation N501Y, enhanced binding affinity to the ACE2 receptor, E484K, enhanced both binding affinity and conferred resistance to neutralising antibodies and K417N abolished key interactions with neutralising antibodies, thereby contributing to immune evasion. These changes made the virus more infectious and enabled it to bypass our immunity. In other words, the mutations would allow the virus to spread faster and more easily, and it could reinfect people.

The scientific data on the mutations in the variants was growing and the challenges we faced were gaining a more distinct outline. But the discourse on the variants was cumbersome because their names did not roll off the tongue. As a result, these variants were widely referred to by their country of first description, which produced unnecessary and, in my view, dangerous stigmatisation. The use of the term 'South African variant' for the 501Y.v2 variant came to trouble me so much that I started politely to correct journalists who used it, especially those representing international news outlets.

I worked with De Oliveira and Loots (of the Department of Science and Innovation) to formalise our objections to the geographic misnaming of variants in a short article published in *Science* in March 2021.[6] While we conceded that mutation-based or lineage names were difficult to say and write, we argued that the use of geographical regions to distinguish variants was inaccurate (there was no way of knowing whether patient zero of the variant had been a resident or visitor to the country in which the variant was discovered). It was also stigmatising and harmful. After South Africa announced its variant, the UK government immediately banned all flights and visitors from South Africa. If this was the consequence of reporting a variant, it could have the effect of disincentivising country-level genomic surveillance and transparent reporting of results.

By February 2021, the 501Y.v1 variant had been reported in 93 countries, the 501Y.v2 variant in 45, and the 501Y.v3 variant in 21. It seemed meaningless to still be referring to variants by country. Nevertheless, the practice continued, making more urgent the anticipated announcement of a standard nomenclature regarding key variants by the WHO. That announcement came at the end of May 2021, but too late for the B.1.617.2 variant of concern (later named Delta) detected in India, which caused havoc in that country in early to mid-2021 and was unfortunately, and nonsensically, labelled a 'double mutant'.

Using letters of the Greek alphabet, the new nomenclature system created new neutral names for two kinds of variants – variants of interest and variants of concern. Variants of interest were new variants that were emerging and had been described, but it was not yet clear if they were going to spread and become dominant. Variants of concern were those variants that displaced past variants as the dominant variant. Importantly, the new labels did not replace the existing scientific names, which conveyed important scientific information for researchers, including genetic lineages, but it was hoped that they would assist in a clearer and less accusatory public discourse.

While the WHO naming system resolved a stigmatisation problem emanating from the variants, we still had to deal with the complex science of mutations and the challenges in interpreting this for policy-makers who desperately wanted to know what the impact of the new variant was going to be. The variants of concern, as the name suggested, were concerning for three reasons: firstly, they may be more infectious and more highly transmissible; secondly, they may be more pathogenic, causing more severe disease; or. thirdly, they may have more immune escape, rendering antibodies from natural infection and/or vaccines ineffective. If the last mentioned occurred, we might end up complicating our potential Covid-19 endgame scenario based on vaccines. But first, we needed access to Covid-19 vaccines in South Africa.

CHAPTER 25

Vaccine rollout fallout

The most powerful weapon against the pandemic, which should have been a public good, became a commodity, while Covax, the world's hope for vaccine equity, struggled to deliver doses timeously. As those in countries awaiting vaccines saw others getting doses, criticism of governments grew.

The emergence of new variants turned out to be just one of the issues that surfaced during my attempt to take an annual break in December 2020. The first shots of a Covid-19 vaccine were being rolled out in wealthier countries like the UK and the US. Yet, discourse had begun about countries being left behind and there was simmering controversy around South Africa's own vaccine rollout.

At that stage, South Africa had signed the required guarantees and completed the process of aligning its systems with those of Covax, the global initiative to ensure vaccine equity for low- to middle-income countries, which was co-led by the Global Alliance for Vaccines and Immunisation, the Coalition for Epidemic Preparedness Innovations and the WHO. South Africa's participation in Covax was self-funded. Our country had a committed purchase for 10% of its population, which was to cover health care workers and the elderly, and the government had entered into negotiations with Pfizer to cover most of the remaining balance. The government's decision to prioritise its vaccine purchases from Covax, while entering into bilateral agreements with pharmaceutical companies, was based on the 17 September 2020 advisory from the MAC.

The idea behind Covax made sense: bringing 184 countries together would create bulk-buying power to push down the price of vaccines. It would also ensure greater equity of access: countries would receive their vaccines in batches and no one single participating country would be substantially ahead of another regarding access to doses. At the time of its formation in April 2020, Covax represented the most rational approach for South Africa, which lacked the resources on its own to secure vaccine supplies through advanced market commitments, particularly prior to vaccine efficacy results. The idea of pooling the resources of self-financing Covax participants and wealthy donor countries in the interests of providing equal access to vaccines for all the world's people, regardless of their status in the world, represented an excellent and much-needed plan. And, with some fundamental modifications to the system, I think it still does.

But Covax failed us. When vaccines were being delivered to wealthy countries that had made advance market commitments, Covax was still waiting for its doses. I am not blaming Covax – while it could have done more to secure vaccine supplies earlier, the situation was beyond its control for the most part. In essence, Covax was at the back of the queue. For countries like South Africa that had put their faith in Covax for the initial doses, political and civil society pressure mounted as the public watched others get vaccines, but there were none for them. While Covax did eventually get its doses – and it has distributed over one billion doses, mostly to the world's poorest countries – it was not able to deliver vaccines when many countries needed doses urgently, as they dealt with new surges of infection in early 2021.

By way of background, it is important to remember that up until Pfizer's announcement of its first vaccine efficacy result on 9 November 2020, there was no way of knowing for certain that any of the candidate vaccines in clinical trials would work against the new coronavirus or how long it would take to secure their regulatory approval. Countries such as Israel, Denmark, Canada and Australia had sufficient resources to take a chance to buy and pay in advance for several vaccines, without any guarantees of their efficacy and gambling that at least one of the candidate vaccines they bought would be effective. Initially, vaccine prices ranged from $10.30

from Covax to $35 per dose from a pharmaceutical company. The cost of the cheapest two doses for 10 million people would be R3.5 billion, with about half this amount required up front to secure an advance market commitment. That is a huge financial commitment for a country to make at a time when it is not yet known if the vaccine paid for is actually going to be effective. In lower- and middle-income countries that could not afford it, the costs of playing this vaccine lottery were simply too high. For most of the world's countries, it was not an option.

This was especially troubling during a period in which new variants were emerging. It was a time that should have brought the world together in its fight against the virus. A virus that spreads is a virus that mutates, something that SARS-CoV-2 had proven as numerous variants popped up around the world. The messaging from the start of the pandemic was that no one is safe until everyone is safe – a philosophy that should have translated into the equitable distribution of vaccines and buy-in to the Covax initiative. But instead, the fear sparked by emerging variants while vaccines were becoming available signalled a splintering global pandemic response.

Since vaccine supply was limited and demand was high at the start of the global vaccine rollout, countries were effectively in competition with each other for a finite number of vaccines, and those with resources were inevitably the winners. It was a market-driven system that oversaw a zero-sum game: the richer countries were able to acquire a disproportionate number of vaccines, draining the global supply at the direct expense of poorer countries. When it came to mRNA vaccines, a particularly anomalous situation prevailed – two companies had a monopoly on this vaccine technology and their executives solely decided the vaccine price and who to prioritise for vaccine doses.

In the midst of this complex terrain, Covax turned out to be the slowest among the five disjointed and separate paths along which the world's countries could pursue their acquisition of vaccines. The five paths that formed part of an utterly broken global distribution system were as follows:

First in line to obtain their doses were countries that invested in developing Covid-19 vaccines. The UK being first out of the starting blocks was largely attributable to its having been one of the countries to actually develop a vaccine – an achievement that put them squarely at the front of the global supply queue, along with other vaccine-developing countries such as the US, Germany, China and Russia. On 8 December 2020, just one month after the first vaccine efficacy results were announced by Pfizer, the UK became the world's first country to embark on its mass vaccination campaign, initially targeting the elderly and vulnerable. China and Russia had started their vaccination programmes even earlier, using locally developed vaccines before the efficacy of these vaccines had been established.

Second were those countries – Israel, Denmark, Canada and Australia – that had used their ample resources to enter into advanced market commitments with vaccine manufacturers. Canada had secured nine vaccine doses per member of its population, the equivalent of enough vaccines to vaccinate each citizen five times over. Canada was not alone; there were other countries with excess secured supplies. Based on an analysis of deals concluded between countries and eight leading vaccine candidates, the People's Vaccine Alliance pointed out that the richer countries – home to 14% of the global population – had bought 53% of the total vaccine stock by November 2020. While wealthy countries such as Canada could afford to buy up more vaccines than they needed before the test results were known (simply to hedge their bets), this was not an option for South Africa. Negotiating advance market commitments was an expensive and risky exercise, given that there was no guarantee at the outset of a successful vaccine.

Third in the distribution queue were countries that accepted vaccine donations from producer countries such as Russia and China. Through a euphemistically called 'vaccine diplomacy' programme, countries like the UAE, Turkey, Morocco, Egypt and Chile obtained vaccines next. Countries making these vaccine donations were likely seeking to exercise regional and global political influence and boost their standing through dispensing vaccines to less-resourced countries, an arrangement described in 'Vaccine diplomacy boosts Russia's and China's global standing', published by *The Economist*, as a 'way to reward old friends and win new ones'.[1]

The fourth group to get vaccines – by far the largest and comprising most of the world's countries – was made up of those nations that had entered into bilateral purchasing agreements with suppliers for approved vaccines. Since these bilateral agreements were entered into after efficacy had been established, these countries had to queue behind the countries that had made advance market commitments with these companies.

Right at the back of the line, pretty much stuck at the start of the obstacle-strewn pathway to vaccines, were the Covax partners, who mainly comprised low- and middle-income countries. Most of them lacked the financial clout to enter into bilateral agreements, let alone engage in advanced market commitments, and so they had little alternative other than to rely on Covax. The Covid vaccine supply chain, based heavily on market forces, ensured a singular outcome: it sent poorer countries to the back of the queue.

The world's most powerful weapon against the pandemic, which should be a public good, was being treated as a commodity, available – in excess – to rich countries, while poor countries went without. It showed how truly flawed the distribution system was. In fact, 'system' was a misnomer because the word implies a certain level of functionality. This 'system' was seriously broken, particularly when you consider that the fill and finish factory for the J&J vaccine based in East London, South Africa, bottled over 30 million doses not for distribution in South Africa, but for Europe, at a time when South Africa did not have Covid-19 vaccines. Further signs of serious imbalances in the system came to light much later when news reports in late 2021 revealed that millions of vaccine doses in the US had gone to waste at a time when many countries had not yet received their first batches. It was not difficult, sitting in South Africa, to interpret the distribution patterns as a form of vaccine apartheid – a crime against humanity.

With the first batch of vaccines still awaited in South Africa, the government's critics grew more frustrated and vocal. We were not alone in this regard. Governments across the world were being heavily criticised for delays in vaccine access. I was taken aback by the invective lashed out against the Australian government for slow access to vaccines. Across Europe, criticism of governments was growing to a crescendo as frustration grew while waiting for vaccines doses to arrive.

Similarly, as South Africans watched the first doses of the Covid-19 vaccines start to be administered to high-risk people in the UK and US in December, sentiment started to shift. Infections in South Africa were rising steadily en route to the peak of our second surge and there was growing impatience. The atmosphere was similar to that which attended the first wave – many people were becoming anxious, feeling helpless and began to tap into the idea of vaccines as a silver bullet, a magical solution that the government was withholding from them, either by omission or commission. These sentiments of distrust, anger and fear were exploited by some political parties and even by some clinicians and scientists by launching a number of broadsides at government through the mainstream media, complaining about the slow vaccine rollout and its over-reliance on Covax.

Some of the concerns of these clinicians and scientists were justified, such as the 'lack of communication', which was 'creating unease'. But criticisms focusing on 'insufficient planning' were off target as planning had begun long before the first vaccine trial results became available. More importantly, some of those doing the criticising were themselves on the MAC and had supported the vaccine MAC advisory on participation in Covax when it was tabled at the MAC, indicating no dissent at the time, providing no alternate advice or offering other solutions to secure vaccines, when they were in a prime position to do so.

While advice on this particular issue fell to the MAC on Covid-19 vaccines, which I attended as an observer, I had some strong views on the subject, all of which were well known. In my view, we had to do what we could to assist Covax, as it was our best hope to ensure equitable access. To bypass Covax at that early stage and negotiate bilateral agreements with pharmaceutical companies would deplete the limited global stock available for distribution via Covax and would undermine Covax, worsening inequity. It would also have the effect of pushing up the price of any vaccine. I was, however, supportive of entering into bilateral agreements early to secure vaccines beyond the 10% that we had secured through Covax. After all, most countries would eventually have to buy vaccines directly, given that Covax was only committing to provide enough vaccines for up to 20% of the population. I found the growing clamour for bypassing Covax and buying vaccines directly from pharmaceutical companies to be seriously misinformed and misplaced, with only a few well-intentioned exceptions.

As criticism of the South African government on vaccine access grew, the government itself contributed to the burgeoning narrative that it had dropped the vaccine ball. Its dealings with Covax were fraught with delays and repeated missed payment deadlines. At one stage, even I questioned whether the government was serious about procuring vaccines when it missed, for the second time, a deadline for payment to Covax. The Covax payment that was due in September 2020 was eventually paid in December 2020 – three months late! The late payment meant that South Africa would not receive vaccines from the first batches Covax procured. This tardiness meant that South Africa fell further back in the queue and was now at the end of the line even within Covax.

Against this backdrop, we were witnessing the burgeoning of 'me-first'[2] attitudes towards the acquisition of vaccination – this perspective also grew in South Africa – spawning the term 'vaccine nationalism', the idea that one country could close ranks, buy up vaccines and beat the virus. Countries that could afford to pay for a position at the front of the queue were leading the 'me-first' charge.

In my view, the idea was founded upon a fundamental misconception of the true nature of a global pandemic. In an interview with Ms Zoe Corbyn from *The Guardian* published in January 2021, I gave voice to these concerns, arguing that it was a 'fundamental fallacy' to believe that one country could be safe when the rest of the world was not.[3] 'None of us are safe if one of us is not. We have mutual interdependence,' I said.

'We need the whole world to be part of Covax: all the drug companies should have committed all their vaccine doses to Covax, which could then equitably provide the vaccine so all health care workers can get vaccinated. It will be terrible if the US is vaccinating low-risk young people, while we in Africa cannot vaccinate health care workers.'

It seemed, however, that not everyone agreed with that stance. In January 2021, a group claiming to all be 'Eminent Scientists', led by a general practitioner with only two published journal articles and zero citations, accused the government of trying to downplay the importance of vaccines and being guilty of 'a frantic cover-up and evasion of culpability'. The article directly questioned South Africa's participation in Covax and accused the government of failing to secure a vaccine supply. It said senior government officials were 'increasingly talking down the prospects for the availability and usefulness of Covid-19 vaccines in South Africa'.[4] Most disturbing to me was their accusation that the government was being irresponsible when it claimed that vaccines were an important part of the Covid-19 response but were 'not a silver bullet'.

The term 'silver bullet' is used as a metaphor to describe 'a simple, seemingly magical, solution to a difficult problem'.[5] Covid-19 vaccines were never going to be a magical solution to the problem of Covid-19, neither then nor now. Many agencies that actively promoted Covid-19 vaccines argued that their value should not be oversold, as it would lead to Covid-19 vaccines being undermined when they could not live up to mythical cure-all hype. While the scientific evidence of the benefits of vaccines was growing rapidly – and there are significant benefits – their shortcomings were becoming evident simultaneously. For example, an AstraZeneca vaccine trial showed a lack of efficacy in preventing clinical Covid-19 illness during the Beta variant wave in South Africa. Well-vaccinated countries – like the Seychelles, which was one of the most vaccinated countries in the world at the time – still struggled during their second wave, having to open field hospitals to cope with the cases. And as it is now widely known, vaccinated individuals can readily get Covid-19, but are at much lower risk of severe disease.

I have always held the belief that vaccines are an essential tool in the fight against Covid-19, with substantial benefits ranging from reducing infections, hospitalisations and deaths to impacting on transmission to unvaccinated individuals. But they are not some seemingly magical solution that is going to wish away the difficult problem of Covid-19. This became even more obvious as new variants like Omicron emerged, with the ability to escape vaccine-induced antibodies. But vaccines are critically important in the Covid-19 response, and I have argued vociferously for vaccine mandates. While vaccines may not be highly efficacious in preventing infection, they are still highly efficacious in preventing progression to severe disease. In a space where new evidence was constantly coming to light about new variants and vaccine efficacy, overstating the benefits of Covid-19 vaccines only served to strengthen anti-vaccine lobbies. I did not really understand why some were so keen on promoting vaccines in this inappropriate manner of a 'silver bullet'. But I can say: it was not about science, eminent or otherwise.

In all my years of standing up for science, I have strongly supported the holding of decision-makers and those in power, like governments and private companies, to account. Activism to achieve this accountability is an important part of democracy. While some critics did well in making valid points that held the government accountable, others, like the voices behind the 'silver bullet' position, seem to have chosen to leverage activist spaces merely to score political points.

Amid this debate was a growing tendency for people to see vaccines as a quick fix, something I felt was a dangerous premise to be setting. Realistically speaking, it would take our country more than a year to reach the WHO target of 70% vaccination coverage – roughly 40 million out of a population of about 58 million – so there was no possibility of the vaccine solving the problem overnight.

Some of the unfounded optimism about the impact of vaccines was driven in part by the mainstream liberal US media. They were so determined to fight the largely conservative anti-vaccine lobby and convince the public to vaccinate that they contributed to a kind of romanticisation of the vaccine and its power to restore normality to our lives. In reality, no vaccine could just simply enable us to go back to normality. The pandemic was a far more complicated foe.

The Lancet COVID-19 Commission Task Force for Public Health

Measures to Suppress the Pandemic, of which I was a member, got together in March 2021 and published an article in the journal *International Health*[6] and subsequently in the Lancet Commission report, where we discussed the role of public behaviour in dealing with the virus on a longer-term basis. Among our contentions was that even with vaccines as an essential public health intervention, human behaviour was key to managing the pandemic. That meant that public health measures such as social distancing, mask-wearing and self-isolation were still critical. The point was that we recognised that while vaccines were a necessary element, they were not sufficient to end the pandemic, or at least wrestle it under control.

The frustration within South Africa over its lack of vaccines led to the narrative that had growing support for the 'me-first' approach. The Democratic Alliance leader in the Western Cape Province spoke about his party's intention to seek independent procurement of vaccines for provincial residents. Around much the same time, Afrikaner civil rights organisation Afriforum and its sister organisation, the Solidarity trade union, indicated their intention to launch a legal bid challenging the national government's monopoly on the procurement of vaccines and named me as one of the respondents. In my answering affidavit, I set out some of the reasons why a piecemeal, market-driven approach to vaccine acquisition and rollout would be bad for everyone. Afriforum and Solidarity did not win this court case.

Their proposal would redirect the world's limited vaccine supply away from programmes that were fostering global equity – Covax – and national equity, the government's national vaccine strategy. That national strategy had been designed to prioritise health workers and other vulnerable groups rather than all the residents of one province. There had also been careful thought given in that strategy to the precise mix of vaccine technology platforms needed to achieve the WHO target of 70% vaccine coverage.

I borrowed the words of WHO Director-General Dr Tedros, who had accused some countries and companies of speaking 'the language of equitable access' but continuing 'to prioritize bilateral deals, going around

Covax, driving up prices and attempting to jump to the front of the queue. This is wrong.'

At the time Dr Tedros made those comments to his executive board on 18 January 2021, more than 39 million doses of vaccines had been administered in at least 49 higher-income countries, while only a handful of low-income countries had received vaccine doses. Aside from the moral and economic arguments in favour of a global equity approach, there were also epidemiological imperatives: Covid-19 was a global pandemic involving a virus that was undeterred by human borders. To achieve viral control in isolation in one province while other parts of the country did not have vaccines was effectively impossible, and the risk of new variants from unvaccinated provinces reaching the Western Cape and bypassing vaccine immunity would be considerable. The same rationale applied in the case of national boundaries, which made it vital for neighbouring countries to receive their due supply of vaccines.

Besides vaccine nationalism leading to poor pandemic control outcomes, I wanted to emphasise the ethical element of the issue as well. My comments to the UK press were picked up in the local media but fell largely on deaf ears as the clamour for vaccines continued to grow louder. It was understandable; cases were rising, the new Beta variant was spreading and leading to pressure on hospitals, and deaths were rising.

A newspaper columnist threw fuel onto the fire by recounting a telephone conversation he had orchestrated with a senior vice-president of commercial vaccines at US pharmaceutical company Moderna, which manufactures an mRNA Covid-19 vaccine. In a column headlined 'Hello, useless ANC. I phoned Moderna and they have vaccines for us', he contended that, unlike the government, he managed to secure an undertaking from Moderna for the possibility of supplying 40 million doses to South Africa with a possible delivery date of mid-2021, all in a phone call with this executive. Little did he know that Moderna had already indicated, both to the government and publicly, that it would not be registering or distributing its vaccine in South Africa. Three years into the pandemic and Moderna has still not sought to license and distribute any of its vaccines in South Africa. Also, the Moderna vaccine is the most expensive of all Covid-19 vaccines, making it an inappropriate choice, especially since South Africa was then awaiting delivery of mRNA vaccines from Pfizer at a fraction of the Moderna price. The article might have been good for newspaper sales, but it exposed a widespread ignorance about the complex process of international pharmaceutical procurement.

Buying vaccines is not like calling to buy pizzas. It involves complex regulatory requirements, cold-chain processes, South African legal requirements and the establishment of injury insurance procedures. For these reasons, only governments can purchase Covid-19 vaccines. While calling to buy vaccines might be good for grandstanding and scoring political points, it cannot actually lead to the purchase of Covid-19 vaccines. Moderna knew that, even if the columnist may not have.

The idea of looking after oneself first is a captivating idea, particularly in a crisis, but in a global pandemic it offers a very short-sighted and morally flawed solution. As Pope Francis had said, we had a 'shared destination' and 'no one is saved alone'.

CHAPTER 26

Variants versus vaccines

As global vaccine stock was a zero-sum game, countries stockpiling doses were draining global supply, diverting doses away from those in need. This undermined the goal of vaccinating as many people as possible, as quickly as possible, to reduce the risk of new variants developing.

While there were many political issues swirling around in relation to the Covid-19 pandemic and the country's response, I was focused on the rapid developments taking place in the realm of research. My task was to focus on the science. The world needed to understand what the new variants would do and scientists across the globe took up this challenge. New data on variants were becoming available at a pace I had never witnessed before.

On 18 January 2021, exactly one month after the televised December webinar at which we had announced the discovery of the new variant in South Africa, we had enough new information for a national televised webinar update to fill in some of the gaps in our knowledge of the new variant. This time I proposed a different format to the minister, comprising eight succinct presentations for the nationally televised webinar. In addition to myself, Tulio de Oliveira and Richard Lessells, I invited Penny Moore, Alex Sigal, Koleka Mlisana, Mary-Ann Davies, an epidemiologist from UCT, and Willem Hanekom, the Director of the African Health Research Institute, to share information about the variant from their various scientific perspectives. I invited speakers who had data to share and who could provide short comments in their area of expertise that would shed light on various aspects of the variant, so that the public could become better informed and get a better idea of what to expect next.

In the webinar, we were able to confirm that the variant was approximately 50% more transmissible – it had taken 107 days during the first wave for the Western Cape to reach its first 100 000 cases and 54 days in the second wave. We could also confirm that reinfections were occurring and that prior infection in the first wave provided little, if any, protection against reinfection. We explained the evidence indicating that the 501Y.v2 variant could escape antibodies generated from previous infection and to some extent those produced as a result of vaccination.

None of this was good news. Such is the science-policy interface; we convey good news sometimes, but we also have to share bad news too. We explained that the mutations were conferring antibody escape that could impact on the efficacy of the vaccines in preventing clinical illness, but we would have to wait for more evidence before being able to determine if the new variant could escape immunity that prevents progression to severe disease.

Clinical evidence on whether vaccines would remain effective against the variant came in early February, when the results from vaccine effi-cacy trials became available. This necessitated another nationally televised briefing, which took place on 7 February 2021. At the minister's request, I participated in this briefing, along with Shabir Madhi, Glenda Gray and Barry Schoub. The results of the AstraZeneca vaccine trial in South Africa were presented by Madhi, who had led this study. The trial showed almost no efficacy of two doses of the vaccine in preventing clinically evident Covid-19 during the Beta variant wave. Since the trial only had cases of mild or moderate disease, there were no data on its efficacy in preventing severe disease and hospitalisation. The trial was a subset of the larger AstraZeneca vaccine trial being led by Oxford University investiga-tors but was analysed, presented and published separately. It had enrolled 2 026 young adults all under the age of 65 (average age of 31 years), which made little sense, given that we needed evidence in the elderly as they were being prioritised for vaccination. At the webinar, Madhi described the disappointing AstraZeneca vaccine trial results as a 'reality check' for South Africa, suggesting that we 'recalibrate our expectations' of Covid-19 vaccines.[1]

The results were all the more disappointing because of the arrival one week earlier of one million doses of the AstraZeneca vaccine from the Serum Institute of India. These had been sourced to stem the rising tide of pressure on the government to bypass Covax and vaccinate health care workers. The South African government used its political connections with the Indian government to jump the queue to get these 1.5 million doses. I later learned that the doses sent to South Africa had originally been earmarked for Covax. It was heart-breaking to learn that our government's purchase of these vaccines directly undermined Covax.

Gray was able to provide more positive results at the briefing. The J&J vaccine trial, which had appropriately included both elderly and young adults, had shown that its single-dose vaccine retained much of its efficacy against the new variant and was effective in preventing both milder and severe forms of Covid-19 illness. Importantly, it was 84% effective in preventing severe disease – a key requirement in assessing the effectiveness of a Covid-19 vaccine.

Shortly after our briefing, Pfizer released the six-month follow-up results of its mRNA vaccine trial. Of the 44 047 people enrolled in this trial, 567 participants, about half of whom were elderly, were from South Africa. The Pfizer vaccine was 100% effective, with a wide confidence interval, in preventing Beta variant infection. All nine infections observed in the four South African sites during the Beta variant wave were in the placebo group, while none of those vaccinated got Beta variant infection. Fortunately, the government had started negotiations with Pfizer in 2020 and had secured several million doses. But these negotiations, which were confidential, much to my annoyance, were very complicated and took a disappointingly long time for our government to finalise, due to Pfizer's onerous requirements. As a result, in early 2021, the Pfizer mRNA vaccine still needed regulatory approval and would only be available in South Africa in several months' time.

Since the South African clinical trial had shown that the AstraZeneca vaccine was not effective in preventing Beta variant infection, Minister Mkhize had a difficult decision to make about the recently arrived one million AstraZeneca vaccine doses. Some were arguing that the AstraZeneca vaccine should be used anyway as it might prevent severe disease, but this was devoid of clinical evidence. I was among those who were hesitant to give health care workers a vaccine when there was clear evidence that it did not prevent Covid-19 and only had a theoretical prospect of preventing severe infection with the new variant.

The day after the webinar, I was asked whether the country would be halting the rollout of the AstraZeneca vaccine at a WHO media briefing hosted by Dr Tedros. After all, the decision and the reasons behind it would have implications for the world; and for Covax, which had signed advance purchase agreements with AstraZeneca and the Serum Institute of India and had plans to distribute nearly 350 million doses in the first half of 2021. At that stage, no decision had yet been taken in South Africa about what to actually do with the AstraZeneca doses. I remarked at the WHO meeting that one option would be to roll the vaccine out in a phased way, vaccinating only a limited number of people and monitoring their hospitalisation rates. Only if it showed protection against severe disease should it be rolled out to the rest of the health worker population. But I acknowledged that this would take a long time and the first phase results would probably only be available months later, by which time other more efficacious vaccines would be available. It was unfortunate that the South African component of the AstraZeneca vaccine trial did not enrol the elderly, as the Brazil and UK sites had done. It became challenging to interpret the conflicting results; while the vaccine was effective in preventing mild and severe Covid-19 in Brazil and the UK, it was not effective in preventing mild infection, but there were no data on severe disease prevention in South Africa. Policy-makers had to decide in the midst of scientific uncertainty as to whether there would be any clinical benefit of the AstraZeneca vaccine against severe disease.

In the end, after mulling over all options, the South African government decided not to roll out the AstraZeneca vaccine and the million doses were sold to the African Union. The move spurred some controversy. Some doctors, scientists and other vocal commentators argued that all available vaccines, including the AstraZeneca vaccine, should be used to protect health workers, even though it was not effective in preventing Beta variant and there were no data on its efficacy in preventing severe disease from this variant. Disappointingly, some scientists were conjuring up exaggerated fictitious numbers of deaths that could be averted to advocate for the use of this vaccine. Differing views are important in science, but some of the advocates for the AstraZeneca vaccine had been involved in its clinical trial and had a vested interest in seeing it succeed. Their disappointment that the vaccine they researched would not be going forward was tangible and was reflected in the vehemence of their criticism of the vaccine policy. Through the editorial pages of the *South African Medical Journal*, Schoub, then head of the vaccine MAC, highlighted the risks inherent in proceeding with a vaccine known to lack sufficient efficacy against the new variant.[2]

Under mounting pressure for vaccines from the public, Mkhize approached both Gray and me to check if we could rapidly pivot to the J&J vaccine for health care workers. I contacted Dr Jerry Sadoff of J&J, as he and I had served on vaccine advisory committees together when he was still at Merck, and I had met with him and his team in April 2020 regarding clinical trials of their vaccine. By the time I reached him, Gray, who had a long-standing relationship with J&J related to HIV vaccines, had already been in touch. She set up a meeting with the company, where we learned that it was in a position to supply, within days, 500 000 doses of the vaccine, which had been manufactured for the clinical trials. J&J was seeking emergency-use authorisation in some countries and was applying for approval in South Africa, but this process would take time. Hence, a phase 3B open-label implementation study was discussed as the best option to introduce the vaccine while regulatory approval was awaited. Regulatory approval to undertake research is a different and faster process than approval to use a medicine outside of a research setting.

Introducing the vaccine through an implementation programme would enable the collection of clinical data to monitor side effects, effectiveness and the progress of what would effectively be a stepped rollout. The vaccine had already been tested for safety, so there was no concern that we were using South African health care workers as 'guinea pigs' – it was simply a matter of getting the vaccines out as quickly as possible. Gray was selected by J&J to lead the implementation study, named Sisonke, and she recruited Dr Linda-Gail Bekker of UCT's Desmond Tutu HIV Centre, Dr Ameena Goga of the MRC's HIV Prevention Research Unit and Dr Nigel Garrett, who heads up vaccine research at CAPRISA, to work on it. In pivoting to a different vaccine, the first doses of the J&J vaccine were administered only a few days later than the originally planned AstraZeneca vaccine rollout start. The J&J rollout had its share of drama at initiation with the SAA jet sent to Europe to pick up the vaccines breaking some aviation rules. Fortunately, the vaccines arrived safely in South Africa. When the Durban allocation of vaccines arrived at the King Shaka International Airport, it was transported to the CAPRISA clinic pharmacy in the city centre, accompanied by several blue-light police vehicles and motorbikes to protect it. The first doses were administered the next day at Prince Mshiyeni Memorial Hospital in Umlazi by a joint MRC-CAPRISA team.

This South African experience with a SARS-CoV-2 variant complicating its vaccine programme also held lessons for the world. The variant had quite simply changed everything in our Covid-19 vaccine plans and was a signal of more uncertainty to come. After the world's initial euphoria over the fact that a vaccine was indeed possible, we were now all in a scientific game of cat and mouse with a mutating virus that was neatly unravelling the hoped-for endgame of universal vaccination and global population immunity.

This fluid terrain, although treacherous, was nonetheless rich in new research opportunities. The global scientific community had learned a great deal about Covid-19, but the new variants had shattered any kind of complacency we might have been experiencing, exposing gaps in research systems and calling for innovative thinking to meet new challenges.

In a series of publications in early 2021, I identified some of the issues I felt needed close attention from scientists in the field as we tackled what had become known as 'variants of concern'.

In a letter to *The Lancet* published on 3 April,[3] I argued that in addition to adequate genomic surveillance, standardised variant nomenclature and a repository of variants and vaccine serum samples, there was a pressing need – in the era of new Covid-19 variants – to establish a Correlate of Protection (CoP) for SARS-CoV-2 infection that would help to remove the obstacles that new variants were placing on global Covid-19 control through vaccination by providing more evidence for decision-making around vaccines.

A CoP is a term used mainly in vaccinology to refer to measurable immune biomarkers, which can predict protection against infection after vaccination or natural infection. A CoP would mean that vaccine efficacy results obtained with pre-existing variants could be translated to newly emerging variants without the need to repeat time-consuming clinical trials for each new immune-escape variant; and it would avoid a situation in which important decisions about vaccines are made without adequate efficacy data – a situation in which South Africa then had very real experience.

'The identification of a Correlate of Protection is too important and urgent to be left to uncoordinated separate studies by individual investigators or vaccine developers,' I wrote. I suggested four key requirements to achieve this aim: all SARS-CoV-2 vaccine developers with existing or completed efficacy trials should commit to transparency and open data sharing; an expert committee (preferably under the WHO) should be appointed to review existing and planned analyses to identify CoPs for each efficacious vaccine; studies to fast-track the identification of an animal model, assay or marker as a CoP should be initiated to address gaps in the correlate research plans; and finally, a central database should be created to collate data for each of the efficacious vaccines, thereby providing larger sample sizes to assess multiple variables as CoPs and to test if a correlate identified in one trial was valid in other trials.

As part of the Lancet COVID-19 Commission Task Force on Public Health Measures to Suppress the Pandemic, I contributed to a report published in March 2021,[4] which tried to make sense of the new reality created by the existing variants of concern and the possible emergence of new ones, particularly for public health leaders trying to manage surges in health care demands, without compromising the care needs of non-Covid-19 patients.

Among our key points, we stressed the fact that no single action was sufficient to prevent the spread of the virus: '… strong public health measures against the virus must be maintained in tandem with global vaccination programs,' we argued. We argued that suppression of infection rates and health system efforts needed to be accompanied by genomic surveillance to identify and quickly characterise emerging variants in as many countries as possible around the world. We were also concerned that existing diagnostic tests may not pick up some new variants and so we recommended monitoring of the ability of diagnostic tests to reliably identify new variants.

In a publication in the *New England Journal of Medicine* in March 2021,[5] reporting in more detail our findings on the clinical, public health and vaccine implications of the variants, De Oliveira and I concluded by noting the importance of genomic surveillance in the early identification of future variants. This was in addition to suppression of viral replication using public health measures and the equitable distribution of vaccines.

It was a message I reiterated when I was asked to give testimony to the US Congressional Committee on Science, Space, and Technology (called a hearing) to discuss how the US federal government could meet national research and surveillance needs to combat the coronavirus as it continued to mutate and produce new variants. Of particular concern was their potential to evade vaccine-induced immunity.

I was in no mind to sugar-coat the truth: 'Expect more variants! No country is safe until every country is safe,' I said at the end of my scientific presentation. Titled 'Covid-19 variants and evolving research needs', the hearing took place virtually on 12 May 2021. The idea was for members of Congress to seek guidance from scientific experts in dealing with the ongoing challenge presented by the variants.

It should be remembered that on 12 May 2021, 36% of the US population was fully vaccinated, with 47% of all Americans having received at least one dose of a vaccine.[6] Like the UK, the US perceived the vaccine as the endgame for Covid-19: about a week earlier, President Joe Biden had set the goal of getting 70% of US adults to receive at least one dose of a Covid-19 vaccine by 4 July 2021. In contrast, by 12 May 2021, less than 1% of the South African population had received a single dose, and our target, 67% of the population by the end of 2021, was looking overly ambitious based on the current vaccination rates. Thus, the US had a significant advantage over South Africa and most other countries in the world. Still, US representatives in Congress correctly recognised a significant threat – variants with immune-escape capabilities – to their neat, vaccine-focused endgame. They were keen to retain a global advantage and stay one step ahead of any mutations.

The US might have been ahead of South Africa in terms of vaccination rates, but, at least in the early days of the pandemic, it had not excelled in SARS-Cov-2 genetic surveillance. In December 2020, at the time the 501Y.v2 variant was reported, the US ranked only 43rd in terms of percentage of cases sequenced among countries with more than 100 reported infections. South Africa, slightly better, stood at position 42.[7] That was not bad for a middle-income country. It was as a result of this capacity that the country was able to detect the world's first significant variant of concern. The detection of these variants carried implications for scientists around the world, prompting a realignment of our collective and still-evolving understanding of SARS-CoV-2.

Mass vaccination for Covid-19 presented a catch-22 situation when it came to the emergence of variants: the scaling up of vaccinations in the context of high transmission rates was certainly the best way to lower transmission rates. However, high transmission rates meant more viral replication and created a higher likelihood of the development of mutations able to escape immune response. The creation of variants in vaccinated people would in turn lead to versions of the virus capable of escaping vaccine immunity, potentially undermining vaccine efficacy. This is no reason not to vaccinate, we just need to be aware that vaccination creates immunity that pressures the virus to evolve to evade this immunity. This very concept is the challenge the world already faces with antibiotic resistance in bacterial infections.

But the limitations of vaccines went further than the potential for escape immunity on the part of the virus. In my written testimony, I argued that inequitable distribution and availability of vaccines around the world as a result of vaccine nationalism had cast doubt on the possibility of achieving control over the virus at a global level. 'There is a mistaken belief by some countries that they can vaccinate their populations and then they will be safe. This simply is not true. There is no endgame that sees one country achieving sustained control of the virus while the rest of the world is dealing with rampant spread. In the Covid-19 pandemic, no one is safe until everyone is safe,' I noted in my congressional testimony.

My position then, as it remains to this day, is that ending the pandemic requires a universal response: a global mechanism such as Covax that invests in the development, manufacturing, procurement and equitable distribution of vaccine candidates as they become available to all member countries, regardless of income level.

At the time I gave my testimony to the US Congress, the vaccination statistics exposed a stark and shameful pattern of inequity: 77% of all vaccine doses had been administered in just 10 countries (the US, China, India, the UK, Brazil, Turkey, Germany, Indonesia, France and Russia). Countries such as Israel – admittedly a small population – had managed to all but stamp out new infections through their vigorous vaccination campaign.[8] Meanwhile, some countries were yet to start their SARS-CoV-2 vaccination programmes. And the average number of people in Africa to have received at least one vaccine dose on 12 May 2021 was only 1.68%.[9]

While I focused on the science in my published articles, policy advice and testimonies, I could not stay silent in the midst of the injustice of vaccine inequity. It was heartening to see so many of my friends and colleagues take up this issue as well. I included a comment on vaccine inequity in most of my media interviews, talks and scientific presentations. At my scientific presentation at the Pasteur Institute conference on global SARS-CoV-2 vaccination, held in Paris over the final days of September 2021, I contended that no one should stay silent when companies and countries that control the supply think that the developing world should be satisfied with leftovers.

I did not see vaccine inequity only as a moral issue. There was a strong scientific argument for an equitable distribution of vaccines as well. As a consequence of the vaccine nationalism and the hoarding we saw in early 2021, only limited supplies of vaccines were available in the market. This had the effect of undermining the objective of systematically vaccinating the highest number of people across the globe in the shortest period of time – and at the same time raising the risk of variants developing, especially in unvaccinated populations with high transmission. It made no sense to me as an infectious disease epidemiologist, and it made no sense to me as a citizen of the world concerned with fairness, justice and universal well-being.

The global state of inequity was thrown into more stark relief in late 2021 when a few wealthy countries such as Israel, France and Germany started rolling out third doses – 'booster shots' – to vulnerable groups in a bid to address the problem of waning immunity. This would mean that people in a poor country would have to wait even longer to receive their first dose.

I was particularly impressed with the WHO's strong stance on this painful situation. In early August, Dr Tedros had called for a moratorium until the end of September on booster shots until at least 10% of the population of every country in the world had been vaccinated.[10] I shared the concern of the WHO, especially as evidence of clinical benefit from boosters was lacking. While there was a strong case to be made for boosters to be given to immunocompromised patients, such as those with HIV, and elderly people, the benefits of boosters to others had not been established at that time. There was, in my mind, no compelling scientific evidence at that time to support the view that waning immunity was having a significant impact on reversing the vaccine benefits of reducing hospitalisation and severe disease.

Because the global vaccine stock was a zero-sum game, countries stockpiling doses for booster shots were draining global supply and diverting doses away from those who needed it. In September 2021, Africa already had a shortfall of 470 million doses and Covax had cut its delivery targets for 2021 because of insufficient supply of doses.[11]

As a scientist, I am trained to deal primarily in facts and evidence. My diction obviously reflects this conditioning to some extent. I have been described more than once in the media as a 'voice of reason'. This is perhaps as it should be – the words of scientists must be based on reason. However, on the issue of vaccine nationalism, the 'voice of reason' seemed to fall on deaf ears. The world's richest countries continued to deftly navigate their way around the deep undercurrents of injustice and greed that threatened to drag us all under the surface.

No matter how many times I challenged the notion of vaccine nationalism, and regardless of the forum in which I did it, I found little real appetite for tackling the 'me-first' imperative among the world's richest nations. The onset of Covid-19 called on all of us to appreciate that each individual person's risk of infection was influenced as much by the actions of others as it was by their own. In much the same way, the antidote to vaccine nationalism was the recognition and appreciation of our mutual interdependence.

We needed an endgame that actually delivered results to the whole world rather than only its richest and most powerful citizens. The Covid-19 endgame clearly involved vaccines, despite the variants, but if those vaccines could not be universally available, did we really have a viable endgame? While we could be proud of the scientific advances and successes that had made the vaccine possible – and so quickly – we were failing in the humanity stakes.

In the world of vaccines versus variants, the virus was not done. Many thought that Delta was as bad as it could get. But a new surprise awaited us – a virus with more than 50 mutations all at once. No one predicted that development. No one prepared for this scenario. South Africa would be ground zero in this battle. The next letter of the Greek alphabet would be needed.

CHAPTER 27

Another new variant – Omicron

*The emergence of Omicron, compounded by the travel bans, created
worldwide anxiety. While it was straightforward for me to estimate
that the fourth wave would occur on 2 December, it was beyond
imagination to anticipate that it would be caused by the
emergence of a super-variant like Omicron.*

'Fact check: Did South African epidemiologist accurately predict
nation's COVID surge?' screamed the headline of an article in US
weekly magazine *Newsweek*.[1] This was in response to the flurry of activity
on social media over the fact that I had publicly predicted the onset of the
fourth wave – to the day – almost four months earlier.[2] On 17 August 2021,
a journalist from Bloomberg asked me persistently whether South Africa
would have a fourth wave and when would it take place. After repeatedly
refusing to answer because I do not generally share my estimations, given
their tentative nature, I relented and told her that I expected the fourth
wave to start on 2 December. I reiterated this December estimate for the
fourth wave when I gave testimony at the Moseneke Commission on the
timing of the elections a few weeks later. In both instances, I was careful
to provide several caveats to the estimation. When the fourth wave of
the pandemic was announced in South Africa on 2 December 2021 by
the new Minister of Health, Dr Joe Phaahla, the accuracy of my prediction got virtual tongues wagging and fuelled inevitable conspiracies about
the pandemic being orchestrated by me. Some even went to the extent
of saying that I was able to predict the wave because I was growing and
spreading the virus.

The truth, of course, was far less interesting: it involved a rudimentary mathematical calculation. I had seen that the inter-wave gap between each of the first three Covid-19 waves was fairly consistent and took place at intervals of between 94 and 99 days. So, all it took was for me to use my experience to project the likely end of the third wave and add 99 days to that date. In respect of the fourth wave, that took us to 2 December 2021. All waves had been driven by new variants, so I also predicted that this would be the case for the fourth wave as well. The fact-check article in *Newsweek* confirmed that I had correctly predicted the fourth wave, providing the rationale behind my prediction and outlining the 'ifs and buts' I stipulated when sharing the estimate, including my comments about the emergence of a new and unknown variant to drive this wave. I was taken aback at the furore this created on social media and the conspiracy theories it engendered.

That new variant turned out to be Omicron – which was first reported in Botswana and brought to the world's attention by South African scientists.

Omicron's arrival was attended by a great deal of hype and panic, which catapulted me back into the media spotlight – not that I had ever left it; it had just taken on a less intense glare. On 30 November 2021, I had received over a thousand mentions – all related to interviews about Omicron.

Once again, I was fitting interviews into little gaps in my regular schedule. Smita Maharaj was turning down many requests from journalists around the world, including countries such as Spain and Brazil, and we were referring many of them to De Oliveira, Lessells and members of the MAC, but still the requests came pouring in. Luckily, Professor Helen Rees, who was a member of the MAC and was very familiar with developments around Omicron, was available to give the South African perspective in several of these interviews; her calm and systematic approach to explaining complex science was what the world needed.

Omicron attracted such frenzied attention in part because it carried so many mutations – a whopping 53 or so, with 30 of them being found in the gene for the spike protein – the key into human cells. The new variant was initially known as B.1.1.529 before the WHO allocated it the name Omicron, skipping over 'Nu' because it would be confusing as it would be mistaken for 'new' when spoken, and bypassing 'Xi' because it sounded like a common surname. It had over twice as many mutations as the virulent Delta variant, which had rapidly become dominant throughout the world. In addition to the unusually high number of changes in the new variant, the fact that scientists did not know what impact all those mutations would have on the behaviour of the virus was a major cause for concern.

Inklings of a significant new variant emerging in southern Africa came from various sources. In Gaborone, virologist Dr Sikhulile Moyo, working in the Botswana Harvard HIV Reference Laboratory, noticed unusual patterns in specimens collected on 9 November 2021, during routine genetic sequencing and uploaded the new genetic data to the international GISAID database. A few days later, a virology laboratory in Hong Kong uploaded the second sequence of this new variant onto GISAID. A UK scientist who is well known in genomics circles noted these two new unusual sequences in a tweet a few days later. But this did not cause alarm, as they were isolated events and the dots had not yet been joined to illuminate their significance.

Around the same time, chair of the South African Medical Association, Professor Angelique Coetzee, started to notice that several of the patients coming to her private practice in Pretoria were presenting with some Covid-like symptoms that did not quite match those associated with the Delta variant. She noted that several of them were university students. She flagged the samples she sent in for testing at the local private virology laboratory. At Lancet pathology laboratory on 4 November, junior technician Ms Alicia Vermeulen noticed something unusual in the ThermoFisher PCR tests she had done for Covid-19 on these swabs; the S-gene was not positive.

The ThermoFisher PCR kit is the only one that tests for three separate genes for SARS-CoV-2; most other kits just test for one gene. When one of the three genes is not positive, the other two positive genes are enough to record the test result as positive, but a negative S-gene result is noted as 'S-gene target failure'. The Alpha variant had a genetic deletion at position 69–70 of the spike protein, which led to S-gene failure. Concerned about the S-gene target failure in her samples, she alerted her manager. After the same anomaly was seen several times, Dr Allison Glass, head of molecular pathology at Lancet Laboratories and a member of the MAC, was informed.[3] Glass, in turn, alerted scientists at the NICD, who raised it with the National Genome Surveillance-South Africa, headed by De Oliveira.

On Tuesday, 23 November, De Oliveira insisted I come down to his office so he could show me a gene sequence on his desktop computer. There was a degree of *déjà vu* about the whole episode. De Oliveira and Lessells had analysed the sequences and were alarmed at the results: the new variant had all the mutations of the previous variants of concern – and more. I could see the problem immediately – to me, it looked like a super-variant. As scientists, we knew that the next step was to verify the data. Out of 100 samples sequenced that day, 76 turned out to be the new variant labelled as lineage B.1.1.529.

Having verified the data, De Oliveira informed Health Minister Phaahla and briefed the WHO. The WHO team recognised the significance of a variant with so many mutations immediately, assigning it the name Omicron. President Ramaphosa was briefed on Thursday, 25 November. On the same day, an online press conference was hurriedly called by the Health minister, who was clearly concerned by the rapid increase in infections. As he told the conference, cases had been rising exponentially over the past four to five days. Reported daily infections rose from 273 on 16 November to 1 200 by 24 November 2021. In addition to Department of Health officials, De Oliveira was supported in the press conference by scientists Penny Moore, Anne von Gottberg and Nicholas Crisp, Deputy DG in the Department of Health in charge of the Covid-19 response. After some technical difficulties, the conference got under way and the announcement of a new variant, amidst a great deal of scientific data, was made. Not unexpectedly, all hell broke loose.

Later that day, the UK announced that South Africa as well as Botswana and four other southern African countries were on the UK Red List and banned all flights to the UK from those countries. The UK was quickly followed by the US and several European Union countries. Southern Africans were justifiably outraged. Travel plans were thrown into chaos. It was easy to believe that the country was being punished for their transparent reporting.

I received the first request for a media interview on Omicron from CNN's Becky Anderson on Thursday evening. I was in Johannesburg at the time because I was due to receive the UNISA Public Servant Award at the UNISA Chancellor's Calabash Award ceremony the following day.

At that stage, very little was known about the impact of the new variant and the significance of its mutations, so it was important to emphasise the uncertainty surrounding what I thought the new variant would do and point to the need for more studies.

Asked by Anderson how worried I was about the new variant, I admitted to being 'quite' worried because of the number of mutations involved but stressed there was a lot we did not know. 'We are not sure if it will be able to evade antibodies and studies are needed, but looking at it, the likelihood is that it will have some level of immune escape and vaccinated people may still get mild symptoms.' We were unlikely to see severe infections increase because of the T-cell response, I said. When Anderson asked, I endorsed the Africa CDC statement in which it discouraged the recently imposed travel bans on the grounds that they had been shown not to 'yield a meaningful outcome' in the past.

'I do agree with it,' I said. 'When dealing with a pandemic like this one, we have to find a way to work with each other; mutual interdependence will enable us to defeat it. If we just shun the rest of the world, we are not going to solve the problem.'

I took the opportunity to explain that Africa was running around seven to eight months behind the rest of the world when it came to Covid-19 vaccine distribution. 'Now we have the challenge of converting vials into jabs ... We will have to face this, but what is important is that we cannot deal with it as Africans, as Europe ... It affects all of us. And it doesn't help that rich countries have stockpiled and when the vaccines are about to expire, they get donated to Africa ... We have got to find a different way. All of us must work together. We've got to help Africa in a way that encourages and builds sustainability because this is not the first variant and it's certainly not the last.'

The emergence of Omicron, compounded by the travel bans, had created a good deal of panic, so much so that by Friday morning a second press conference was being planned by the Department of Health. Throughout the day, I took more interviews with international media networks and national media houses from my hotel room in Johannesburg. Between interviews, at around mid-afternoon, I received a call from Minister Phaahla, who said he wanted me to attend the second presser. Perhaps it would help to have a familiar face on screen to explain what we knew about the new variant to calm nerves down. If it did not clash with my UNISA commitment, it would be fine, I explained. He called again that evening while he was attending a briefing on the new variant. I was at the Houghton Hotel where the Chancellor's award ceremony was just kicking off and so could not join him in the briefing. I stepped out of the dinner venue and into the hotel kitchen, and from this noisy spot I shared with the minister my three cardinal rules for communicating bad news to the public: start by reminding people that the new variant was expected, and that we found it because we have been actively looking for it through our surveillance; secondly, that we have dealt with new variants before and can deal with this one too, conveying information with clarity and confidence so that the public can feel some confidence, even if the science might be a little difficult to follow, that the authorities know what they are doing and there is no need for panic; and thirdly, tell people what the path forward might look like as this helps reduce uncertainty.

On Monday morning, yet another press conference was called. Minister Phaahla asked me again to make a presentation – speaking now as a scientist as I was no longer the chair of the MAC. In my presentation, simply titled 'What we do and don't know about the Omicron variant', I was concerned to place the recent events around the variant in context. I methodically went through an overview of the information we had about Omicron and what we could likely expect from it. I tried to reassure people by reminding them that we had seen variants before and had managed their impact. And we could do so again. It was also important to acknowledge the way in which the variant had been detected and South Africa's important role in sharing this information with the rest of the world. All that we needed now was an equally successful response.

The fallout from the country's initial announcement of Omicron – which had a direct impact on the economies of South Africa and its neighbours – prompted some commentators to suggest that it would have been wiser for South African scientists not to communicate to the public about it until they had more information about what we were in for. I don't agree with that argument; there is nothing to be gained from delaying information of such important public interest. I also believe the travel bans were inevitable and would have happened regardless of the way in which the announcement was made because governments around the world needed to show politically that they were taking some action in the face of a crisis.

The Omicron variant indeed turned out to be more transmissible but produced less severe disease. Regardless of the variant's features, the fourth wave still presented an epidemiological challenge. It was set to push up the official global tally of approximately 5 million deaths and, importantly, the excess death count, which was estimated to be around 16.8 million at that time – a concerning figure that dramatically changed the mortality patterns in regions afflicted by under-reporting, such as Africa, Russia and parts of Central America.

Regardless of the palpable pandemic fatigue that had set in around the world, there was no indication as to whether Omicron would be the last variant the world would see. Uncertainty on the emergence of new variants remained. Indications were that Omicron would continue mutating, creating new sub-variants of itself, leading to more waves of infection, which would quickly spread around the world in spite of travel bans and other knee-jerk measures. In a discussion I had with Dr Sandile Buthelezi, who was by then DG of the National Department of Health, after his important leadership role as CEO of the South African National AIDS Council, I raised the issue that the uncertainty made it difficult to plan and so we needed a plan A and a plan B – perhaps even plan C. In his usual thoughtful way, he took it in his stride, saying that we will need to find a way to be ready for this highly variable future.

On the vaccine front, trying to keep one step ahead of Omicron had seen two broad approaches, development of variant specific boosters and research on variant-proof vaccine candidates. Several research groups have been working on the development of coronavirus vaccines that can prevent infection caused by both known and future variants of concern, which are effective against pre-emergent sarbecoviruses (lineage B of genus betacoronavirus) that have the potential to cause human infection. The goal of this approach is to obviate concerns around vaccine-escape variants. Although this line of innovation represents a significant challenge for medical scientists – it is sobering to remember that it has not yet been possible to develop a single vaccine to combat seasonal influenza strains – research indicates the feasibility of a pan-sarbecovirus vaccine strategy.[4]

While pan-coronavirus vaccines are still in development, antiviral treatments hold the prospect of being variant agnostic so that they would remain effective against all variants. While we wait for real safe and effective treatments for Covid-19, purveyors of miracle treatments have found fertile ground to exploit.

CHAPTER 28

Miracle treatments

In desperate times, people clamour for a cure – any cure. Some
politicians, doctors, pharmacists and others exploited this situation,
promoting unproven treatments like hydroxychloroquine, convalescent
plasma, artemisinin and ivermectin, all of which were
subsequently proven to be ineffective.

While the world waited for science to deliver a safe and effective treatment for Covid-19 in 2020 and 2021, desperation mounted, creating fertile ground for snake-oil salespeople seeking to make a quick buck, overnight 'experts' craving attention and politicians desperate to boost their political standing. And, in the case of hydroxychloroquine, they were helped by bad science, specifically a flawed observational study about the benefits of the drug for Covid-19 patients conducted in Marseille, France, and published online in the *International Journal of Antimicrobial Agents*, which is generally known to be a reputable journal.[1]

The findings were endorsed by the Minister of Health of France. After some high-profile tweets about the study findings, the issue was quickly picked up by American right-wing media and President Trump, who wasted no time in describing the drug as 'one of the biggest game-changers in the history of medicine'. Showing scant concern for the regulatory processes that are critical to ensuring scientific standards, President Trump announced that his government had bought a 'tremendous amount' of hydroxychloroquine to treat Covid-19 patients.

In reality, the Marseille study design was of such dubious quality that, two weeks after its online publication, the International Society of

Antimicrobial Chemotherapy, which publishes the *IJAA*, issued a statement in which it said that the group's board 'believes the article does not meet the society's expected standard'.[2]

But the damage had been done and the notion that a miracle cure was out there started to gain traction. Demand for the drug skyrocketed and lupus patients – among those who had a legitimate need for the drug, along with people with rheumatoid arthritis – were unable to get hold of it for their treatment.

Under pressure from President Trump, the US Food and Drug Administration (FDA)[3] issued an Emergency Use Authorization (EUA) on 28 March 2020, allowing doctors to prescribe hydroxychloroquine to hospitalised Covid-19 patients. Three months later, the EUA was revoked as it was becoming clearer that the drug did not work and could cause serious side effects.

Thankfully, sense – and science – prevailed. Several clinical trials subsequently published in the *New England Journal of Medicine* and elsewhere showed more definitively that hydroxychloroquine was ineffective and in fact could be life threatening when repurposed for Covid-19 patients. After that, hydroxychloroquine started to disappear from public debate.

The allure of a cure-all is difficult to resist in desperate times. Another untested remedy swam into view, again buoyed by President Trump's endorsement. In August 2020, an EUA was issued by the FDA for convalescent plasma as a Covid-19 treatment, based on research by the Mayo Clinic. The research had not been peer reviewed and there had been no clinical trials. The EUA was announced in an FDA statement at the White House on the eve of the Republican National Convention, with the headline 'Another achievement in administration's fight against pandemic'.[4]

Within months, the usefulness of plasma was being widely questioned, as no solid evidence of its benefit was emerging from studies. In April 2021, *The New York Times* reported that the use of plasma in hospitals had all but ended owing to a growing acknowledgement of its lack of efficacy.[5]

In South Africa, convalescent plasma was not administered outside of clinical trials and never gained traction to the extent it did in the US, where it was directly supported by the Trump administration, which, according to *The New York Times*, awarded more than US$800 million to entities involved in the collection and administration of plasma.

South Africans are by no means immune to the seduction of wonder cures. In fact, no one is. Shortly after President Trump started to promote hydroxychloroquine, Madagascar's president, Andry Rajoelina, began to champion an unproven herbal remedy made from the *Artemisia annua* plant, which contains the compound artemisinin – used to treat malaria – as a treatment for Covid-19. Among the many emails that came through to my inbox during South Africa's first Covid-19 wave were several from people pushing artemisinin and still others blaming me for 'depriving' people of a miracle remedy for Covid-19.

I had spoken out vociferously against the practice in Madagascar, where the president had arranged for people to receive his self-proclaimed miracle cure without regulatory approval. On 10 July 2020, the MAC submitted an advisory to the Department of Health, making it clear that the 'lack of clinical evidence for both interferons and *Artemisia annua* precludes their use in the treatment of Covid-19 outside a clinical trial setting'.

While artemisinin is a groundbreaking and effective treatment for malaria, the science in support of artemisinin as a Covid-19 treatment was entirely absent at that time, although a number of studies were under way in Europe, the US, Mexico and South Africa. None of these studies provided evidence warranting further consideration of artemisinin for Covid-19 treatment.

The reference to interferon in the 10 July 2020 advisory was the advice the MAC provided when the South African military bought interferon for AIDS treatment from Cuba. The Cuban interferon story had an earlier chapter before the military purchased it from Cuba to treat Covid-19. The former mayor of Ekurhuleni, Mzwandile Masina, announced in his state of the city address that he would be using the city's emergency funds to procure a coronavirus vaccine in March 2020, before Covid-19 vaccines even existed. It turned out that the 'vaccine' he was referring to was actually interferon alfa-2b, manufactured by joint Cuban–Chinese company ChangHeber.

Gauteng's Provincial Health Minister Bandile Masuku had earlier that day, at a provincial government briefing, endorsed the procurement of the Cuban-made drug as treatment for patients with Covid-19. Masuku acknowledged the source as a statement issued the day before by the National Education, Health and Allied Workers' Union (NEHAWU).

NEHAWU claimed that this interferon 'has cured more than 1 500 patients from the [SARS-CoV-2] virus and has been used by the Chinese National Health Commission to combat respiratory diseases'.[6] NEHAWU went on to say, 'The Cuban pharmaceutical industry gave a guarantee on Saturday [14 March 2020] that … Interferon alfa-2b has been proven to be very effective in fighting the virus.' It was intriguing to hear that NEHAWU, a trade union active in the health sector, was allegedly colluding with the Cuban pharmaceutical industry in punting a fake cure for Covid-19.

In the midst of the frenzy to capitalise on this 'miracle cure', Masina, Masuku and NEHAWU were plugging interferon interchangeably as a vaccine or a cure, clearly oblivious to the difference. There was no evidence at that or any other time that interferon is effective either in preventing or treating Covid-19. Their attempts to spin a tale got even weirder when Masuku's spokesperson said that doctors in Gauteng would use guidelines as set out by the WHO, even though the WHO did not recommend interferons for Covid-19 treatment.

My daughter Aisha wrote an article shortly after this debacle started, exposing the players involved in buying this supposed vaccine. Looking closer at this matter, it is hard not to ponder what exactly was going on, as those involved in the purchase could not be buying it because they had seen the evidence that it was an effective treatment. They had little knowledge of the medication and whether it was a vaccine or cure for Covid-19. Perhaps some other reason for this purchase was at play.

Opening a weekly Sunday newspaper on the morning of 6 December 2020, I came across an article about a clinical pharmacologist at the Durban University of Technology (DUT), referred to only as 'the professor' by the newspaper.[7] He claimed that he had developed a successful treatment for Covid-19, dubbed HIM20, which was based on the suppression of cytokines.

He said that the research was conducted under the auspices of IM Chemical Corporation, a company that turned out to be owned by him. I was naturally intrigued by the claims but rather concerned that the journalist of the piece had adopted a wholly uncritical approach to the claims being made, failing to interrogate the notion that a clinical drug trial could be conducted without the necessary approvals. There was no evidence of fact-checking and the story relied entirely on a single source. Even the headline was incorrect in its claim that the pharmacologist had developed the 'first' anti-Covid treatment – because in fact there were two other approved treatments available at the time. This was not my first encounter with shoddy journalism in the local newspapers, though I have generally found the quality of stories in South African newspapers to be quite good.

Not a little alarmed, I called the journalist to ask him to put me in touch with the unnamed 'professor', which he did, after seeking permission from the 'professor' himself. I contacted the 'professor' to get more information, expressing my reservations about the story and its claims. During our phone call, he shared his name, Dr Ismail Mohamed Mall, and contact details, including email address, explaining that he had no objection to his name being known. I explained to Mall that I was keen to read the protocol, see the primary analysis of the data and know whether or not the trial had been given the requisite approval by the ethics committee of the university to which he was affiliated – in this case DUT – and by SAHPRA. All studies of new medications and existing medications being repurposed for a new illness require approvals from the relevant authorities. In this way, people are protected from unscrupulous researchers doing unethical research on patients, using them as guinea pigs.

After my amicable telephonic conversation with Mall, I sent him some questions by email, which received no response, in spite of his promise to send me replies within days. From my own subsequent investigation, I established that Mall had a PhD in pharmacology but was only a part-time lecturer at DUT, where he was neither a professor nor an associate professor. I could find no evidence that he had secured a research protocol or that he had undertaken a scientifically valid research study. The study was not registered, as required by Department of Health, in any of the clinical trial registers. I confirmed with SAHPRA CEO Dr Boitumelo Semete-Makokotlela that it had not been submitted to the medicines regulator for approval. DUT likewise confirmed that there had been no application from Mall for ethics approval at that institution. After reviewing the details of his study, it seemed that he had not conducted a clinical trial but had conducted what seemed to be more like a 'clinical intervention' in Covid-19 patients with an unapproved medicine outside the ambit of a clinical research protocol.

I experienced flashbacks to the 1997 announcement by perfusion technician Olga Visser about her 'discovery' of the fake AIDS cure Virodene, which was actually a harmful chemical solvent. Virodene was tested in a group of AIDS patients without any approval and then announced by Visser, with the support of politicians in South Africa, as a miracle cure for HIV. That announcement had also been made through the media, without any peer-reviewed scientific presentation or publication, by individuals with questionable academic standing. Was HIM20 another case of false therapeutic claims stemming from unethical studies without regulatory approval? It turned out to be so.

Conveying falsehoods about discovering a new treatment or cure in the midst of a pandemic is a serious problem. Not only did such a study have the potential to physically harm its trial participants, but the spreading of unsubstantiated claims about HIM20's beneficial effects for Covid-19 carried the risk of sowing confusion, raising false hope or encouraging a false sense of security in patients taking untested treatments. It was also illegal in terms of the State of Disaster Act, which, in its regulations, criminalises misinformation.

Armed with what I had gleaned from my own enquiries, I informed the Health minister and SAHPRA, who instituted an investigation. I also contacted, for the second time, the journalist who wrote the article to provide him with the outcomes of my investigations into HIM20. He, in turn, informed his editor about my now-substantiated concerns and conveyed my request for a retraction of the article and a public correction of its misstatements.

A number of weeks passed, and no action was taken by the newspaper to retract the article. On 10 January 2021, over a month since the initial article had appeared, a follow-up piece appeared in the same newspaper. It did little to assuage my disquiet. In fact, the second article made things worse. The journalist used his second article to give the 'professor' the opportunity to respond to my concerns without clearly explaining my concerns. In this second article, Mall stated that he had used his own resources to conduct the research – as if self-funding somehow absolved him of any need to seek official approval for a clinical study. All research, whether public or private, must be submitted to the appropriate bodies for approval – and anyone with a PhD in a medical discipline, like he had, would have known that.

The article went further to quote Mall's attorney, Mr Reeves Parsee, who gained notoriety for his unsuccessful defence of convicted fraudster Shabir Shaik.[8] In the quote, he said, '… any suggestion that this was a new drug or medication administered without approval was mischievous and misplaced.' He then proceeded to state, 'No protocol was submitted to anyone.' This confession by Mall's attorney that the research was not submitted for approval made it unequivocal that his 'study' had violated several fundamental scientific and ethical guidelines and rules for the conduct of therapeutic research. The cherry on top was the final quote in the article that the treatment method had 'yielded excellent results, and the combination of the drug and therapeutic method is safe and acceptable'. It seemed that they were not aware that unethical research can only be invalid, never excellent.

The second article in my view put us back to square one when it came to misinforming the public. I felt I had no option at that point but to approach the Independent Media Ombudsman, a move that resulted in a published apology from the newspaper editor on 21 February 2021, in which it was conceded that the original article contained untruths and that the editorial staff had failed their own reporting standards.[9] There was no retraction, however, and both articles remain available online, the second happily perpetuating the primary falsehood of the first.

I felt that I had done what I could to mitigate the possible damage caused by these articles. Fortunately, HIM20 failed to gain a foothold in the public consciousness or as a commercial product, as far as I am aware. Perhaps this was because it did not have high-profile political support like Virodene did.

In the midst of burgeoning fake treatments, the despair around a Covid-19 cure remained tangible. When the second, larger Covid-19 wave started to swell, and public desperation along with it, anti-parasite drug ivermectin became the new miracle cure – and because it had a number of local champions from within the medical fraternity, the drug gained real traction within our borders. My neighbours sheepishly let me know many months later that they had paid R6 000 for a course of ivermectin – which surprised me because ivermectin is a very cheap medicine. Clearly, I was treading on toes and undermining those trying to make a quick buck from ivermectin. Again, I received several calls and emails from people – much more vociferous in their tone – admonishing me for failing to see the benefits of ivermectin. Some of it bordered on hate mail. I even received correspondence from attorneys for Dr Naseeba Kathrada, a doctor who runs a slimming business and promoted ivermectin for Covid-19 treatment long after the WHO recommended against its use.

Both ivermectin and artemisinin are excellent drugs in their own right and share an interesting link. In 2015, the Nobel Prize in Physiology or Medicine was awarded jointly to three people: William C Campbell and Satoshi Ōmura for their discovery of ivermectin as a treatment for the parasite that causes river blindness and lymphatic filariasis; and Chinese pharmaceutical chemist Tu Youyou, for her discovery of artemisinin as a treatment for malaria. As the Nobel Prize committee indicated, both these drugs have had a global impact, resulting in improved human health and reduced suffering, particularly in the developing world.

So, the problem is not with the drugs themselves, but the purposes for which they are being used. What made ivermectin attractive was that it was reasonably priced and had been used widely in humans for many years – although for very different purposes. Ivermectin as a 'miracle cure' for Covid-19 had been actively championed in the US by Dr Pierre Kory, a lung and ICU specialist in that country. At the invitation of Republican senators, on 8 December 2020, Kory attended a meeting of a US senate committee looking into early outpatient Covid-19 treatment, where he claimed that data showed the 'miraculous effectiveness' of the drug. His false claims gained traction, not just in the US but in several other countries as well. The footage of his senate testimony was later removed by YouTube in accordance with its Covid-19 misinformation policy and Kory is reported to have said he regrets using hyperbole.

The reality is that not a single peer-reviewed clinical trial in a reputable journal has shown ivermectin to be effective against Covid-19, as I pointed out in Chapter 14. The WHO guidelines on Covid-19 treatment have a specific recommendation against the use of ivermectin. Despite this, Kory found support among some South Africans, including general practitioners and pharmacists, many of whom were prescribing and distributing ivermectin, even though it was not then registered for human use in South Africa. Not surprisingly, there were even a few from the Nelson Mandela Medical School who supported Kory and wrote articles with him in support of this fake treatment. He was given media space in South Africa when he was interviewed by Independent Online newspapers.

Concerned about the safety of the drug at uncontrolled doses as well as the risk of sub-standard or falsified products finding their way onto a thriving black market, the MAC weighed in with another ivermectin advisory on 11 January 2021. The MAC reiterated the lack of evidence about the drug's efficacy in Covid-19 cases as well as the processes that needed to be followed before a drug can be registered. 'Premature support of a medicine with unproven safety and efficacy information is difficult to justify,' our advisory noted. 'The argument that medicine found to be safe in other conditions can be used for Covid-19 before the arrival of adequate Covid-specific safety and efficacy data is not sound. For example, while chloroquine and azithromycin are both individually safe medicines, their use in severely ill Covid-19 patients with multiple comorbidities is now associated with emerging signals of possible harm.'

In the absence of sufficient evidence to support the efficacy of ivermectin, we were defending not only science but the regulatory governance, which served an absolutely vital function in ensuring the medications available to the public were safe and were being used for the purposes for which they were intended.

Interestingly, even the original manufacturer, Merck, cautioned that there was no scientific basis from pre-clinical studies for a potential therapeutic effect against Covid-19. In a statement on 4 February 2021, the drug manufacturer said there was no 'meaningful evidence' for clinical activity or clinical efficacy in Covid-19 patients and noted a 'concerning lack of safety data in the majority of studies'. On 25 January 2021, the NEMLC Covid-19 sub-group also released the results of a rapid review of ivermectin, in which they concluded that there was insufficient evidence to recommend it for prophylaxis or treatment of Covid-19. They said the drug should not be used for Covid-19 treatment except in clinical trials – basically the same position as the WHO.

SAHPRA, the authority in South Africa that controls the registration of new or repurposed drugs, got its own team of experts to conduct a review of the available data, and they reached the same conclusion as the MAC and the NEMLC review groups: there simply wasn't enough evidence to support the use of ivermectin for Covid-19 treatment or prevention.

SAHPRA had every right to be cautious. It has a statutory function as a 'guardian' of the safety of the South African public. However, for its stance on ivermectin, SAHPRA was accused of standing in the way of people having access to treatment – either for reasons of administrative inefficiency or for more nefarious reasons related to vested interests of the kind touted on social media. No application for registration of the drug had at that stage been lodged – largely because there was no hard evidence to support its efficacy in Covid-19 treatments. And SAHPRA had already indicated that it would welcome and even fast track an application for a randomised controlled trial – the gold standard in drug efficacy testing.

The inappropriate use of ivermectin was not limited to South Africa and the US. It was widespread. On 12 May 2021, the state of Uttarakhand became India's third state, after Goa and Karnataka, to announce that it would be administering ivermectin as a prophylaxis against severe Covid-19 to all adults, irrespective of their Covid-19 status. With daily infection rates during India's Delta wave sitting at around 400 000 in early May 2021, authorities were under massive pressure to take action.

In South Africa, the clamour continued, with substantial pressure and legal action by clinicians who were using and promoting ivermectin wanting SAHPRA to register the drug for human use. This eventually resulted in the regulator allowing 'compassionate use' of the drug in terms of Section 21 of the Medicines and Related Substances Act, 1965. Compassionate use is meant as an interim measure until more data from trials become available. Section 21 is a well-known mechanism to give individuals access to potentially life-saving drugs that are not yet registered. It requires a special application by the treating physician on behalf of a named patient, along with the payment of a fee. Consideration of the application can take time, which is why the Section 21 provision was deemed by critics of the regulator to be too restrictive and basically unfit for purpose in the case of Covid-19 cases, which often required urgent treatment.

This dissatisfaction culminated in four court cases being brought against SAHPRA and the government. The first of these was brought by a Pretoria-based general practitioner, Dr George Coetzee, two of his patients and AfriForum, a lobby group for white Afrikaner interests. The second was by the African Christian Democratic Party and a group called Doctors for Life. The third was by the 'I can make a difference' doctors and medical practitioners group and a group of pharmacists.

On 9 April 2021, based on an out-of-court settlement, the Pretoria High Court issued a single order, giving doctors the right to initiate treatment with ivermectin at the same time as a Section 21 application for an individually named patient was submitted to SAHPRA (although there was an obligation to report patient outcomes). The order permitted licensed health care facilities to hold bulk stock of the drug to avoid delays in access and it permitted the 'compounding' of medicines containing ivermectin as an active ingredient. Compounding is the process whereby active ingredients in a registered medication are used by pharmacists (under prescription from doctors) to create a new medication that is tailored to the needs of specific patients. It meant that pharmacists could make up small batches of medicine containing ivermectin for Covid-19 patients provided it had been prescribed by a doctor. This would not require filing a Section 21 application.

Despite the fact that SAHPRA made no admission of liability and reiterated its position on the lack of evidence in support of ivermectin, it nonetheless contributed a total of R1.75 million towards the applicants' costs in order to put an end to what, in SAHPRA's view, could be protracted litigation. The applicants portrayed this outcome as a victory for ivermectin. Although I was shocked that the regulator seemed to concede so readily, going all the way to the point of contributing to the applicants' costs, in reality it achieved a change in SAHPRA procedures. Several months later, SAHPRA withdrew this Section 21 mechanism for ivermectin when demand for ivermectin dwindled, as both patients and doctors came to appreciate first-hand the treatment's lack of efficacy.

But the damage was done. Doctors had been dishing out ivermectin willy-nilly.

In a case relating to the dismissal of an employee for refusing a Covid-19 vaccination, I learned from an affidavit filed by the employee that a certain Dr Rapiti, whom I have never met, had prescribed ivermectin, together with vitamin D, fluvoxamine and chloroquine for thousands of his Covid-19 patients. In my affidavit on the case, I argued that this constituted quackery! I noted that the WHO guidelines *strongly* recommend *against* chloroquine and hydroxychloroquine, recommend *against* ivermectin and have *no recommendation* for vitamin D for the treatment of Covid-19. I pointed out that he was not prescribing any of the WHO-recommended medications, systemic corticosteroids and interleukin-6 receptor blockers like tocilizumab. By deliberately choosing not to treat his patients with scientifically proven medicines and using medicines that were specifically recommended against, he had deliberately mistreated more than 3 000 patients. His actions may have constituted medical malpractice.

His supporters leapt to his defence on social media, showering me with abusive comments but providing no evidence to challenge my points. It highlighted for me how a lack of knowledge can foster almost religious fervour for an unproven medication in the midst of a pandemic. The most up-to-date meta-analysis, published in BioMed Central in July 2022, included 25 randomised control trials comprising 6 310 patients.[10] Of these 25 trials, 14 compared ivermectin with placebo and 9 compared ivermectin plus the standard of care with just the standard of care. Two studies compared ivermectin to an active comparator. Ivermectin did not show an effect in reducing mortality or mechanical ventilation. This lack of efficacy was consistent when comparing ivermectin vs placebo, and ivermectin plus standard of care vs standard of care. In summary, there is no doubt that ivermectin is not effective in treating Covid-19.

In a *New England Journal of Medicine* editorial, I wrote with Dr Nikita Devnarain on ivermectin and fluvoxamine, we captured some of the problems that emerge when medical practitioners become charlatans promoting ineffective treatment despite evidence to the contrary. If this matter was not dealt with now during Covid-19, I said, I was concerned about what doctors may do in promoting and selling fake cures when the next pandemic came along – the professional bodies needed to set some ground rules to deal with this.

At times, it felt like I was in a pinball machine, lurching from one bogus treatment to the next. Each new miracle-cure claim required a careful assessment of the available data, a clear set of arguments on why the treatment was not authentic and a strategic approach to countering the misinformation that accompanied each claim. Clearing up falsehoods was becoming as consuming as conveying the facts. But the miracle cures were just the tip of the iceberg when it came to misinformation. The mis- and disinformation in Covid-19 became a pandemic in itself, acquiring a new term, 'infodemic'.

CHAPTER 29

The disinformation bandwagon

Disinformation was rife, ranging from denial of the pandemic, downplaying its seriousness, challenging the efficacy of interventions to undermining vaccinations. Every one of us, I believe, can fight mis- and disinformation by being a myth-buster and an ambassador of science.

In a 1710 essay titled 'The art of political lying', the famous Anglo-Irish satirist Jonathan Swift wrote: 'Falsehood flies, and the truth comes limping after it; so that when people [he actually said 'men', but I am taking the liberty of being PC instead] come to be undeceived, it is too late; the jest is over, and the tale has had its effect.' Here, Swift captures the allure of manufactured lies, the easy attraction that we humans experience when we come across an idea that seems to explain the unexplainable and satisfies a thirst for clarity to reduce our anxiety about the unknown. It's only human to want to avoid uncertainty by grasping at narratives that help us make sense of the world. But, as Swift notes, falsehoods can have an impact that lingers long after they are revealed to be untrue. Because of their natural advantage – their ability to fly – it is often impossible for truth to catch up with falsehoods, particularly when aided by today's world of digital communication networks.

The Covid-19 pandemic facilitated various kinds of falsehoods or, to put it more bluntly, lies. Some of these lies were the result of misinformation (which refers to the unintentional spread of inaccurate information, that is, getting the facts wrong), but many of the Covid-19 falsehoods were disinformation. Disinformation is defined as the intentional dissemination of false information to deliberately mislead people, that is, information designed actively to deceive. I had become familiar with the concept of disinformation during the apartheid years as the National Party government lived off its ability to use disinformation. The AIDS pandemic, like the Covid-19 pandemic, had its share of disinformation. There was the famous incident when the then Soviet Union launched a disinformation campaign, known as Operation Infektion, to propagate the notion that the US invented AIDS. The KGB propaganda department, known as the 'Special Disinformation Office', attained notoriety for this campaign. I learned at the time that the word 'disinformation' is a translation of the Russian word 'dezinformatsiya', which had been derived decades earlier from the name of this very office.

In the past, state intelligence agencies and their front organisations routinely used a combination of both truthful and false information to further a political agenda, sometimes referred to as propaganda. Using some kernels of truth in the narrative helped boost their credibility. The same combination is now being used by a range of others – lay individuals, non-profit organisations and business entities – to spread disinformation, which affects our ability to promote public health, address climate change, sustain a stable democracy and much more. South Africa had been the victim of this tactic to destabilise its democracy when the British company Bell Pottinger mounted a disinformation campaign on 'white monopoly capital' to create racial disharmony as a smokescreen for corruption during the Zuma era. Covid-19 generated several Bell Pottinger-like mini-campaigns on public health measures like masks and vaccines, predominantly through social media.

I was intrigued to come across a study by researchers at Cornell University that showed the extent of misinformation in the media in the early stages of Covid-19.[1] An analysis of over 38 million English-language media articles published in print and online around the world from January to late May 2020 found that over 1.1 million individual articles (a total of 1 116 952 – just under 3%) mentioned misinformation about Covid-19. The articles covered stories about misinformation, stories that sought to counteract the misinformation, as well as those stories that repeated misinformation. What was even more shocking was that a single individual – President Trump – was found to be responsible for over one-third – 37.9% – of those cases of misinformation.

The study found that most prevalent misinformation concerned miracle cures (at 26.4%). As I pointed out in the previous chapter, I had many miracle cure challenges to repudiate during the pandemic, but the first one that I had to deal with was denialism. In the early days of the pandemic, denialism often took the form of a likening of Covid-19 to influenza. People dismissed the significance of the new virus by saying it was 'just another flu' and persisted with this idea even when it was clear that Covid-19 was much more severe and serious. For a period at the beginning of the pandemic, President Trump was one of the most notable proponents of this fallacy. In subsequent recorded interviews with journalist Bob Woodward, he admitted to knowing it was much worse than the flu, but claimed that he had been right to downplay its severity.

In South Africa, there were a few groups that also perpetrated this 'flu' falsehood. One group in particular, known by the acronym Panda, lobbied vigorously against Covid-19 restrictions by promoting disinformation. The group was co-founded by an actuary and senior executive of Sanlam, a life assurance company created by Afrikaner farmers during apartheid. It specialised in attacking scientific information, arguing that PCR tests were inaccurate, case numbers were exaggerated, death data were erroneous and excess death calculations were flawed. It occasionally produced their own analyses, including one that indicated that the lockdown restrictions led to 30 times more deaths than the pandemic itself.[2] Its report making this claim has been described as 'deeply flawed' and a 'complete sham masquerading as science'.[3]

A well-researched exposé in the *Daily Maverick* titled 'Kung-Flu Panda: Dodgy analytics or pandemic propaganda?'[4] outlined the links that this organisation had with several controversial British and Canadian Covid-19 disinformation groups and even with 'Cambridge Analytica, the controversial data-firm exposed for using fake news and disinformation to support the Donald Trump presidential campaign'. To spread its message more widely, this organisation was aided and abetted by a local business news website, which already had an arguably poor reputation for its journalism, but stooped even lower when it published a three-part article by Panda targeting me. Riddled with falsehoods, the three articles followed the disinformation playbook with only a thin veil of pretence as an exposé.

In its spurious arguments on deaths from lockdowns, I could see echoes of the AIDS denialists who contended that the antiretroviral treatment for HIV was likely to kill more people than HIV itself. As in both AIDS and Covid-19, arguing that the government's intervention measures were unwarranted, its disinformation was designed to create controversy and divide people, causing ructions in the midst of a pandemic, when solidarity and co-operation were needed.

Among the many Covid-19 denialists I had to deal with, there was a 'blast from the past' – Dr David Rasnick, who submitted an affidavit in a South African legal matter, denying the existence of the Covid-19 pandemic. Rasnick, an American biochemist, gained infamy for his support for President Mbeki's AIDS denialism, as a participant in the Mbeki AIDS Panel in 2000. When Covid-19 struck, Rasnick had another opportunity to ply his brand of denialism, arguing that the symptoms of Covid-19 were actually flu, as they are the same as the symptoms of seasonal influenza and that the Covid PCR test was 'fraudulent'. He argued that if the tests stopped, so would the pandemic. It reminded me about how little children are sometimes told to close their eyes to make something scary disappear. If only pandemics could be eliminated so easily …

In 2021, disinformation ratcheted up a few notches when South Africa was about to embark on a vaccine rollout. Besides the conspiracy theories about 5G and computer chips in the vaccines, there was a more insidious challenge. Ostensibly persuasive disinformation was doing the rounds on social media that the mRNA vaccine would denature a person's DNA. The arguments stemmed from misinformed claims by medical professionals that the vaccine was manipulating human genes, that it was not a vaccine but gene therapy.

A common refrain I heard was that the vaccines were developed too quickly. This must, in their view, have been the result of shortcuts that were taken, compromising the information on safety. I could understand this concern as the vaccines were developed, tested, approved, manufactured and distributed in record time – time frames that I had not considered possible barely a few months earlier. This concern needed factual reassurance, I felt. Since journal articles publishing each vaccine trial usually included data on the frequency distribution of individual side effects, I could quote the actual rate of common side effects to illustrate the fact that these had been measured in the trial, and that regulatory approval usually comes with a requirement to monitor long-term safety. Honest and verifiable assurance was also my approach on some of the other reasonable vaccine concerns, ranging from the lack of information on long-term safety, side effects and efficacy as new variants emerged.

Every now and then I would be flooded with queries about a particular side effect of the vaccines. This would follow when someone who had developed some severe side effects after being vaccinated shared their experiences on social media, and these were being amplified by bots to create the impression that severe side effects, like Guillain-Barré syndrome, were common. This false impression led some to think that getting the vaccine was worse than getting the disease, with little appreciation that all medications have rare side effects, but their benefits outweigh the risks. Trying to address this barrage could be a full-time job. I would investigate the concern only occasionally as there were too many to do them all. Sometimes, I found out that the side effect being reported was real, but mostly I found that they were just made up. I could sometimes spot the made-up ones from little tell-tale signs, but this was long after they had already been 'forwarded many times' on WhatsApp.

Vaccine hesitancy was not new in South Africa. Small groups of individuals have taken a position against vaccinating their children and some have promoted anti-vaccine sentiment. In Covid-19, vaccine hesitancy grew markedly, with estimates ranging from 8% to 24% of the population at different times during the pandemic. Unlike the situation in the

US, where vaccine hesitancy is politically partisan, this was not the case in South Africa. With somewhere between one in four and one in 10 people being vaccine hesitant across the political spectrum, this was a different problem from the one the country had in the past. Vaccine hesitancy took many different paths in South Africa, but social media was a common factor. Instagram, WhatsApp, Twitter and Facebook were the main social media platforms being used to disseminate incorrect information about Covid-19 vaccines. Given their role in disseminating disinformation in the name of free speech, social media platforms have some culpability for the consequences. Yes, we do need to actively protect free speech, but I have difficulty categorising disinformation as free speech. There is a fine line when free speech leads to harm to others, including death when not vaccinated. In anticipation that social media will play a major role in disseminating important information during the next pandemic, some action is required as soon as possible to address the problem of disinformation on social media.

A further disinformation challenge reared its ugly head every now and then, namely, the origins of the virus. I was very familiar with this issue, having spent a lot of time countering the origins of disinformation and the consequences of Operation Infektion. Several people were sending me videos of interviews on the origins issue such as right-wing US television broadcasts where individuals with little knowledge of virology and the origins of past epidemics espoused grand theories about how Chinese scientists made the virus in collaboration with American researchers doing gain-of-function research. I became concerned when I learned that a survey conducted in 15 African countries on behalf of the Africa CDC found that 27% of the over a thousand respondents believed that SARS-CoV-2 was man-made.[5] It perpetuated the narrative that the West was responsible for problems in Africa, absolving local leaders for failing to act in limiting the spread of the virus. This was *déjà vu*. I had had to refute very similar arguments in HIV more than two decades before.

Exasperated by the irrepressible flow of misinformation, I agreed to an interview with Sally Burdett on eNCA on 13 January in an attempt to help dispel some of the myths about Covid-19 generally, and vaccines in particular. I made a distinction between three types of vaccine hesitancy: those individuals who are uninformed; those who are misinformed; and those who are decidedly anti-vaccination and are often responsible for spreading misinformation, helped along by social media.

Again, I used the opportunity of a live television broadcast to remind everyone of their responsibility to provide the most accurate information possible about vaccines. I said, '… they must make up their own minds (about getting vaccinated), but if they are not sure, it's our job, all of us – the media, the public, community-based organisations, government and private sector – to ensure that we promote the most accurate information on vaccines for people to make an informed decision. Every one of us who understands vaccines has to talk to others about it. We are all agents of change and can play that role …'

It was essentially the same message I had given shortly before in a student webinar. At the close of my keynote address, I urged students to remember their role as ambassadors of truth and science in the context of misinformation. As custodians and generators of knowledge, I said, they should all be challenging fake news and conspiracy theories when they encountered them. If they are not challenged, social media, which amplifies mistruths, will ensure that such falsehoods grow and spread to the detriment of public trust in science.

In taking up this challenge of repudiating disinformation on denialism, vaccines, viral origins, fake treatments and others, I had become a target. I was regularly challenging myths and conspiracy theories in the broadcast media, press interviews, webinars and my writings. This led to a substantial backlash against me – attacks, insults, 'lock-him-up' tweets and death threats. I knew that I would be a prime target of the anti-vaxxers because of my high profile. But the attacks went deeper. They targeted my wife and daughters too. Quarraisha was also included in a three-part article attacking me. Safura's job was under threat when her boss was called by a research funder concerned about her role in Covid-19 vaccines. Aisha was receiving hate mail and hate tweets. I had never been so naïve as to think that the opposition would make it a clean fight. Fortunately, my family members never bent under the threats and pressure. They remained steadfast in their resolve. They were not going to stop standing up for science.

I personally found that the way to deal with the attacks, political machinations and misinformation during the pandemic was to understand their context and source – and simply to stick to the science. When faced with this situation, ask yourself: What is the evidence? What does it say? How does it say it? Should we have confidence in it? My personal challenge when it came to public communication was often – How do I promote an evidence-based approach without inflaming controversy? I tried to adopt this approach with ivermectin and vaccines but paid the price of severe opprobrium from some quarters. Naturally, I would do the same again. I also took this line on the issue of schools reopening and again I paid the price in the currency of political mud-slinging. South Africa is fortunate to have many scientists who are skilled in communication and who have taken up the challenge of refuting myths and disinformation. We need to go one step further. Every one of us, I believe, can be a myth-buster and an ambassador of science.

CHAPTER 30

The Good, the Bad and the Complicated

*Making policy based on science, despite its limitations, was a better
option than the alternatives of politicians making pandemic decisions
based on political advice, financial reasons, expediency or, worse, for
personal gain. But there are more shades of grey in science
than black and white.*

'The meaning of science in an age of Covid-19' was the somewhat
grandiose title of the Nobel-Inspired Lecture organised by the
Swedish Embassy and the South African National Research Foundation
in October 2020. Both countries had decided to invite their chief Covid-
19 scientists to do presentations that year. So, I joined Dr Anders Tegnell,
Sweden's state epidemiologist, for the event, which is held each year during the week of the Nobel prizes.

The lecture was held just after the announcement that Harvey J Alter,
Michael Houghton and Charles M Rice had won the Nobel Prize in
Medicine for their discovery of another novel RNA virus: hepatitis C. The
blood-borne virus had eluded isolation for over a decade and its identification enabled the development of anti-viral drugs that can now cure the
disease. Since I had done my doctoral research on viral hepatitis, I was
familiar with their research contributions and was moved by their success.
Theirs was a truly inspiring discovery, symbolising the capacity of science,
among other things, to save lives, improve well-being and serve the greater
good.

The Nobel Prize shines a light on the best outcomes and meanings of
science. But, as I explained in my Nobel-Inspired Lecture, in addition to

positive spin-offs for science during the Covid-19 pandemic, there were other, less-desirable implications for the meaning of science. You could say we had the Good (those positive spin-offs), the Bad and the Complicated.

My apologies to Italian film director Sergio Leone, whose 1966 movie *The Good, the Bad and the Ugly* inspired the analogy in my choice of lecture title. I got the idea of using a variation of the movie title from an article my daughter Aisha had written on Covid-19 vaccines the previous month, titled 'The good, the bad, and the promise of the frontrunners', as we patiently waited to learn whether the vaccines worked. In the 1960s, I lived in Lorne Street in central Durban, about 100 metres from the Shah Jehan cinema, which was the largest and grandest movie theatre in the city at that time. Low-budget cowboy movies made in Italy, referred to as spaghetti westerns, were standard fare on Saturdays in this movie house. I was a regular patron. The Leone classic *A Fistful of Dollars* was my first movie in the genre, followed by *For a Few Dollars More*. The trilogy starred a young Clint Eastwood as a poncho-wearing, unshaven, justice-seeking gunslinger. But I digress – back to the Nobel-Inspired Lecture.

I'll begin in reverse – with the Complicated.

'Follow the science' became a common refrain in South Africa and around the world during Covid-19. While it certainly promoted the importance of evidence-based decision-making, it also had the effect of elevating science to a point at which it could justify the curbing of individual freedoms. Comparisons were made frequently in the media between the progress of those countries perceived to be 'following the science' (for example, South Korea) and those perceived to be thumbing their nose at science (for example, Brazil).

All of this was done without a full appreciation of the challenge of scientific uncertainty. In reality, there was very little science to go on at the time the lockdowns were instituted. In fact, the lockdowns were implemented mainly because of the uncertainty regarding the severity of the infection. How do you have an evidence-based approach when there is no evidence? At best, we could extrapolate from SARS-CoV-1 and MERS, where the case fatality rates were 11% and 36% respectively, and early data from China indicated case fatality rates of 2.3%, going as high as 14.8% in the elderly. Fortunately, the SARS-CoV-2 case fatality rate turned out to be around 1%.

Some have argued that we should never have instituted lockdown, given the lower mortality rate of SARS-CoV-2, which became evident only after the fact. Looking at a situation or decision with the benefit of hindsight is very different to looking at it at the time when uncertainty is rife. It's the 'Monday morning coach' phenomenon: where smart alecs know exactly how the soccer should have been played and how their team could have scored several goals, when they discuss the match on Monday morning, ignoring the fact that the coach did not have this hindsight of how the opposition was going to play at the time of the match on Sunday. When we look at evidence with hindsight, we need to be careful about unfairly criticising decisions and actions taken. At the time that these decisions were made, or actions were taken, there may have been very little to go on. At the 2022 Euroscience Fair, I learned at a session attended by the chief Covid-19 scientists of several countries that such critics have a name in Belgium – 'Captain Hindsights'. These are after-the-fact know-it-alls who use the benefit of hindsight to criticise decisions that were appropriate at the time they were made.

When science is put on a pedestal, it is difficult to avoid making bigger claims than it can meet. Expectations are high, including that the scientists know the answers. Under Covid-19, we saw an opening up of scientific knowledge and we saw science assuming a new importance in daily decision-making. It became a guiding light, a demystifier.

But in reality, science is about uncertainty in the midst of data or lack thereof, the contestation of ideas, and differing interpretations; and science is not necessarily value-free. Scientific conclusions are views, interpretations of evidence and with substantial uncertainty. There are more shades of grey in science than black and white.

Having said all that, science is more objective than the alternatives. I sometimes felt that science was put on this pedestal for decision-making by the public during Covid-19 because the alternatives were too ghastly to contemplate. We would much rather have politicians making decisions based on scientific advice than on political advice, financial reasons, expediency or, worse, for personal gain. At least if you stick to the science, chances are you'll be okay. When it comes to communication, it became clear that we needed to be able to communicate to the public about insecurities regarding evidence. To make mistakes is human and if mistakes are made, it is important to self-correct. That is an integral part of the scientific process.

Among the 'Good', we can rank the greater role for science in decision-making and the rapid democratisation of science, which started with the discovery of a novel coronavirus spreading rapidly around the globe. Overnight, science moved out of musty university libraries and rarefied laboratories and into living rooms and workplaces. Real-time data on Covid-19 statistics became available to anyone with a cell phone and an internet connection. The effect on science was truly transformative – and unlike anything I have witnessed in my lifetime. Instead of being something conducted behind the scenes by a small band of experts, science had become a common pastime. In particular, epidemiology and its language became the order of the day, with terminology such as 'case fatality rate' and the 'R_0' being bandied about over family dinner tables. Every day new information about the disease and its transmission was coming to light, creating a massive amount of information. A positive effect of this democratisation was a form of empowerment – people had the ability to take greater control over their lives and protect themselves from the virus.

Importantly, this access to information served as a bulwark against the flip-side of information overload: the propagation of conspiracy theories, fake news, fear-mongering and general misinformation that tend to surface during pandemics. This 'Bad' was well known to those of us working in HIV/AIDS in South Africa, as we had first-hand experience of the way that denial, stigma and conspiracy theories tend to spread during epidemics, exposing pre-existing social fault lines.

One of the most tragic pieces of misinformation that gained traction during the HIV pandemic was the idea that having sex with a virgin would cure men of HIV. It took many years of concerted effort, even after antiretroviral treatment started to be administered, to divest some people of that erroneous and damaging belief. Other conspiracies were related to the origins of the HI virus: many people believed, for example, that HIV was made by American scientists as a means to decimate African and homosexual populations. There was even a book postulating that American scientists put the HIV they created into polio vaccine vials used in vaccination programmes in West Africa to spread this virus. There was no shortage of crazy ideas during the early days of the AIDS pandemic. Kooky conspiracy theories on viral origins of HIV were rife.

SARS-CoV-2 fared no better on the conspiracy front. In fact, it was arguably worse, given the increased prominence of social media and digitisation. The conspiracies followed a similar playbook to those we had seen in the past, particularly around HIV. For example, like HIV, the origins of the coronavirus were, and continue to be, the subject of major speculation, despite little or no evidence to support such speculation. To this day, some people believe that the virus was deliberately manufactured in a Chinese laboratory. For those who were sceptical about the Chinese having the capacity to make such a virus, the conspiracy was expanded to say that American scientists worked with the Chinese laboratory to make the virus, with further embellishments that the US government's NIH funded the American scientists to work with the Chinese to make this virus.

Others believe that Bill Gates engineered Covid-19 as a premise for a global vaccination programme that would see all vaccinees injected with tracking microchips. Still others believed that 5G caused Covid-19, a belief that triggered attacks on several cell phone towers across Europe in early 2020.[1] South Africans took a little longer to latch onto the 5G theory, but, in early 2021, four cell phone towers in KwaZulu-Natal were torched shortly after an ANC councillor sent out a voice note on social media and WhatsApp groups, in which he linked 5G to Covid-19.[2]

As I elaborated in the previous chapter, alongside an explosion in reputable scientific information, the Covid-19 pandemic became a giant

Petri dish for the breeding of misinformation, so much so that the WHO issued a warning about what they called an 'infodemic' – an information overload, including false or misleading information causing confusion and risk-taking behaviours that can harm health, create mistrust in health authorities and undermine the public health response.

With the infodemic leading the way on the 'Bad' spin-offs for science that occurred during Covid-19, we saw the eclipsing of scientific evidence to promote personal agendas and unproven treatments.

It was disappointing to observe several cases of South African professionals, including scientists, crossing the line – presenting speculation as fact – and in the process raising the risk of eroding public trust in science, not only trust in an individual scientist, but in science generally. Among these scientific transgressions was a very early suggestion downplaying the novel coronavirus, saying that it was 'just like flu' or that it was unlikely to gain a foothold and spread in South Africa because of the country's warmer climate. This notion was widely reported in the national media, even though there was absolutely no evidence to support it. Other unsubstantiated assertions included speculation that hundreds of thousands of people with HIV would die, owing to the fact that their immune systems were already compromised; that non-pharmaceutical interventions were not useful in the public health response; and that herd immunity had been achieved in the South African population after the first wave.

In October 2020, the notion that South Africa was at or close to achieving herd or population immunity after the first wave started to gain traction in certain scientific circles. For example, a scientist was widely quoted as saying that South Africa had achieved herd immunity.[3] The claim at that time was that 'a high proportion of the population infected' seemed to be based on the findings of a seroprevalence survey conducted among 2 700 pregnant women and HIV-positive patients attending public health sector facilities in Cape Town, which suggested that between 27% and 40% of people living in high-density settings had SARS-CoV-2 antibodies and, as a result, likely had some degree of immunity. (This was obviously before the second variant had been detected.) Some even argued that the stringent lockdown had exacerbated rather than mitigated the spread of the virus in high-density settlements, a postulation that encouraged a UK newspaper to report a story in October 2020 that drew an unfortunate conclusion that poverty and overcrowding may have been beneficial in helping communities reach herd-immunity protection from Covid-19.

Meanwhile, in reality, we had insufficient evidence about the extent of population immunity, based on antibody prevalence or a combination of antibody prevalence plus public health measures. For one, the Cape Town seroprevalence study was too small to draw conclusions on the state of immunity nationally or even in Cape Town itself. Mary-Ann Davies, the UCT epidemiologist who did the studies, was clear about the limitations of her data; she told a provincial government press briefing that the study could not tell what proportion of the wider population had been infected.

Population immunity is a tricky concept and estimating a threshold of immunity – that point at which the number of people in a population who are immune is great enough to stop the spread of the disease – is almost impossible, given the variables at play. These variables include, but are not limited to, the advent of new variants, individual human behaviour, the kind of vaccine being administered, as well as the length of immunity conferred, either naturally or through vaccination. For all these reasons, herd-immunity estimates are usually calculated when an epidemic is over or close to over. Attempts to measure it earlier lead to premature, inaccurate estimates.

In the midst of all the media coverage about population immunity, Minister Mkhize called me. 'Can it be true, Slim,' he asked, 'that we have herd immunity?'

I had little hesitation in telling him the hard truth: that there was no way to know this at this early stage of the pandemic. High seroprevalence rates, even if accurate, do not necessarily directly translate to herd immunity. Anyone making herd-immunity claims was doing so with insufficient evidence to support the claim. We were both concerned about a false sense of security setting in among the wider public. Even if we had some level of herd immunity, taking a more relaxed approach to infection control would be disastrous. My advice was reinforced when Barry Schoub addressed the issue at a subsequent MAC meeting attended by the Health minister and took the same approach, arguing that we did not have enough data on immunity levels throughout the country and any claims about us having herd immunity under those conditions could be very dangerous.

The hope that the first waves had led to herd immunity were not unique to South Africa. At around the same time, there were reports coming out of Brazil[4] and the following January from India[5] about possible herd immunity. A study of blood donors in the Brazilian city of Manaus, published in the journal *Science*, reported 76% prevalence of SARS-CoV-2 antibodies in October 2020, following its first wave. This led to several claims, including by several scientists, that Manaus had reached herd immunity through natural infection. These turned out to be premature when the Gamma variant wave ripped through Manaus, leading to a devastating second wave, as described in *The Lancet*.[6] The reports of herd immunity being achieved following the first wave led to greater complacency, and were followed, tragically, by a sudden and dramatic spike in infections, owing to the appearance of a new variant: the Beta variant in South Africa, the Gamma variant in Brazil and the Delta variant in India.

So, as far as possible, I tried to avoid dabbling in speculation and stuck to the science. On the rare occasions I did indulge in speculation, I tried to make it very clear that it was speculation – not fact. I was always concerned to be measured in my comments, to say what I knew to be true based on the available evidence, and to honestly acknowledge the limits of our collective knowledge about Covid-19. As a result, it was difficult for anyone to challenge the scientific veracity of my comments or my assessments. But some still tried.

In May 2020, a political commentator argued in a column that my claim that a 'severe epidemic' was 'inevitable' was wrong and gave the government an excuse to abdicate its responsibility to protect people.[7] He argued that 'a science' followed by Western countries that was anti-lockdown was promoted by South African scientists and so not everything to contain the virus was done in our country, as was the case in South Korea. If they could contain the virus, why couldn't we? he asked. He went on to argue that the science on Covid-19 was 'not as clear as we are told' and that people should stop treating 'even renowned scientists as if they are all-knowing' and ask them 'hard questions'.

I couldn't agree more about asking scientists hard questions. I had spent many hours answering lots of hard questions. Science, as I hope to have illustrated in this book, is in fact often not 'clear cut' and senior scientists, me included, are not all-knowing (and should never present themselves as such), and we definitely deserve hard questions.

However, scientists do know some things. One is that in epidemiology, suppression, containment and mitigation of disease are part of a continuum. When designing a response to a pandemic, it is impossible to single out either containment or suppression as separate goals – because the game plan according to which you reach those goals have many elements in common. They are not two distinct choices; you aim for both, obviously hoping for containment as the first prize, but knowing in reality you are more likely to reach suppression. And that reality was reflected in our 'flatten the curve' strategy: fewer cases, not zero cases. Rather than a manifestation of defeatism, ours was the most realistic strategy available considering the information we had about the virus and its spread in other parts of the world. Now that we have hindsight on the SARS-CoV-2 variants, the political commentator turned out to be wrong! While a few countries, mostly island nations, did manage to contain some of the SARS-CoV-2 variants, no country has been able to contain more transmissible variants like Omicron. Every country that chose containment has had to abandon their 'Zero Covid' policies, including South Korea. The last country that had a containment approach was China, which opened its borders and abandoned its mass testing and lockdown strategy in the midst of a massive, devastating Omicron BA.5 wave in 2022 that is estimated to have caused up to a million deaths in that country.

Moving beyond views on the politics of science with little epidemiological understanding of viral transmission dynamics, we as scientists advising on the pandemic response have a job to do and have to accept that we will be subject to criticism, whether ill-informed or not.

Looking back at the Good, the Bad and the Complicated in the Covid-19 pandemic, there are many lessons we can take forward as we prepare for future pandemics. One of those lessons for me personally is about leadership and the importance of knowing when to step down. When I stepped down from the MAC, there was substantial speculation in the media about the reasons. Although I had publicly stated my main reasons for stepping down, articles were written suggesting that I was stepping down because I was disenchanted with the government's response to the pandemic. Nothing could be further from the truth. There were five reasons behind my decision.

Firstly, I felt that I had made my important contributions and that it was time to move my focus back to HIV. After all, good leaders should know when to go. The failure of leaders to recognise this is common in Africa when individuals want to hold onto positions of authority. I also felt that the South African response had reached a point where a vaccine focus was more important. The work needed a year later had become different – a shift in focus to vaccines and variants and no longer on public health measures. I felt that other capable people were in place to continue the good work and rise to even greater heights. Just as I had confidence in the first MAC, I had a high level of confidence in the revised MAC. Also, the vaccine-related advice was in the capable hands of Schoub and the Vaccine MAC, making my contributions less critical.

Secondly, I cannot serve on committees half-heartedly. My attention, a year into the pandemic, had been shifted to assisting the continental response to Covid-19. I had been drawn into so many activities at a continental level and global level that my available time for the MAC had diminished drastically.

Thirdly, Covid-19 became all-consuming, and I was losing focus of my life's work on HIV. I had to find a better balance in the attention I was devoting to Covid-19 compared to HIV. I was involved in several HIV studies and needed to rededicate myself to our research on HIV prevention. In particular, I had an important study on bnAbs that needed a lot more time and effort.

Fourthly, while I was stepping down from the MAC to free up some time to devote to continental and global Covid-19 activities as well as my HIV research, I was still active in providing science advice and continuing my educational role within South Africa. I just did not feel that continuing to devote the large amounts of time that participation in the MAC required was still justified, given the multiple calls on my time. In stepping down from the MAC, I was not deserting my scientific roles – just my MAC leadership role – to assume a broader leadership role in providing science advice to several governments, the Africa CDC and various international bodies.

Fifthly, by deprioritising time for committee work, I freed up time to focus on a bigger contribution – providing weekly epidemic intelligence. Since early in the pandemic, I have sent out an email every week monitoring the pandemic and providing new insights on Covid-19. These epidemic intelligence reports are sent out to several subscribers across the world late on Sunday night so that they get to read it first thing on Monday morning. The weekly epidemic intelligence reports are also available on the CAPRISA website.[8] This weekly intelligence report started off as a set of slides on the evolving epidemiology of Covid-19 and over time included a narrative over and above the slides. Also, I could then dedicate some time to help the WHO Hub for Pandemic and Epidemic Intelligence, which is located in Berlin and is led by Dr Chikwe Ihekweazu, who led the Nigeria CDC previously.

With these epidemic intelligence reports, we can help avoid repeating the mistakes of the past. In South Africa, we have built up a rich repository in our scientific institutional memory, based on our experiences of past epidemics and pandemics. How we tackle the next one will be the test of how much we have benefited from the past and how much resilience we have developed in tackling future pandemic threats.

Lessons for the future

CHAPTER 31

Contemplating the paths forward

As uncertainty on the emergence of new variants remains, the availability of antiviral treatments that are agnostic to variants increase hope for the best-case endgame scenario. As we pursue 'living smartly with the virus', tackling treatment inequity is the next major challenge.

In facing a future with Covid-19, a question mark loomed large: how many more variants of concern is the world likely to witness? How would the SARS-CoV-2 pandemic ultimately play out? What does the endgame look like? In 2022, I cobbled together a viewpoint piece to provide a perspective on potential endgame scenarios:

Best-case scenario: There are no more variants of concern and, as a result, no serious new waves. Additional mutations come at a high 'fitness' cost for the Omicron variant and so do not confer on the virus major new characteristics. As a result, the virus is unable to continue to mutate to advantage. With widespread natural infection and high vaccine coverage and boosters, life in most countries returns to a semblance of normality relatively quickly, although low endemic transmission continues. Treatment that is agnostic to variants becomes widely available, minimising the threat posed by new variants.

Worst-case scenario: New variants of concern (including those exhibiting vaccine-escape abilities) continue to emerge, owing in part to, and occurring alongside, patchy and low vaccine coverage throughout the world. Pi, Rho and Sigma (the next letters in the Greek alphabet) emerge over the next few years. In order to address the ongoing pandemic and the waves of infection these will spawn, heterologous boosters will need to be developed and administered on an ongoing basis. Poor countries cannot keep up with repeated new boosters. Treatment does not become widely available, and its efficacy is diminished by emerging drug resistance. Public health measures – masks, social distancing and hand hygiene – continue to be a part of daily life.

Middle-of-the-road scenario: The Omicron variant continues to mutate with some advantages, producing a series of new sub-variants, including more infectious and immune-escape mutants, ushering in modest new outbreaks but no major new waves. Omicron then ultimately exhausts its ability to mutate without fitness cost. Vaccines continue to remain effective in reducing hospitalisation against new Omicron sub-variants. Treatment retains its efficacy across sub-variants and there is progressively increasing access in poor countries. The public learns to live smartly with the virus, and this leads to an eventual return to normalcy and low endemic transmission.

Each of these scenarios will be impacted to some extent by the fact that the world is moving into what I call the *third era* in our pandemic response, one in which effective treatment is added to the Covid-19 response toolbox. In 2022, such a treatment, a combination of nirmatrelvir with ritonavir, was sold by Pfizer under the commercial name Paxlovid. Other treatments, like remdesivir and molnupiravir, were also available but were substantially less efficacious.

The *first era* of the Covid-19 response was characterised by lockdowns and public health interventions such as mask-wearing, sanitising, social distancing and testing/isolation in 2020. Then came the *second era*, which added effective vaccines to the public health interventions in 2021. The *third era* added effective treatment to existing vaccines and public health interventions in 2022. Like vaccines, the antiviral drugs are set significantly to shift the clinical impact and trajectory of the pandemic, reducing viral replication and thereby reducing the risk of progression to severe disease, hospitalisation and death, as well as the risk of infecting others.

To grasp the potential benefits of treatment, the results of the clinical trial of the protease inhibitor Paxlovid are worth reviewing. A total of 774 patients were randomised to receive five days of either Paxlovid or placebo within three days of being diagnosed. The results were published in the *New England Journal of Medicine* and were impressive.[1] There was an 89% reduction in risk of Covid-19-related hospitalisation or death, compared with placebo. Only 1% of patients who received Paxlovid were hospitalised through day 28, compared to 6.7% of placebo recipients. In the overall study population through day 28, no deaths were reported in patients who received Paxlovid, as compared to 10 deaths in those who received placebo.

Since the original Paxlovid clinical trial was limited to unvaccinated individuals, a key question was whether the benefits also applied to vaccinated individuals. A large analysis that included 567 560 patients, of which 146 256 (around a quarter) received Paxlovid, reported that the benefits of Paxlovid in reducing the risk of hospitalisation were present in both vaccinated and unvaccinated individuals, with unvaccinated individuals deriving a greater benefit.[2] In this analysis, the benefits of Paxlovid in reducing hospitalisation was evident in all age groups above 18 years, but the scale of the benefits gets progressively lower going from the elderly to the young. The report stated, 'Fully vaccinated patients over age 50 who were treated with Paxlovid are about three times less likely to be hospitalized than those not treated with Paxlovid.'

With its high efficacy in reducing hospitalisation and death, Paxlovid could make an important difference in the hospital burden related to Covid-19. Available as pills, the treatment can be taken at home by individuals diagnosed with Covid-19, thereby deflecting potential pressure on hospitals. The treatment has the significant advantage of being effective against all variants of Covid-19. Used in conjunction with public health measures *and* vaccinations, the treatment era of the Covid-19 response is set to see disease become a manageable condition for high-risk patients.

Paxlovid enables a 'test-and-treat' approach in the third era of the pandemic response. The availability of treatment, as it did in the case of HIV, will therefore transform the way in which the disease is viewed – not only by medical scientists and practitioners, but by all of humanity.

While Paxlovid has been shown to be effective in clinical trials and in real-world implementation studies, there are significant limitations or concerns related to this treatment. The first is that people need to have tests for Covid-19 to diagnose their SARS-CoV-2 infection in order to qualify and know that they need to take Paxlovid. And after testing, they need to start treatment within three days for maximum benefit. As the advantages of Paxlovid gain traction, Covid-19 testing rates may improve because of the availability of treatment. We certainly saw this with HIV – when treatment became available, willingness to test and testing rates rose.

Second, Paxlovid gained media attention when President Biden took this treatment when he had Covid-19. Dr Fauci also took it when he had Covid-19. Both of them experienced rebound, a phenomenon where a person tests positive or gets symptoms after they've completed treatment and tested negative. This means viral replication starts again shortly after the antiviral effects of the drug wear off. In 2022, the FDA asked Pfizer to investigate whether a longer course could avert the problem of rebound.

Third, there are many routinely used medicines that are metabolised by the enzyme pathway that is inhibited by Paxlovid – this drug-drug interaction requires checking for concomitant medication and adjustment of dosages or even temporary stoppages of other medications. While the list of medicines that could interact with Paxlovid is quite long, this problem is, however, not as big as it may first appear. According to the Infectious Diseases Society in the US, of the 100 or so drugs where drug-drug interactions are possible, only two – rivaroxaban and salmeterol – produce severe interactions. Patients taking either of these two drugs should avoid Paxlovid. For the others, either dose reductions or temporary stoppages will suffice when taking Paxlovid.

A fourth concern is around drug resistance, which is a challenge for every new antibiotic or antiviral and is not grounds for not using an effective treatment. Several other antivirals are being tested for SARS-CoV-2 infection. As other antivirals demonstrate efficacy in treating Covid-19, treating patients with a combination of two or more antivirals will reduce the risk of resistance in future.

The fifth challenge is cost. The price of Paxlovid in the US at the end of 2022 was $53 per dose, that is, $530 for a course of treatment. At that time, this cost was fully covered by the government in most developed countries, including the US and Canada, and Paxlovid is provided free for all patients. Generic versions of Paxlovid have been manufactured by pharmaceutical companies in India and they sold Paxlovid at the end of 2022 in their restricted markets for about $2 per pill, or $20 for a course of treatment. It is anticipated that these costs should drop when widespread use leads to large volume production by generic manufacturers.

As the use of Paxlovid has expanded in wealthy countries, solutions have systematically emerged to overcome these challenges, enabling the widespread use of Paxlovid. But, access to Paxlovid was almost non-existent in poor countries by the end of 2022. Given our experience with vaccine access, there is good reason to expect that access to treatment will to some extent be determined by the same social and economic disparities that gave rise to and entrenched patterns of global vaccine inequity. Covid-19 vaccines threw those disparities into stark relief and there is nothing to suggest we will not see those disparities play out again in the rollout of Covid treatments, particularly in the beginning when the drugs will be in short supply.

In a press release on 18 November 2021, Pfizer announced that it had concluded a US$5.29 billion agreement with the US government for the sale of 10 million treatment courses to that country, pending FDA authorisation. The company also announced it had entered into advance purchase agreements with several other countries. Wealthy countries bought up initial stocks of Paxlovid from Pfizer – as they had done with Covid-19 vaccines. But supply did not seem to be an obstacle for treatment, as the capacity to manufacture the tablets did not have the same constraints as vaccine manufacturing. The lack of willingness and commitment of lower- and middle-income countries to provide treatment is the major obstacle. Treatment equity will not simply happen by itself. It will require advocacy and activism to challenge pharmaceutical companies, health care providers and governments to do more for universal treatment access.

There are good grounds for optimism on supply and cost. The UN-backed non-profit Medicines Patent Pool (MPP) entered into a licensing agreement with Pfizer that will allow companies to produce generic versions of both drugs – a move that will improve global supply and affordability. The deals allow the sale of generic Paxlovid in 95 countries.[3] Most of the countries included in this licensing deal are low- and middle-income countries in Africa and Asia.

The MPP's origins – as an organisation seeking to expand affordable HIV treatment around the world in the form of antiretroviral drugs – are salutary in this regard and could herald a similar treatment trajectory for Covid-19.

As new-generation vaccines and effective pharmaceutical combination treatments, the prospect of bringing the pandemic under control seems more realistic now than at any other time during the pandemic. By 'under control', I am referring to a time when the virus continues to spread and outbreaks continue to occur, but these will be mild infections, rather than a disease capable of causing serious illness, death and disruption to lives and livelihoods. On 5 May 2023, the WHO declared the end of the public health emergency of international concern (PHEIC), marking a major milestone in the pandemic. We continue to live in the midst of the pandemic with Covid-19 infections, hospitalisations and deaths still occurring, albeit at a much a lower level. The end of the PHEIC recognises that the world has entered into a new phase of the pandemic, where massive waves of infection are a much lower threat.

Viral control is not a short-term reality. SARS-CoV-2 is likely to remain a human infection for a long time. Hence, we need a simpler and more immediately applicable approach to dealing with Covid-19. Simply 'living with the virus', in my view, is somewhat defeatist as it conveys a passive approach where we would just let the virus do what it wants and accept its consequences. I did not see that as a constructive or appropriate approach. I chose 'living *smartly* with the virus'. There are five strategies that comprise living smartly with the virus.

Be fully vaccinated

Being fully vaccinated is an essential first step to living smartly with the virus, the goal being to be fully vaccinated, however that is defined in each country. From the immunological evidence available, three doses are needed to reach the peak antibody levels, while subsequent booster doses help raise waning antibody levels to the peak levels that were achieved following the third dose. Since antibodies wane after a few months, and high antibody levels are needed to stave off infection with new variants, boosters are advisable.

Know your epidemic

Knowing the level of community transmission enables a person to adjust their risk appetite accordingly. This approach is fundamental to mitigating the risk of HIV infection and the maxim 'know your epidemic – know your response' is a core element of AIDS prevention programmes. In Covid-19, if the cases are high or rising, going to a large indoor gathering like a wedding would be inadvisable. However, if cases are low, the chance that there will be an infected person in the audience is substantially lower, and so attending an indoor gathering like a wedding would be much less risky.

Prefer the outdoors

When getting involved in group activities or going to places involving interactions with people, preferably do these outdoors. For example, when eating at a restaurant, choose the outdoor option if there is one. The risk of infection is much lower outdoors.

Mask up in poorly ventilated indoor settings

When entering poorly ventilated settings where windows are closed, often for the inclement weather, and large numbers of people are in close proximity, a mask can help mitigate some of the risk of infection in that setting. Using a mask in these selected times, putting it on only to mitigate the highest risk settings, is minimally disruptive of normal routines.

Protect yourself – protect others

The use of rapid Covid-19 tests has made establishing infection status simple and quick. Those who feel that they have been exposed or are feeling ill, should test themselves. Those who test positive need to do three key things: first, mitigate the risk of infecting others through self-isolation; second, self-monitor changes in clinical status such as oxygen saturation with home pulse oximeters; and third, initiate treatments like Paxlovid as soon as possible after diagnosis to limit spread to others and reduce progression to severe disease.

With these five strategies, a person can live smartly with the virus in a way that the risk of infection is mitigated, the risk of progression to severe disease is diminished, and the risk of infecting others is assuaged, thereby slowing the spread of the virus and aiding the control of the pandemic.

CHAPTER 32

Learning from the past to prepare better for the next pandemic

To better prepare for the next pandemic, South Africa should heed the key lesson from Covid-19 of the need for a well-resourced pandemic preparedness plan supported by decisive political leadership that strengthens good governance and fights corruption.

Covid-19 was not the first coronavirus outbreak that the world has had to confront, and it is unlikely to be the last. But the key to battling future pandemics lies in following the wise words of Colin Powell, 'There are no secrets to success. It is the result of preparation, hard work, and learning from failure.'

In mid-2015, an outbreak of MERS in South Korea infected 186 people and left 38 dead. The South Korean government managed to suppress the outbreak after two months, but still faced public criticism for its handling of the episode. Chief among concerns was the government's lack of transparency, exemplified in its initial refusal to identify the hospitals in which MERS patients were being treated. Another concern was based upon what South Koreans perceived as a lax approach on the part of the national health ministry to contact tracing: when it emerged that an infected patient had attended a function in Seoul that attracted over 1 500 people, the ministry announced that it would only conduct 'passive surveillance' of all those who had attended the event. That half-hearted action did not go down well and led to the mayor of Seoul stepping in to announce at a meeting at the Seoul City Hall on 4 June 2015 that municipal authorities would take responsibility for contacting every individual who had attended the event and ensure their isolation[1] – which was exactly what they did.

In the first two weeks of June, thousands of schools were shut down across the country, hundreds of thousands of foreign visitors cancelled planned visits, and South Korea's Central Bank cut interest rates by 0.25 percentage points to stem the economic impact of the contagion.[2] The fallout went far beyond the economy: public perceptions of a poorly handled crisis were reflected in a sharp drop in support for South Korea's president at the time, Park Geun-hye,[3] and, later that year, they cost Health Minister Moon Hyung-pyo his job.

The brush with MERS shook things up in South Korea, prompting a massive investment by the government in rapid and extensive diagnostic testing and high-tech contact tracing capabilities. The latter included legal measures that authorised health authorities to access patients' credit card transaction histories and location data from cell phones so as to be able to trace prior movements and identify likely viral exposure. The country also introduced an emergency-use authorisation programme, along the lines of the system that exists in the US, to allow the temporary production and use of test kits in an emergency situation and when there was no other authorised product domestically available.[4] All of these measures would be expected to supplement the conventional interventions such as mask-wearing, social distancing and hand hygiene.

The results were positive: the next time a novel viral outbreak came its way – SARS-CoV-2 – South Korea was far better prepared, so much so that President Moon Jae-in eschewed the option of a wholesale lockdown of the sort that was in place in China, just across the Yellow Sea from South Korea, in favour of selective and temporary closures of businesses as and when necessary.

The early Covid-19 outbreak in South Korea was both swift and severe. In February 2020, South Korea was second only to the US in terms of countries with the highest number of Covid-19 cases. The first surge was linked to a large secretive religious grouping called the Shincheonji Church of Jesus, which held meetings of up to a thousand people at a time, all of them sitting and chanting in close proximity. The authorities took radical but effective action: approximately 9 000 people who had visited the church premises in the city of Daegu were identified through church records. A stringent system of testing and tracing kicked off and all of those churchgoers were ordered to self-quarantine.

The Daegu outbreak was successfully contained, but there were subsequent surges. In December 2020, new daily infections exceeded 1 000 before dropping back to half that number, which was roughly where the country still sat at the end of March 2021. Each outbreak was identified and tackled head-on, using the testing, tracing and quarantine system. In this way, small fires were extinguished and a runaway blaze prevented.

In 2020, South Korea was frequently held up to the world as a relative success story – an example of human ingenuity, learning and application prevailing over an existential threat. In an interview with Bloomberg, the health director for epidemiological investigations at the Korea Disease Control and Prevention Agency, Park Young Joon, spoke of the recognition by his agency of the need 'to approach this [pandemic] in a very scientific way'.[5] That scientific approach, underpinned by the government's financial resources and decisive leadership (as well as co-operation from the public, particularly when it came to surveillance and mandatory quarantine), played a meaningful role in the country's handling of the pandemic. Scientific capacity and insight, combined with astute political leadership, was able to produce some impressive results.

Parallels were frequently drawn between the pandemic responses of South Korea compared with the US. Both countries had reported their first cases on the same day, 21 January 2020, and both were reluctant to shut down their economies. But, unlike Korea, the US was slow to get out of the starting blocks and consistently came off second best in the media. The comparisons irritated President Trump enough for him to petulantly declare in late March 2020 that the US had done more testing for Covid-19 in eight days than South Korea had done in eight weeks. While President Trump's figures turned out to be only slightly wrong, they were still a serious misrepresentation because they were based on raw numbers and failed to take into account population size.

South Korea has 52 million people, not a small nation by any measure, but smaller than the US at 328 million. On a per capita basis, the US still lagged a long way behind South Korea – and other nations – when it came to testing.[6] The fact that South Korea had started its testing process much sooner than the US made a big difference in limiting the spread.

It clearly helped that South Korea had some past experience of epidemics such as SARS, H1N1 and MERS. The same was true for other countries perceived to have had some success in their handling of the crisis, including Singapore, Vietnam and, to some extent, Japan. But in other parts of the world, like the US and the UK, the idea of a pandemic that necessitated major adjustments to daily life and economic activity seemed difficult to digest for many leaders. At root, among some leaders, there was a sense of denial, a resistance to learning from science – or being led by science – rather than their own political acumen or agenda.

In the UK, Prime Minister Johnson boasted about shaking hands with coronavirus patients at a time when the public health messaging was encouraging people to avoid contact, while President Trump repeatedly told Americans that the virus would 'miraculously disappear' and they could get back to work.

President Trump's bungling of the US response drew much of the world's attention, particularly as the country consistently topped the list of Covid-related deaths from late March 2020 and well into 2021. But there were several others in positions of power who, like President Trump, essentially refused to accept the threat posed by the coronavirus pandemic, and, concomitantly, the science available to drive a national response.

In Africa, the Tanzanian president, John Magufuli, sported the title of the continent's most prominent Covid-19 sceptic up to his death in March 2021. President Magufuli went so far as to discourage the use of the term Covid-19 and told his people that prayer, steam inhalation and herbs would save them.

In Brazil, President Jair Bolsonaro became a poster child for the kind of poor leadership that can cause real damage. He challenged the expertise of his own health authorities, referred to Covid-19 as 'little flu' and told his people to 'stop whining'. By the end of April 2021, Bolsonaro's obsession with keeping the economy running at any cost had contributed to a death toll of 400 000, and he was facing a congressional inquiry into his government's handling of the pandemic.

In other countries such as Belarus and Turkmenistan, which have their own brand of megalomaniac leaders, concerns were raised about the deliberate under-reporting of official statistics; and in countries such as Myanmar and Thailand there were concerns about the use of Covid-19 restrictions to harass political opponents or to silence critics.

Reflecting on these wide-ranging experiences of political leadership during Covid-19, I pondered on one of the most politically fraught decisions in the South African Covid-19 response – instituting a lockdown. It was a brave decision. Some may say that it was a foolhardy decision. The scientific evidence says otherwise.

There was substantial evidence for social distancing as a Covid-19 prevention measure from a March 2020 study based on a South Korea call centre. An article in the *Journal of the American Medical Association* that showed how extensively a Covid-19 patient could contaminate a hospital room reinforced the efficacy of hand hygiene and surface-decontamination procedures.[7] We were also then starting to become aware of the role of super-spreader events and the effect of poor ventilation from a study on infections among members of a choir in Skagit county in Washington in March, published in the *Morbidity and Mortality Weekly Report*.

But these measures would not be enough. Even more drastic action was needed.

The government feared that if they failed to take early action, South Africa would end up in the same position as New York and Italy where hospitals were being overrun by Covid-19 patients. The government also knew that it could not rely solely on voluntary behaviour change – partly because in crowded township conditions, where a large proportion of our population lives, social distancing and hygiene measures such as hand-washing and sanitising were extremely difficult, if not impossible. So, a lockdown was the best measure available at the time and, as I said, I supported it then as it reduced the spread of the virus, flattening the curve and delaying the first surge. By 1 April 2020, 86 countries throughout the world had instituted some form of lockdown, so the steps taken in South Africa were being implemented across the world.

As I said previously, I was not aware of 'lockdown' as a term in epidemiology or disease control prior to the Covid-19 pandemic. Yet, lockdowns came to define the South African Covid-19 response. Part of the reason for this was a nomenclature problem.

From President Ramaphosa's initial announcement of the stay-at-home stringent lockdown in March 2020, to the lighter restrictions we experienced, as the public perceived it, the severity of the epidemic and of South Africa's response to it could be understood through the shifts and changes to various 'lockdown levels'. The problem was that South Africa's terminology when it came to Covid-19 restrictions was incorrect and confusing. No matter what the measure was, during the state of disaster, the government, media and the public referred to Covid-19 measures as 'lockdown'. From restrictions on movement to the infamous ban on the sale of cooked chicken – all of it was part of South Africa's 'lockdown'. This baffling terminology led me to try to draw a distinction between lockdowns and other restrictions by calling the actual lockdown a 'stay-at-home' lockdown or a 'stringent' lockdown, just to avoid confusion about what I was referring to when I spoke about lockdowns.

In truth, however, there are three things that must be present for the measure to constitute a lockdown. First, the country's borders must be closed. Second, there must be a stay-at-home order that limits people's ability to leave their homes. Third, infected persons must be isolated. Against these criteria, only the first nine weeks – being the five weeks of Level 5 and the four weeks of Level 4 – of South Africa's Covid-19 response actually constituted a lockdown. The remaining time under the state of the disaster consisted of varying degrees of what are more appropriately called 'restrictions' or 'public health measures', as there was definitely no lockdown in the country beyond the initial nine weeks.

When the President announced the Level 5 lockdown, there was no way to know whether it would actually work to reduce transmission of the virus in South Africa – and by how much. If any intervention had a chance of flattening the curve, a lockdown would be top of that list. But would three weeks actually be enough? The success seen in China with this approach created a positive precedent, but whether we could replicate that in South Africa was the question.

The complexity of implementing a lockdown was apparent from the outset and consistently we were forced to consider the benefits of implementing a lockdown against the substantial cost. Lockdowns were not purely about public health but about changing the very operation of society and, without question, there would be resistance to this. Nothing could have illustrated this more clearly than the news that, within 24 hours of Ramaphosa's announcement, a fringe group of anti-science conspiracy theorists had launched a challenge to the lockdown in the Constitutional Court. This case was easily dealt with.

Lockdowns have a simple premise: they reduce social interaction and thus minimise opportunities for the virus to spread. The difference between lockdowns and other measures, such as social distancing, is that lockdowns result in marked reductions in the risk of the virus spreading, particularly to vulnerable groups such as the elderly, and thus do not just prevent infections but prevent deaths. While the South African lockdown contributed to flattening the curve, the cost was high as it constrained economic activity across both supply chains and individual livelihoods. The adverse economic effects of lockdowns were felt disproportionately by low-income groups and informal workers. Lockdowns are also a blunt and broad tool – one has to lock down entire communities even when the virus may be spreading mainly in one or two areas.

There were also significant social costs to the lockdowns. Existing societal problems were exacerbated. South Africa's already high rates of gender-based violence increased, and the long-term effects of the pandemic on mental health are continuing to reveal themselves more than three years later. There were also major disruptions to critical social safety nets such as the National School Nutrition Programme, which feeds over nine million learners and which was stopped when school closures occurred. These disruptions in schooling, which persisted for two years, compromised the education and development of many learners, particularly the poorest.

Unfortunately, the Covid-19 lockdown also led to disruptions in the provision of other health care services. Elective surgeries, chronic disease care and long-term treatments were interrupted. The effects of reductions in routine childhood vaccination were seen in 2022 when measles outbreaks started occurring, due to a drop in measles vaccine coverage.

Given the pros and cons, there is no simple answer to the question of when lockdowns should be used. Simply ruling them out of order or simply supporting their uncritical use are equally unintellectual approaches to dealing with the scientifically complicated and politically charged question of whether to use lockdowns in future. Drawing on the lessons from the use of lockdowns in Covid-19, we can be better informed about when lockdowns should be used in future pandemics, recognising that each pandemic and the virus causing it are going to be different.

The lockdown conundrum has sometimes been reduced to choosing lives versus livelihoods. Implementing lockdowns can reduce viral spread and save lives while leading to substantial costs, including jobs, income, social isolation and lost schooling. While not implementing a lockdown may yield short-term economic benefits, the resulting high levels of infection and deaths can negatively affect the economy in serious ways, as people change their behaviour on their own accord to negatively impact on the economy in response to high rates of infection.

As I previously explained, the benefits of reduced transmission through lockdowns disproportionately benefits high-risk groups, especially the elderly, while the costs are most acutely felt by the young by impacting on their schooling, jobs and social activities. This is perhaps one of the many shortcomings that emerged in the economic analyses of lockdowns, as gains are often measured in terms of money or financial gains where the lives of the elderly offer less value in disability-adjusted life years and quality-adjusted life years analyses because they are considered to have little financial benefit.

But perhaps one of the biggest difficulties in undertaking this cost-benefit analysis of lockdowns is that the impact of lockdowns is hard to measure. There are no control groups that can be used to understand the ways in which lockdowns change behaviour, particularly in light of the fact that people will change their behaviour to reduce movement and risk of infection as cases rise, irrespective of whether a lockdown is in place. Even cross-country comparisons are challenging because lockdowns are implemented differently in each country and compliance with lockdown measures varies.

After explaining what we do and don't know about lockdowns, what is the punchline, you wonder. Lockdowns should be part of the arsenal of tools we use to fight an infectious disease, including pandemics. They can make a massive difference if a country acts early and hard – in other words, puts stringent lockdowns in place and puts them in quickly. China and New Zealand provide the clearest evidence of just how much infections can be halted if early and strict lockdowns are put into place – with infections reducing to zero in instances with good compliance. But they should be used judiciously and must be accompanied by a social security network to mitigate some of their negative impacts. In future pandemics, flattening the curve to buy time is going to be vital. With the availability of mRNA technology, vaccines may become available within 100 days! Existing panels of antiviral drugs can be tested in laboratories rapidly and promising candidates tested in platform trials within months. Having the full array of tools at our disposal is going to be important to slow down infection rates initially as we await vaccines and treatments, which we can reasonably expect to become available within 6–12 months.

As I think back to the Covid-19 lockdown more than three years after it was implemented, I am once again struck by the remarkably brave decision, which was appropriate, given the evidence we had at the time. South African courts have confirmed this finding in favour of the government's decision in numerous challenges against the lockdown. While hindsight is 20-20, there remains value in reflecting on both the benefits and the costs associated with lockdowns. As South Africa demonstrated, they remain powerful tools in our armamentarium for novel public health threats.

An evidence-based approach to lockdown decision-making is becoming possible as studies make their findings available. For example, a group of scientists attached to the Complexity Science Hub in Vienna published a fascinating study in *Nature* that used several statistical methods to rank the effectiveness of 4 500 Covid-19 governmental interventions around the world in reducing R_0 during the first wave.[8] The study found that the most effective interventions included 'curfews, lockdowns and closing and restricting places where people gather in smaller or large numbers for an extended period of time'. This included the cancellation of small gatherings (closures of shops, restaurants, gatherings of 50 people or fewer, mandatory home working and so on) and, interestingly, the closure of educational institutions.

Importantly, the study also found that no single intervention represented a silver bullet: no measure on its own could decrease R_0 to below one. Instead, a combination of measures that was tailored to the local context in specific countries and a country's 'epidemic age' was required. The timing of interventions was critical. Lockdowns have the biggest benefits when used early and hard. This and other studies will be invaluable for decision-makers. In the absence of a vaccine or treatment for an infectious disease, there is evidence-based guidance available, according to which a government can more sensitively balance the curtailment of freedoms with the imperative to save lives.

Among its myriad lessons beyond lockdowns, this pandemic highlighted five key elements.

First, the importance of decisive political leadership, leadership that has the interests of its people at heart but is also open to scientific advice. In instances where denial has characterised a leadership response, we have seen consistently poor outcomes. Good leadership is not a panacea – the challenges facing a country in the midst of a devastating pandemic like Covid-19 are simply too great or too complicated – but it's a solid foundation from which to launch any potentially effective response. Good leadership encompasses wisdom, honesty, empathy and openness that enhances good governance, minimises corruption and motivates people to follow the steps taken by government in its pandemic response. A critical element of effective leadership in a pandemic situation is decisiveness as speed is of the essence in dealing with a fast-spreading respiratory infection. Prevarication, endless consultations and dilly-dallying have no room in a pandemic response.

Second is a fit-for-purpose legal and financing framework for a pandemic response. Pre-existing laws providing the authorities with specific powers and provisions to act are essential, especially legal provisions for testing, quarantine, surveillance, disinformation control, border controls and vaccination. Financing provisions and controls need to be in place in advance so that they can be activated with urgency in response to a pandemic threat.

Third is business continuity planning, especially to enable essential businesses to continue operating in the midst of a pandemic so as not to compromise food production, health care and supply chains, among others. In particular, the business continuity plan needs to include steps to avoid supply chain disruption, which can negatively affect health care access and provision at a time when it is most needed.

Fourth is a social security network that includes food security for the most vulnerable in our society who are even further disadvantaged in a pandemic setting. Fifth is a pandemic preparedness plan, which is elaborated below.

All of the above five elements, based on the lessons emanating from the experiences of Covid-19, will require strengthening the capacity of the state. South Africa has witnessed, over the past two decades, a systematic erosion in the ability of the state to deliver on its promises, leaving well-laid plans as nothing more than ideas on paper, with limited capacity to actually convert them into effective programmes on the ground. Going forward, it is clear that South Africa will need to do better to strengthen its epidemic response capacity. Even in well-resourced countries, the Covid-19 pandemic has shown that there is no room for complacency and lots of room for improvement.

Recognising the likely origins of Covid-19 as a zoonosis and the increasing impact of climate change, pandemic preparedness plans need to build on the fundamental interconnectedness and interdependence of animals, humans and plants, as well as their shared environment. This 'one health' paradigm involves a fundamental dismantling of traditional barriers between all scientific disciplines and sectors in the surveillance, identification and management of pandemics.

Strengthening South Africa's pandemic response capacity is not simply about adding more infrastructure. It also means investing in its people. It needs high-level teams of epidemiologists, virologists, infectious disease specialists, mathematical modellers, behavioural scientists – a cadre of highly qualified individuals. As I explained at a Research and Innovation Dialogue hosted by Universities South Africa in June 2021, higher education institutions and research institutes will be central to the development of human capital needed to deal with the next pandemic.

The main activities of the country's pandemic preparedness plan should include: a) surveillance, epidemiology and laboratory activities linked to scientific and biotech infrastructure for the development of diagnostics, vaccines and therapeutics; b) medical countermeasures such as diagnostic tests, vaccines, therapeutics and respiratory devices; c) health care system preparedness; d) communications and public outreach; and e) regional and international co-ordination.

The NICD and the NHLS, with some support from private and academic laboratories, are responsible for pandemic-related surveillance, epidemiology and laboratory activities in South Africa. A dedicated team at the NICD, focused on these activities, is an essential component of the plan. As such, a dedicated team should be housed in a well-resourced Epidemic Response Unit within the NICD, with clear lines of authority as to who is responsible for the individual activities for pandemics. The Epidemic Response Unit will need to manage surveillance, provide guidance to the government and draw on all government departments to ensure actions are informed by a comprehensive multi-sectoral approach.

In order to ensure co-ordination across all the different surveillance data collection systems, the data from their various sources would need to be integrated into a single national system held by the NICD. This would include the systems to collect numbers of tests and phylogenetic information from public and private medical laboratories, information on emergency room visits and admissions from public and private hospitals, death notification data from the Home Affairs Department, and information on uptake or vaccines and treatments from pharmacies and other ad hoc provision points. A single integrated repository for surveillance is essential to provide analyses that are needed to guide the response.

The NICD's Epidemic Response Unit would need to have on their books a team of academics based at universities so as to be able to draw in this additional capacity when needed at short notice, because it would be difficult to establish this kind of surge scientific capacity fully in-house. The Epidemic Response Unit also needs to link directly to one or more biotechnology hubs that have the capacity and experience in developing some of the diagnostics, vaccines and therapeutics needed as medical countermeasures during the pandemic. Covid-19 has exposed vast global inequities in access to essential medical technology supplies. To correct this imbalance, South Africa needs a sustained effort in strengthening local capacity to manufacture diagnostic kits, medicines and vaccines.

South Africa did not invent any novel technologies during the Covid-19 pandemic, but local scientists played an important role in assessing new diagnostics developed elsewhere through a partnership involving the Foundation for Innovative New Diagnostics, CAPRISA and the Africa CDC. While this is an important contribution to the ACT-Accelerator's work, South African biotech companies need to be able to develop local diagnostic tests. The WHO had set up the Access to COVID-19 Tools (ACT) Accelerator as a global collaboration to accelerate development, production and equitable access to COVID-19 tests, treatments and vaccines.

Whereas SARS-CoV-2 vaccines were developed and manufactured by just a handful of pharmaceutical companies, there are vast capabilities throughout Africa to manufacture vaccines at international standards. Companies like Biovac and Aspen in South Africa, the Pasteur Institute in Senegal and Vacsera in Egypt have the potential to rapidly adapt to start making SARS-CoV-2 vaccines if provided with funding, intellectual property rights and know-how. The WHO's mRNA vaccine technology transfer hub in South Africa has produced a candidate mRNA vaccine, which needs to complete the various clinical trial phases of testing.

When I was asked what my one regret was during Covid-19, I explained that I should have put more effort into local manufacture of vaccines. Since no one else in the country was attempting to develop a Covid-19 vaccine in 2020, I should have brought a team together to work on it. Even if we did not succeed, we would have been able to galvanise interest and capacity to make vaccines in South Africa again.

Historically, several African countries have developed and manufactured vaccines for human and animal use. Until three decades ago, South Africa, for example, manufactured BCG, diphtheria-tetanus-pertussis and oral polio vaccines, making it self-sufficient for its local needs. The changing vaccine landscape, with more stringent regulatory requirements and advancing technology, made the costs of producing small vaccine quantities prohibitively expensive and weakened local production, leaving constrained capacity on the continent. Procurement shifted to a handful of large-scale vaccine producers in China, India, South Korea and elsewhere that could produce vaccines at substantially less than the local production cost in Africa.

While the country made little contribution to vaccine development until the WHO hub was established, South Africa had a huge competitive advantage in testing vaccines, stemming from the capacity built over the years to test HIV vaccines in this country. Clinical trials of Covid-19 vaccines from Pfizer, Moderna, J&J, AstraZeneca, Sanofi and others have been conducted in South Africa, a strength that South African scientists need to leverage more actively for post-trial access to successful vaccines.

With regard to local manufacture of new drug treatments, generic pharmaceutical companies have well-developed capabilities and capacities to undertake the tableting process for new treatments in South Africa, but there is no local active product ingredient manufacturing capacity.

An important initiative during Covid-19 was the establishment of local capacity to manufacture ventilators at the South African company Defy, which usually makes household appliances.

The Covid-19 pandemic highlighted the risks attached to South Africa's (and indeed, Africa's) reliance on other countries for diagnostics, vaccines and therapeutics. Increasing local investments in science and technology to build self-sufficiency in these areas needs to be part of the country's long-term plan as a step towards self-reliance. Essentially, South Africa needs to continue building its technology-testing capacity but also the capacity to move beyond testing technologies made by others to producing technologies ourselves.

Health care system preparedness will need substantial effort in South Africa. While some health care providers remain islands of excellence, many facilities have deteriorated due to either ineptitude or corruption in multiple levels of management within the health system. The public health service has been deteriorating steadily over the past two decades, due largely to widespread incompetence. Many of those appointed to lead public health care facilities have failed and simply presided over the decline in their services, leading to the downward spiral of poor leadership, which in turn leads to poor performance and low morale, and where high performers leave, thus worsening the services. In the midst of incompetence, corruption thrives. Tembisa Hospital's R1-billion corruption scandal, which Babita Deokaran was assassinated for exposing, is a case in point. And the rot goes all the way to the top; a string of Gauteng MECs (the equivalent of provincial ministers of health) had to step down in disgrace: Dr Qedani Mahlangu for the Life Esidemeni scandal, Dr Brian Hlongwa for corruption charges and Dr Bandile Masuku for PPE corruption charges. Masuku's role in PPE tender fraud was detailed in a Special Investigating Unit report. Similarly, the Digital Vibes corruption, involving National Minister of Health Mkhize, his family and colleagues, was detailed in a report by the Special Investigating Unit, which is playing an increasingly important role in uncovering and reporting on corruption by politicians in charge of health care. South Africa needs to appoint honest and capable health leaders to guide our country's efforts to strengthen the health system and implement national health insurance as a step towards universal health care, which could go a long way to building health care preparedness for the next pandemic. Similarly, trustworthy and competent health care facility leaders are needed to strengthen the health system in preparation for future pandemics.

South Africa has generally done well in communications and public outreach, ranging from providing daily data on cases and deaths to widespread access to Covid-19 educational materials to the President's 'family meetings'. Disappointingly, communications activities during the pandemic were marred by corruption, just as we had witnessed with PPE procurement. We need to learn from these experiences, consolidating the positive learnings, wiping out opportunities for communication corruption, and use the collective experiences to build a better official communications plan for the next pandemic.

And finally, the pandemic preparedness plan needs to stipulate how South Africa will co-ordinate its pandemic response with the other countries in the Southern African Development Community region, the African continent (especially the Africa CDC and the African Union) and globally through the WHO. The symbiotic relationship South Africa developed during the Covid-19 pandemic with the Africa CDC played a major role in enabling continental genomic surveillance and wider sharing of information and resources. Similarly, collaboration with the WHO has been helpful in building local pandemic response capacity.

No country in the world or its leaders can claim to have made zero mistakes in its Covid-19 response, and the five elements I outlined above, including the pandemic preparedness plan, are key to learning from our past successes and failures to be better equipped and organised for the next pandemic.

If we are to succeed in doing better in our next pandemic response, the words of Benjamin Franklin ring out: 'By failing to prepare, you are preparing to fail.'

CHAPTER 33

Science – the universal language of fellowship

As humanity, rising to the challenge of future pandemics lies in working together. Just as science has had a huge impact on the pandemic through global collaboration, so, too, governments across the world now need to join forces to predict, prevent, detect, assess and respond to pandemics.

My science hero has been Isaac Newton since I was in high school. Newton is someone whom I have admired because of the elegance of his work. His contribution was profound as it helped us understand the world. My personal admiration for Newton initially stemmed from his 'aha' moment when he developed his theory of gravity when an apple fell from a tree, which was an amazing accomplishment given that millions of other people observed falling apples with no revelations or ground-breaking discoveries resulting. As Louis Pasteur stated, 'Chance favours only the prepared mind.'

It turned out that this epoch-making situation occurred because of a pandemic! The bubonic plague led to the temporary closure of Cambridge University in 1665, forcing Newton to return to his childhood home, Woolsthorpe Manor. It was in the manor's orchard that he witnessed an apple drop from a tree onto the ground, and not on his head, as the ficti-tious version would have you believe. Newton had personally told his friend William Stukeley that this observation caused him to ponder why apples always fall straight to the ground (rather than sideways or upward) and inspired him to develop his law of universal gravitation.

For me, the apple event was just the hors d'oeuvre; the entrée was his three laws of motion; 1) an object will not change its motion unless a force acts on it; 2) the force of an object is equal to its mass times its acceleration; and 3) when two objects interact, they apply forces to each other of equal magnitude and opposite direction. In three simple rules, and a bit of maths, Newton managed to make sense of the world, initiated the Scientific Revolution – and laid the bedrock of modern physics – and that, to me, made him the greatest of all scientists. He was elected as a Fellow of the Royal Society in 1672, becoming its president in 1703, until he died 24 years later. And that is how the seeds of my dream were planted – to achieve the pinnacle recognition in science, Fellowship of the Royal Society.

As a young researcher, I had been impressed to learn that once scientists joined the ranks as a Fellow of the Royal Society, they dropped all post-nominal letters – the list of academic qualifications that traditionally follow one's name – in favour of just three short letters: FRS – Fellow of the Royal Society. These three letters superseded all others. To me, it seemed to be an understatement at its most elegant. To those in the know, it signalled a kind of apotheosis of scientific recognition. I was genuinely inspired to dream that I could perhaps one day reach that summit – and I am still humbled to this day to have achieved it.

I was elected a Fellow of the Royal Society in 2019, joining an assemblage of about 1 700 scientists from the UK and across the world who have made a 'substantial contribution to the improvement of natural knowledge'. Among the Fellows of the Royal Society are scores of Nobel laureates and many of the world's great scientists, such as Albert Einstein, Charles Darwin, Dorothy Hodgkin, Sigmund Freud and Stephen Hawking. The highlight of my induction as a Fellow was signing the bulky book that every past Fellow had signed – and I peeked in its back pages to get a glimpse of Newton's signature from 350 years ago.

Shortly after that hot summer day when Bernie Fanaroff FRS and I were inducted in the hallowed halls of the Royal Society building in London, the pandemic struck, bringing with it significant challenges, for the world, for the country, for colleagues, friends and family and also for me personally. It has not been an easy time and there have been many new problems to confront. Amid the battles to ensure that evidence remained at the forefront of our pandemic response, there have been many late nights, long calls and Zoom meetings and sacrifices made by all.

But getting to this point has been made possible by the support that comes from working in teams and global collaborations. Among these teams, the most important is the personal and professional partnership I have with my wife and fellow scientist Quarraisha. She has been a steadfast presence by my side for about 35 years, and it is a partnership that I relied on heavily during the pandemic, for her expertise, innovative thinking and support.

Then there is CAPRISA, which was founded in 2002 specifically as a multi-institutional collaboration. It started with five local and international partner institutions: the University of KwaZulu-Natal, the University of Cape Town, the University of the Western Cape, the National Institute of Communicable Diseases and Columbia University in New York. What began as a group of eight scientists with an idea to establish a research organisation focused on HIV prevention and treatment has grown into an world-class institution of more than 300 people and hundreds of global collaborators from South Africa and around the world.

I stress the contribution of collaboration to emphasise that science by its nature thrives on collaboration. By bringing together people from different disciplines, with different expertise and perspectives, especially if they come from different parts of the world and represent different cultures, a cauldron is created for new ideas and greater success. There are parallels here with findings by scientists who study the evolution of human intelligence. Studies suggest that a leap in early human capacity for artistic expression and culture may be linked to a simultaneous increase in human interaction as a result of greater population density and human migration. The same principle applies to science: the more the collaboration, the more the innovation.

The idea of science as universal is an alluring one, even if it is contested and faces valid criticisms about a historical and even current lack of inclusivity. I believe people have managed science and its benefits poorly in some cases, but on its own science is a powerful tool for everybody. When used correctly, science should be viewed in a global context for its enduring contribution to human progress and its power as a basis for mutual understanding.

Dr Mukhisa Kituyi, a Kenyan politician who served as secretary-general of the United Nations Conference on Trade and Development, wrote in 2020 that the pandemic had 'not only raised the expectations we have of science, it has also accentuated the fact that global challenges require global solutions'.[1] As Kituyi argued, international collaboration in health and science has in the past contributed towards breakthroughs and advancements that would not have been possible if countries had been working alone. These include the eradication of smallpox, the more recent containment of Ebola and, of course, ongoing efforts to find a vaccine for HIV/AIDS. Even in the earliest stages of the Covid-19 pandemic, international collaboration was evident, for example in the collaboration between Australian and Chinese scientists that produced the first genome sequence of SARS-CoV-2.

While science has shown what is possible through global collaboration, political co-operation has struggled to keep up. No one knows this better than WHO head Dr Tedros, who has consistently warned against the problems of a 'me-first' approach to a global problem. Dr Tedros sounded suitably impatient when he announced in March 2021 that the 'world cannot afford to wait for the pandemic to be over before it starts planning for the next one'.[2] His warning was a preface to some promising news: an announcement that the WHO and 25 countries, including South Africa, the UK, France and Germany, had agreed to work towards an international pandemic treaty. The proposal had progressed well to reach a first draft of the treaty by the end of 2022. While the final version may only be approved in 2024, this global treaty is intended to secure countries' political commitment to building a 'more robust international health architecture' to protect future generations.

The initiative gives expression to the reality that no single government can address a global pandemic alone. Governments need to work as part of a team to predict, prevent, detect, assess and respond to pandemics in a co-ordinated way. While the concept of pandemic preparedness involves a good measure of scientific capacity, in the case of a global pandemic it also requires us to confront and deal with inequity. For example, the ACT-Accelerator and its vaccine pillar Covax will need substantial additional support to ensure timeous universal and equitable access to safe and affordable vaccines, medicines and diagnostics.

Most of us in global health appreciate that, as humanity, our greatest hope in mitigating the impact of future pandemics lies in working together. Infectious diseases do not respect political borders. All of us, regardless of our nationality, are its targets. I hope that the pandemic treaty, reminiscent of the kind of binding agreements signed in the wake of past world wars, will go some way to plugging a gap in global leadership and solidarity that has been evident in uneven country-specific pandemic responses across the world. My further hope is that it signals an era of global leadership that oversees a universal health system built on solidarity that will serve all countries with justice, transparency and equity.

Albert Einstein wrote that whatever science produces in the hand of a human [he actually said 'man', but I have taken the liberty of updating his time-bound language] depends entirely on the nature of the goals alive within them. He went on to say: 'Once these goals exist, the scientific method furnishes means to realize them. Yet it cannot furnish the very goals. The scientific method itself would not have led anywhere, it would not even have been born, without a passionate striving for clear understanding.'

In that striving for clear understanding, science represents one of the most powerful tools we have to help change the world for the better.

That is an idea worth standing up for.

Scientific publications

Scientific publications and commission reports from
1 January 2020 to 31 December 2022

A. The Covid-19 response

1. **Abdool Karim SS.** The South African response to the pandemic. *New England Journal of Medicine* 2020; 382(24): e95.

2. Abdool Karim Q, **Abdool Karim SS.** COVID-19 affects HIV and tuberculosis care. *Science* 2020; 369(6502): 366–368.

3. Sachs JD, **Abdool Karim SS,** Aknin L, Allen J, Brosbøl K, Barron GC, Daszak P, Espinosa MF, Gaspar V, Gaviria A, Haines A. Lancet COVID-19 Commission statement on the occasion of the 75th session of the UN General Assembly. *The Lancet* 2020; 396(10257): 1102–1124.

4. **Abdool Karim SS,** Kelemu S, Baxter C. COVID-19 in Africa: Catalyzing change for sustainable development. *PLoS Medicine* 2021; 18(11): e1003869.

5. Sachs JD, **Abdool Karim S,** Aknin L, Allen J, Brosbøl K, Barron GC, Daszak P, Espinosa MF, Gaspar V, Gaviria A, Haines A. Priorities for the COVID-19 pandemic at the start of 2021: Statement of the Lancet COVID-19 Commission. *The Lancet* 2021; 397(10278): 947–950.

6. Skegg S, Gluckman P, Boulton G, Hackmann H, **Abdool Karim SS,** Piot P, Woopen C. Future scenarios for the COVID-19 pandemic. *The Lancet* 2021; 397(10276): 777–778.

7. Baxter C, Abdool Karim Q, **Abdool Karim SS.** Identifying SARS-CoV-2 infections in South Africa: Balancing public health imperatives with saving lives. *Biochemical and Biophysical Research Communications* 2021; 538: 221–225.

8. Lee J-K, Bullen, C, **Abdool Karim SS,** Bush S, Colombo F, Gaviria A, Lavis J, Lazarus J, Lo Y-C, Michie SF, Norheim OF, Reddy S, Sáenz Madrigal SdR, Rostila M, Smith L, Thwaites J, Were MK, Xue L. SARS-CoV-2 variants: The need for urgent public health action beyond vaccines. March 2021; 1–4. https://covid19commission.org/commpub/blog-post-title-three-88hdx.

9. **Abdool Karim SS,** Devnarain N. Time to stop using ineffective Covid-19 drugs. *New England Journal of Medicine* 2022; 387(7): 654–655.

10. **Abdool Karim SS.** Communicating in the midst of a pandemic. *Public Understanding of*

Science 2022; 31(3): 282–287.

11. Sachs JD, **Abdool Karim SS**, Aknin L, Allen J, Brosbøl K, Colombo F, Barron GC, Espinosa MF, Gaspar V, Gaviria A, Haines A. The Lancet Commission on lessons for the future from the Covid-19 pandemic. *The Lancet* 2022; 400(10359): 1224–1280.

12. Lee J-K, Bullen C, Amor YB, Bush SR, Colombo F, Gaviria A, **Abdool Karim SS**, Kim B, Lavis JN, Lazarus JV, Lo Y-C, Michie SF, Norhei FP, Oha J, Reddy KS, Rostila M, Sáenz R, Smith LG, Thwaites JW, Were MK, Xue L (The Lancet COVID-19 Commission Task Force for Public Health Measures to Suppress the Pandemic). Institutional and behaviour-change interventions to support COVID-19 public health measures: A review by the Lancet Commission Task Force on Public Health Measures to Suppress the Pandemic. *International Health* 2021; 13(5): 399–409.

13. **Abdool Karim SS**, Benamar T, Bhutta Z, Buss P, Cui W, Hotopf M, Low N, Sáenz R, Sarmiento RF. Call for global health data sharing framework for global health emergencies: A communiqué of the Inter-Academy Partnership. February 2022; 1–10. https://www.interacademies.org/publication/call-global-health-data-sharing-framework-global-health-emergencies.

14. Jassat W, **Abdool Karim SS**, Mudara C, Welch R, Ozougwu L, Groome MJ, Govender N, Von Gottberg A, Wolter N, Wolmarans M, Rousseau P, the DATCOV author group, Blumberg L, Cohen C. Clinical severity of COVID-19 patients admitted to hospitals during the Omicron wave in South Africa: A retrospective observational study. *The Lancet Global Health* 2022; 10(7): e961–e969.

15. Lazarus JV, Romero D, Kopka CJ, **Abdool Karim SS**, Abu-Raddad LJ, Almeida G, Baptista-Leite R, Barocas JA, Barreto ML, Bar-Yam Y, Bassat Q, Batista C, Bazilian M, Chiou ST, Del Rio C, Dore GJ, Gao GF, Gostin LO, Hellard M, Jimenez JL, Kang G, Lee N, Matičič M, McKee M, Nsanzimana S, Oliu-Barton M, Pradelski B, Pyzik O, Rabin K, Raina S, Rashid SF, Rathe M, Saenz R, Singh S, Trock-Hempler M, Villapol S, Yap P, Binagwaho A, Kamarulzaman A, El-Mohandes A, COVID-19 Consensus Statement Panel. A multinational Delphi consensus to end the COVID-19 public health threat. *Nature* 2022; 611(7935): 332–345.

B. Covid-19 variants

16. **Abdool Karim SS**, De Oliveira T. New SARS-CoV-2 variants – clinical, public health, and vaccine implications. *New England Journal of Medicine* 2021; 384(19): 1866–1868.

17. **Abdool Karim SS** and Abdool Karim Q. Omicron SARS-CoV-2 variant: A new chapter in the COVID-19 pandemic. *The Lancet* 2021; 398(10317): 2126–2128.

18. **Abdool Karim SS**, De Oliveira T, Loots G. Appropriate names for COVID-19 variants. *Science* 2021; 371(6535): 1215.

19. **Abdool Karim SS**. Vaccines and SARS-CoV-2 variants: The urgent need for a correlate of protection. *The Lancet* 2021; 397: 1263–1264.

20. **Abdool Karim SS**, Baxter C. Impact of SARS-CoV-2 variants of concern on Covid-19

epidemic in South Africa. *Transactions of the Royal Society of South Africa* 2021; 77(1): 101–104.

21. Fontanet A, Autran B, Lina B, Kieny MP, **Abdool Karim SS**, Sridhar D. SARS-CoV-2 variants and ending the COVID-19 pandemic. *The Lancet* 2021; 397(10278): 952–954.

22. Jassat W, **Abdool Karim SS**, Ozougwu L, Welch R, Mudara C, Masha M, Rousseau P, Wolmarans M, Selikow A, Govender N, Walaza S, Von Gottberg A, Wolter N, Terrence Pisa P, Sanne I, Govender S, Blumberg L, Cohen C, Groome MJ, DATCOV author group. Trends in cases, hospitalization and mortality related to the Omicron BA.4/BA.5 sub-variants in South Africa. *Clinical Infectious Diseases* 2023; 76 (8): 1468–1475.

C. Global inequity in Covid-19

23. **Abdool Karim SS**, Were MK, Pate M, Agata N, Awandare G, Amor RB, Bishaw T, Maaroufi A, Nkengasong JN, Omaswa F, Sall A, Sachs J, Sidibe M. Urgent appeal for 300 million doses of COVID-19 vaccines for Africa. 2021 June; 1–3. https://covid19commission.org/commpub/urgent-appeal-for-300-million-doses-of-covid-19-vaccines-for-africa.

24. IJsselmuiden C, Ntoumi F, Lavery JV, Montoya J, **Abdool Karim SS**, Kaiser K. Should global financing be the main priority for pandemic preparedness? *The Lancet* 2021; 398(10298): 388.

25. Sachs J, **Abdool Karim SS**, Aknin L, Boone L, Brosbøl K, Barron GC, Daszak P, Espinosa MF, Gaspar V, Gaviria A, Haines A, Hotez PJ, Koundouri P, Bascuñán PL, Lee J-K, Pate M, Frenk J, Polman P, Ramos G, Reddy KS, Serageldin I, Shah R, Thwaites J, Vike-Freiberga V, Wang C, Were MK, Xue L, Zhu M. Enhancing global cooperation to end the COVID-19 pandemic. February 2021; 1–27. https://covid19commission.org/enhancing-global-cooperation.

26. **Abdool Karim SS**, Sikazwe I. Building on Pasteur's legacy: Producing vaccines in Africa. *The Lancet* 2022; 400(10369): 2164–2166.

27. Hunter DJ, **Abdool Karim SS**, Baden LR, Farrar JJ, Hamel MB, Longo DL, Morrissey S, Rubin EJ. Addressing vaccine inequity: Covid-19 vaccines as a global public good. *New England Journal of Medicine* 2022; 386(12): 1176–1179.

28. Lazarus JV, **Abdool Karim SS**, Van Selm L, Doran J, Batista C, Ben Amor Y, Hellard M, Kim B, Kopka C, Yadav P. COVID-19 vaccine wastage in the midst of vaccine inequity: Causes, types and practical steps. *BMJ Global Health* 2022; 7(4): e009010. doi: 10.1136/bmjgh-2022-009010.

29. Abdool Karim S, Abdool Karim Q, **Abdool Karim SS**. COVID-19: The challenge of global vaccine inequity. *Social Research: An International Quarterly* 2023; 90(1): 75–109. https://www.muse.jhu.edu/article/887093.

D. Collaborative SARS-CoV-2 virological and immunological studies

30. Cele S, Jackson L, Khoury DS, Khan K, Moyo-Gwete T, Tegally H, San JE, Cromer D, Scheepers C, Amoako DG, Karim F, Bernstein M, Lustig G, Archary D, Smith M, Ganga Y, Jule Z, Reedoy K, Hwa SH, Giandhari J, Blackburn JM, Gosnell BI, **Abdool Karim SS**, Hanekom W, NGS-SA, COMMIT-KZN Team, Von Gottberg A, Bhiman JN, Lessells RJ, Moosa MS, Davenport MP, De Oliveira T, Moore PL, Sigal A. Omicron extensively but incompletely escapes Pfizer BNT162b2 neutralization. *Nature* 2022; 602(7898): 654–656.

31. Cele S, Karim F, Lustig G, San JE, Hermanus T, Tegally H, Snyman J, Moyo-Gwete T, Wilkinson E, Bernstein M, Khan K, Hwa S, Tilles SW, Singh L, Giandhari J, Mthabela N, Mazibuko M, Ganga Y, Gosnell BI, **Abdool Karim SS**, Hanekom W, Van Voorhis WC, Ndung'u T, Lessells RJ, Moore PL, Moosa MS, De Oliveira T, Sigal A. SARS-CoV-2 prolonged infection during advanced HIV disease evolves extensive immune escape. *Cell Host & Microbe* 2022; 30(2): 154–162.

32. Khan K, Lustig G, Bernstein M, Archary D, Cele S, Karim F, Smith M, Ganga Y, Jule Z, Reedoy K, Miya Y, Mthabela N, Magula NP, Lessells R, De Oliveira T, Gosnell BI, **Abdool Karim SS**, Garrett N, Hanekom W, Gail-Bekker L, Gray G, Blackburn JM, Moosa MS, Sigal A; COMMIT-KZN Team. Immunogenicity of SARS-CoV-2 infection and Ad26.CoV2.S vaccination in people living with HIV. *Clinical Infectious Diseases* 2022; 75(1): e857–e864.

33. Khan K, Karim F, Cele S, Reedoy K, San JE, Lustig G, Tegally H, Rosenberg Y, Bernstein M, Jule Z, Ganga Y, Ngcobo N, Mazibuko M, Mthabela N, Mhlane Z, Mbatha N, Miya Y, Giandhari J, Ramphal Y, Naidoo T, Sivro A, Samsunder N, Kharsany ABM, Amoako D, Bhiman JN, Manickchund N, Abdool Karim Q, Magula N, **Abdool Karim SS**, Gray G, Hanekom W, Von Gottberg A, COMMIT-KZN Team, Milo R, Gosnell BI, Lessells RJ, Moore PL, De Oliveira T, Moosa MS, Sigal A. Omicron infection enhances Delta antibody immunity in vaccinated persons. *Nature* 2022; 607: 356–359.

34. Khan K, Karim F, Ganga Y, Bernstein M, Jule Z, Reedoy K, Cele S, Lustig G, Amoako D, Wolter N, Samsunder N, Sivro A, San JE, Giandhari J, Tegally H, Pillay S, Naidoo Y, Mazibuko M, Miya Y, Ngcobo N, Manickchund N, Magula N, Abdool Karim Q, Von Gottberg A, **Abdool Karim SS**, Hanekom W, Gosnell BI, COMMIT-KZN Team, Lessells RJ, De Oliveira T, Moosa MS, Sigal A. Omicron BA.4/BA.5 escape neutralizing immunity elicited by BA.1 infection. *Nature Communications* 2022; 13(1): 4686.

35. Pooley N, **Abdool Karim SS**, Combadière B, Ooi EE, Harris RC, El Guerche Seblain C, Kisomi M, Shaikh N. Durability of vaccine-induced and natural immunity against COVID-19: A narrative review. *Infectious Diseases and Therapy* 2023; 12(2): 367–387.

Publications in scientific journals about Salim S. Abdool Karim

1. Joubert M. From top scientist to science media star during COVID-19: South Africa's Salim Abdool Karim. *South African Journal of Science* 2020; 116(7/8). https://doi.org/10.17159/sajs.2020/8450.

2. Nordling, L. Our epidemic could exceed a million cases: South Africa's top coronavirus adviser. *Nature* 2020, 583(7818): 672. https://doi.org/10.1038/d41586-020-02216-5.

3. Joubert M, Guenther L, Rademan L. Expert voices in South African mass media during the COVID-19 pandemic. *South African Journal of Science* 2022; 118(5–6): 1–6. http://dx.doi.org/10.17159/sajs.2022/12480.

4. Kimmie-Dhansay F, Shea J, Amosun S, Swart X, Thabane L. Perspectives on academic mentorship, research collaborations, career advice and work–life balance: A masterclass conversation with Professor Salim Abdool Karim. *African Journal of AIDS Research* 2022; 21(1): 86–91. https://doi.org/10.2989/16085906.2022.2047078.

5. Joubert M, Guenther L, Metcalfe J, Riedlinger M, Chakraborty A, Gascoigne T, Schiele B, Baram-Tsabari A, Malkov D, Fattorini E, Revuelta G. 'Pandem-icons': Exploring the characteristics of highly visible scientists during the Covid-19 pandemic. *Journal of Science Communication* 2023; 22(1): A04. https://doi.org/10.22323/2.22010204.

Scientific committee appointments

Covid-19 scientific and policy committee appointments from
1 January 2020 to 31 December 2022

1. Member of World Health Organization's Science Council

Invited to serve on the nine-member WHO Science Council by WHO Director-General Dr Tedros. The announcement was made at the inaugural meeting of the Council on 27 April 2021. Chaired by Dr Harold Varmus, the council provides scientific advice and guidance, including the identification of current and new technologies that will impact global health. It also provides strategic advice to the WHO on science, research and innovation in relation to the future impact of scientific developments. Dr Tedros explained that the council is part of the organisation's deep-rooted transformation embarked upon four years ago '… to strengthen WHO's scientific work, so that we are not just keeping up with the latest scientific developments but staying ahead of the curve and harnessing the best science for global health'. 'Individually you each represent scientific excellence in your domain,' said Dr Soumya Swaminathan, Chief Scientist at the WHO.

2. Chair, Ministerial Advisory Committee on Covid-19 (later Co-Chair) of the South African Ministry of Health

Appointed the overarching Chairperson (and later Co-Chair) of the Ministerial Advisory Committee on Covid-19 (MAC) that was established by Minister of Health Zweli Mkhize. This committee initially comprised 51 professionals from a diverse range of scientific and medical backgrounds to provide high-level advice on Covid-19 to the Minister of Health and the National Department of Health. After the first six months, the MAC was changed, removing employees of the NDoH or its entities and making it smaller. Served as Chair for the first six months and then as Co-chair for the next six months before stepping down.

3. Commissioner, Lancet COVID-19 Commission

Appointed as one of 28 commissioners to the Lancet COVID-19 Commission 'created to help speed up global, equitable, and lasting solutions to the pandemic'. Commissioners were 'leaders of health science and delivery, business, politics, and finance from across the world'. As volunteers, the commissioners 'work together towards a shared and comprehensive outlook on how to stop the pandemic and how best to promote an equitable and sustainable recovery in the shared belief that effective solutions can be found on the basis of global cooperation, social justice, sustainable development, and good governance that builds on public trust'.

4. Commissioner, African Union Commission on Covid-19

Appointed to serve as a commissioner on the Commission on African Covid-19 Response established by President Ramaphosa in his capacity as the African Union Champion on Covid-19. The 14-member commission is chaired by the President and deputised by the Director of the Africa Centres for Disease Control and Infection (Africa CDC), initially Dr John Nkengasong and later Dr Ahmed Ogwell Ouma. Members of the commission represent a cross-section of society, including civil society, academia, the continental scientific community, the public health sector, the medical fraternity, the private sector, and development finance institutions. In the invitation, President Ramaphosa said, 'I look forward to working with you as part of a team that will produce a report presenting a broad perspective on the impact of Covid-19 and the different response efforts.'

5. Member of the Steering Committee, Africa Task Force for Coronavirus

Appointed to serve on the Steering Committee of the Africa Task Force for Coronavirus in early 2020 by Dr John Nkengasong, Director of the Africa CDC. The task force was established by the Health ministers of the African Union when they approved the African Continental Strategic Plan for the Covid-19 pandemic. The plan established the task force to spearhead the continent's efforts to strengthen member state capacities in preparedness and response to Covid-19. The steering committee was responsible for ensuring effective development and implementation of the continent-wide strategy.

6. Member of the WHO COVID-19 Global Vaccination Strategy Advisory Group

Appointed by the WHO to serve on the COVID-19 Global Vaccination Strategy Advisory Group. This advisory group was established by the WHO to inform country targets and global vaccination goals for 2022 in light of key uncertainties, promote an equitable approach to vaccinations globally as part of broader pandemic control strategy, and inform global policy-making and access efforts, investments by financial/donor institutions, R&D groups and manufacturers, and country planning and work.

7. Elected Vice-President of the International Science Council and a Member of the Council's Oversight Committee on the Covid-19 Outcome Scenarios Project

Elected Vice-President for Outreach and Engagement of the International Science Council (ISC). The ISC is the Global Voice of Science, with its unique global membership that brings together over 200 international scientific unions with national and regional science academies and research councils. In addition, appointed to the committee providing oversight of the ISC's Covid-19 endgame project. This outcome scenarios project outlines a range of scenarios over the mid- and long term. The scenarios aim to assist in understanding the options the future may hold for Covid-19.

8. Member, Physicians for Human Rights Advisory Council

Appointed to the inaugural Advisory Council of Physicians for Human Rights (PHR). PHR shared in the 1997 Nobel Peace Prize for its leading role in the International Campaign to Ban Landmines. PHR investigates and documents human rights violations, gives a voice to survivors and witnesses, and supports reconciliation by ensuring that perpetrators can be held accountable for their crimes. It uses the core disciplines of science, medicine, forensics and public health to inform its research and investigations and strengthen the skills of frontline human rights defenders. The Advisory Council of PHR, chaired by Dr Kerry J Sulkowicz, the immediate past chair of the board of directors of PHR, advises on human rights research and advocacy capacity, to build a more powerful voice of health professionals working to protect human rights.

9. Chair, National Academy of Medicine (NAM) Interest Group on Global Health, Infectious Diseases, Microbiology

Invited to serve as Chair of the NAM Interest Group on Global Health, Infectious Diseases, Microbiology by NAM President, Dr Victor Dzau. The US National Academy of Medicine (NAM) is a non-profit organisation of eminent scientists in health that works outside of government to provide objective advice on matters of science, technology and health. The key purpose of the interest group is to bring together NAM members from different disciplines and sections to address interdisciplinary issues on pertinent scientific and policy issues related to infectious diseases.

10. UNESCO – The Next 50

Invited by the Assistant Director-General for Culture of UNESCO, Ernesto Ottone, to participate in meetings in observation of the 50th anniversary of the World Heritage Convention ('The next 50: World Heritage as a source of resilience, humanity and innovation'). The events titled '50 minds for the next 50' sets out to have important thinkers of our time from the arts, sciences, humanities and culture explore the future of World Heritage and heritage from an interdisciplinary perspective. In his invitation, Mr Ottone outlined, 'Your unparalleled expertise in the field of health will surely provide a unique perspective and a long-lasting impact on the future of World Heritage and heritage at large.'

11. Director of the Global Virus Network – CAPRISA Centre of Excellence

CAPRISA was appointed a Global Virus Network (GVN) Centre of Excellence with Professor Salim Abdool Karim as its Director. In making this appointment, GVN President, Dr Christian Bréchot, and the GVN Co-Founder and Director, Dr Robert C Gallo, explained, 'It is clear that your inspired clinical and epidemiological HIV-AIDS/TB and SARS-CoV-2 expertise, strong training programs, and global collaborations with world virology centers, will play an important part of the overall GVN mission of working to prevent and treat viral infections, and to prepare for still undiscovered viruses with pandemic potential.'

12. Co-Chair of the Consortium for COVID-19 Vaccine Clinical Trials of the Africa CDC

Appointed as Co-Chair of Africa CDC's Consortium for COVID-19 Clinical Trials (CONCVACT). As part of the Africa Joint Continental Strategy for COVID-19, the Africa CDC convened a high-level conference on the development and access to Covid-19 vaccines that resulted in the establishment of the Africa CDC CONCVACT. CONCVACT aims to dismantle the most critical barriers to clinical trials in Africa. In the letter of invitation to serve as the consortium's co-chair, Dr John Nkengasong, Africa CDC Director, said, 'In recognition of your outstanding expertise and leadership in fighting the ongoing pandemic on the continent, the Africa CDC would like to formally invite you as a co-chair to help lead efforts to achieve the objectives of CONCVACT.'

Awards

Awards and recognition from 1 January 2020 to 31 December 2022

1. John Maddox Prize for Standing up for Science

The Maddox Prize recognises individuals who stand up for sound science and evidence. Professor Salim Abdool Karim and Dr Anthony Fauci, Director of the National Institute of Allergy and Infectious Diseases (NIAID) in the US, were jointly awarded the prestigious 2020 John Maddox Prize for Standing up for Science. The prize is a joint initiative of the Sense about Science charity, and the scientific journal *Nature*. According to the judges, Abdool Karim and Fauci were chosen 'for going beyond the line of duty as government advisers on health and had communicated the complex and changing science of Covid-19 to the public and policymakers, in the midst of international uncertainty and anxiety'.

2. The Fourth Hideyo Noguchi Africa Prize for Medical Research

On 28 August 2022 the government of Japan awarded the Fourth Hideyo Noguchi Africa Prize in the Medical Research category to Salim and Quarraisha Abdool Karim in recognition of the 'Abdool Karims' global contributions in HIV/AIDS prevention and treatment, capacity development of African scientists and unwavering scientific leadership in the Covid-19 response in Africa'. The Hideyo Noguchi Africa Prize, which is one of the most prestigious by Japan, was established in honour of an outstanding Japanese medical scientist, Dr Hideyo Noguchi (1876–1928), and 'aims to honour individuals or organizations with outstanding achievements in the fields of medical research and medical services to combat infectious and other diseases in Africa, thus contributing to the health and welfare of the African people and of all humankind'. The announcement was made at the high level 8th Tokyo International Conference on African Development (TICAD 8), held jointly with African heads of state and governments under the African Union and the government of Japan, in Tunisia.

3. John Dirks Canada Gairdner Global Health Award by the Gairdner Foundation

The John Dirks Canada Gairdner Global Health Award recognises the world's leading researchers who have used rational, scientifically based research to improve the well-being of those facing health inequalities worldwide. Professor Salim Abdool Karim, together with Professor Quarraisha Abdool Karim, received the 2020 John Dirks Canada Gairdner Global Health Award. Chair of the Foundation explained, 'The Gairdner Foundation prides itself on our ability to celebrate and recognize leading scientists from around the world and we are excited to have you included in our Gairdner family of laureates.'

4. VinFuture Special Prize for Innovators from Developing Countries

The VinFuture Prize celebrates the power of science and technology to solve global problems. Professor Salim Abdool Karim, together with Professor Quarraisha Abdool Karim, were jointly awarded the prestigious inaugural VinFuture Special Prize for Innovators from Developing Countries, in recognition of their groundbreaking research on HIV prevention by the VinFuture Foundation in Vietnam. The Abdool Karims have 'tirelessly championed the importance of science in defining the HIV and Covid-19 response', said Ms Bongiwe Ntuli, Chair of the CAPRISA board. 'South Africa is blessed to have such world-class scientists whose research is making the world a better place.'

5. Honorary Fellowship by the College of Pathologists in Virology from the Colleges of Medicine of South Africa (CMSA)

The Senate of the CMSA awarded Professor Salim Abdool Karim with the Honorary Fellowship of the College of Pathologists in Virology. In conferring this award, the President of the CMSA, Professor Flavia Senkubuge, explained, 'We believe that you have not only distinguished yourself in the incredible work that you do nationally, regionally, and internationally, but certainly we recognise your enormous achievements in scientific leadership and knowledge generation in virology, strategy, and policy formulation. We further remain inspired by your seminal contributions regarding global health issues such as the HIV/AIDS epidemic and more recently the COVID-19 pandemic.'

6. Conference on Public Health in Africa (CPHIA) 2021 Lifetime Achievement in Public Health Award

The inaugural CPHIA highlighted the contributions of scientific research to the emergency health response in Africa. At CPHIA 2021, African policy-makers, scientists, public health experts, data experts and civil society representatives shared progress, best practices in public health interventions and the latest innovative research on the Covid-19 pandemic. In recognition of his contribution to science, research and development in Africa, Professor Salim Abdool Karim was awarded the CPHIA 2021 Lifetime Achievement in Public Health Award at the closing ceremony of the first international CPHIA, hosted by the African Union and the Africa Centres for Diseases Control (CDC).

7. UNISA Chancellor's Calabash Award by the University of South Africa (UNISA)

The UNISA Chancellor's Calabash Awards recognise extraordinary South Africans who have made significant contributions in shaping humanity and have shown exemplary achievements and service to our society. Professor Salim Abdool Karim received UNISA's Chancellor's Calabash 2021 Public Servant Award. The awarded was presented by the Chancellor of UNISA, His Excellency Dr Thabo Mbeki, at the Chancellor's Awards Dinner in November 2021.

8. Clarivate Web of Science Highly Cited Researcher

Each year, Clarivate Web of Science™ identifies the world's most influential researchers – the select few who have been most frequently cited by their peers over the last decade. In 2020, less than 6 200 (about 0.1%) of the world's researchers in 21 research fields and across multiple fields earned this exclusive distinction. Professor Salim Abdool Karim was ranked among an elite group of the world's most highly cited researchers, who have exceptional research influence, 'demonstrated by the production of multiple highly-cited papers that rank in the top 1% by citations for field and year in the Web of Science™'.

9. 500 Years of the Straits of Magellan Award by the Chilean government

At the opening session of the 2020 Science Forum South Africa, the Chilean ambassador to South Africa, His Excellency Francisco Berguño presented the commemorative '500 Years of Magellan Award' from the government of Chile to Professor Salim Abdool Karim and Professor Quarraisha Abdool Karim for their research achievements and scientific contributions. According to Ambassador Berguño, Chile commemorates the occasion through the recognition of innovators who, through their research or actions, have contributed to providing solutions to global needs. In conferring this award, Berguño said, 'This initiative also seeks to recognise innovation and entrepreneurship, with the aim of building a better world together …'

10. Ranked among the 100 most influential Africans

Professor Salim Abdool Karim was named one the 100 most influential Africans in 2020 by the Paris-based publication *Jeune Afrique*. He was ranked 63 in a list comprising leaders of major companies, sportsmen, artists, scientists and politicians. The publication's ranking is based on three broad categories: influence/or the ability to shape public opinion, media exposure and popularity on social networks and the dynamics of each individual's journey. 'Salim Abdool Karim became one of the main faces of the fight against Covid in South Africa, and on the continent' and for gaining worldwide recognition for his Covid-19 work.

11. The Sunday Times Top 100 Honorary Award for contributions to the South African Covid-19 response

A special honorary award was bestowed for the first time in the history of the Sunday Times Top 100 Companies to Professor Salim Abdool Karim in recognition of his commitment in guiding South Africa in the response against the Covid-19 pandemic. The Sunday Times Top 100 Companies Awards is one of the most prestigious and highly anticipated events on the South African business calendar, where leaders of industry are honoured. Professor Karim's 'ability to translate complex science into easily understandable language resonated with a nation in a high state of anxiety in the early days of the lockdown', the award stated, 'and he quickly become a popular – and even more importantly – a trusted and credible figure'.

12. Honorary Doctorate: DSc (honoris causa) by Rhodes University

Rhodes University conferred upon Professor Salim Abdool Karim the degree of Doctor of Science (DSc) (honoris causa) in recognition of his outstanding scholarly achievements and distinguished contributions in HIV prevention and treatment and for his leadership in guiding South Africa's response to the Covid-19 pandemic. He was commended for 'his commitment to science advocacy and enormous contribution to the public understanding of science. He has led the South African public to an understanding of the Coronavirus, how it causes Covid-19 and the measures of preventing infection ... He has a gift to explain complex science clearly so that members of the community are able to understand their involvement in containing or spreading the epidemic, without being patronising. As members of the South African public, we are grateful for the time and effort that he has spent doing research and keeping us informed during the pandemic.'

13. Honorary Doctorate DSc (honoris causa) by McMaster University

McMaster University in Canada conferred upon Professor Salim Abdool Karim and Professor Quarraisha Abdool Karim an Honorary Degree (DSc) in recognition of their professional achievements. Dr David Farrar, President and Vice-Chancellor of McMaster University, congratulated the Abdool Karims for their scientific accomplishments.

Media

Media coverage from 1 January 2020 to 31 December 2022

A. Overview of Salim Abdool Karim's media coverage from 1 January 2020 to 31 December 2022 from the Meltwater Media Intelligence Report and Newsclip

The summary analysis below is from the Meltwater Media Intelligence Report and Newsclip Surveillance*. It emanates from tracking and monitoring media coverage of 'Salim Abdool Karim' on local and global online platforms, local print media, local broadcast media and social media platforms. News sources include major news outlets, trade publications, local and regional journals and weekly newspapers, as well as television and radio transcripts.

Summary analysis of Salim Abdool Karim's online, print, television and radio media coverage from 1 January 2020 to 31 December 2022 (36 months):

❑ 2 865 print media articles (~3 per day)
❑ 3 210 broadcasts (TV and radio) (~3 per day)
❑ 13 249 online articles (~12 per day)
❑ Average: ~18 media stories on TV, radio, online or in print, each day for 36 months
❑ 61% of print, broadcast and online media coverage is from outside South Africa –
  ▪ Top 5 countries: United States, United Kingdom, Vietnam, India and Canada
❑ ~58 192 social media mentions (~53 per day)

Meltwater is the world's first international online media monitoring company – it was founded in Norway and is headquartered in the USA with offices across Europe, North America, Asia/Pacific, Australia and Africa. The Meltwater Media Intelligence Report and Newsclip service provide a line listing of all print articles, online articles, radio broadcasts and television appearances that involve or mention Salim Abdool Karim.

B. A selection of Salim Abdool Karim's print, online and broadcasting media coverage from 1 January 2020 to 31 December 2022

Print and Online Media

1. **Andrew Harding**, Coronavirus: South Africa braces for the worst, *BBC*. 19 March 2020. https://www.bbc.com/news/world-africa-51949125.

2. **Rudolph Nkgadima**, South Africans bow to a great mind at work, *Daily News*. 15 April 2020. https://www.pressreader.com/south-africa/daily-news-south-africa/20200415/-281659667171039.

3. **Sarah Evans**, Slim: The life, times and education of Salim Abdool Karim, *News24*. 16 April 2020. https://www.news24.com/news24/Analysis/slim-the-life-times-and-education-of- salim-abdool- karim-20200416.

4. **Zimasa Matiwane**, Salim Abdool Karim: The man outsmarting Covid-19, *Sunday Times*. 19 April 2020. https://www.caprisa.org/DBFile/Files/23958d21-3fd8-480a-af06-7eca0851d453/Sunday%20Times%20%20Outsmating%20corona%2019%20April%202020.pdf.

5. **Ivan Fallon**, Coronavirus in South Africa: 'The biggest issue is not the outbreak – it's hunger', *The Times*. 26 April 2020. https://www.thetimes.co.uk/article/coronavirus-in-south-africa-the-biggest-issue-is-not-the-outbreak-its-hunger-tdqmmmg96.

6. **Gezzy S Sibisi**, In expert hands, *YOU* magazine. 30 April 2020. https://www.caprisa.org/DBFile/Files/5779ef3c-0549-4d97-915d-28442e309001/You%20-%20You%20-%2030%20Apr%202020%20-%20p.15.pdf.

7. **Nicci Botha**, #OnTheFrontLine with the Abdool Karims, *BizCommunity*. 4 May 2020. https://www.caprisa.org/DBFile/Files/2ab52584-b9ba-4b64-bcce-3e6373e53367/OnTheFrontLine%20with%20the%20Abdool%20Karims%20-%20Bizcommunity%20-%204%20May%202020.pdf.

8. **Salim Abdool Karim**, Covid-19: Sailing a ship while building it, *Sunday Times*. 31 May 2020. https://www.timeslive.co.za/sunday-times/opinion-and-analysis/2020-05-31-covid-19-pandemic-sailing-a-ship-while-building-it/.

9. **Kuben Chetty**, Convert anxiety to action, *Pretoria News*. 29 June 2020. https://www.pressreader.com/south-africa/pretoria-news-weekend/20200620/281479278669583.

10. **SANews**, Karim warns of possible second wave as COVID-19 cases decline, *South African Government News Agency*. 26 August 2020. https://www.sanews.gov.za/south-africa/karim-warns-possible-second-wave-covid-19-cases-decline.

11. **Andrew Harding**, Coronavirus in South Africa: Relief, pride and the 'new normal', *BBC*. 19 September 2020. https://www.bbc.com/news/world-africa-54207503.

12. **Suthentira Govender**, Did South Africa get it right when tackling the pandemic, *Sunday Times*. 20 September 2020. https://www.timeslive.co.za/sunday-times/news/2020-09-20-did-sa-get-it-right-when-tackling-the-coronavirus-pandemic/.

13. Q&A with Professor Salim Abdool Karim, *Gavi, the Vaccine Alliance*. 5 October 2020. https://www.gavi.org/vaccineswork/qa-professor-salim-karim.

14. **Lynette Dicey**, A steadfastly honest path, *Sunday Times*. 15 November 2020. https://arenaevents.africa/events/sunday-times-top-100-companies/wp-content/uploads/2021/01/Sunday-Times-Top-100-Supplement-2020.pdf.

15. **Cristina Serra**, COVID-19 and South Africa: Communication is key, *TWAS*. 18 November 2020. https://twas.org/article/covid-19-and-south-africa-communication-key#:~:text=Building%20trust%20in%20scientists%20and,Karim%20at%20ESOF%20in%20Trieste.\.

16. **Karen Singh**, Abdool Karim receives international award for standing up for science, *The Mercury*. 15 December 2020. https://www.iol.co.za/mercury/news/professor-abdool-karim-and-dr-anthony-fauci-receive-international-award-for-standing-up-for-science-ec5c121d-fa9b-45bb-b915-492b886d2ec0.

17. **Witness Reporter**, South Africa's Karim, U.S.'s Fauci honoured for work during Covid-19, *The Witness*. 16 December 2020. https://www.news24.com/witness/news/south-africas-karim-uss-fauci-honoured-for-work-during-covid-19-20201216.

18. **The Presidency**, President congratulates Prof Salim Abdool Karim on John Maddox Prize, press statement. 17 December 2020. https://www.presidency.gov.za/press-statements/president-congratulates-prof-salim-abdool-karim-john-maddox-prize.

19. **Haru Mutasa**, South Africa facing isolation amid fears over new COVID strain, *Al Jazeera*. 12 December 2020. https://www.aljazeera.com/news/2020/12/22/south-africa-says-virus-variant-driving-resurgence.

20. **Zoe Corbyn**, Salim Abdool Karim: 'None of us are safe from Covid if one of us is not. We have mutual interdependence', *The Guardian*. 10 January 2021. https://www.theguardian.com/world/2021/jan/10/salim-abdool-karim-none-of-us-are-safe-from-covid-if-one-of-us-is-not-we-have-mutual-interdependence?CMP=Share_AndroidApp_Other.

21. **Andrew Harding**, Hogging Covid vaccines endangers all nations, warns South Africa expert, *BBC*. 27 January 2021. https://www.bbc.com/news/world-africa-55825559.

22. **Zakiyah Ebrahim and Kyle Cowan**, 'Calling it the SA variant is a stigmatising approach' – Prof Salim Abdool Karim on 501Y.V2, *News24*. 4 February 2021. https://www.news24.com/news24/southafrica/investigations/covid19/calling-it-the-sa-variant-is-a-stigmatising-approach-prof-salim-abdool-karim-on-501yv2-20210204.

23. **Ivan Fallon**, Variant? What Covid variant? South Africa shrugs off infections to hit the beach, *The Times*. 7 February 2021. https://www.thetimes.co.uk/article/variant-what-covid-variant-south-africa-shrugs-off-infections-to-hit-the-beach-bgxqlpwx0.

24. **Chris Smyth and Tom Whipple**, Concerns have been raised about the vaccine's effectiveness against the South African coronavirus variant, *The Times*. 8 February 2021. https://www.thetimes.co.uk/article/autumn-jab-to-ward-off-mutant-coronavirus-strains-x6sd0mgvk.

25. **Laura Spinney**, What can we learn from Africa's experience of Covid? *The Guardian*. 28 February 2021. https://www.theguardian.com/world/2021/feb/28/what-can-we-learn-from-africa-experience-of-covid-death-toll-paradox.

26. **Tebogo Monama**, Covid-19 one year on: 'First wave was like Kilimanjaro, the second like Everest' – Prof Karim, *News24*. 5 March 2021. https://www.news24.com/news24/

southafrica/news/covid-19-one-year-on-first-wave-was-like-kilimanjaro-the-second-like-everest-prof-karim-20210305.

27. **Carlos Amato**, South Africa's voice of reason. *The Witness*. 9 March 2021. https://www.caprisa.org/DBFile/Files/63c93713-e307-4e22-8ef1-d7c5ab0c9e66/South%20Africas%20Voice%20of%20Reason%20The%20Witness%209%20March%202021.pdf.

28. **Kuben Chetty**, We acted bravely: Prof Abdool Karim reflects on SA's Covid-19 milestones and challenges, *IOL*. 14 March 2021. https://www.iol.co.za/news/politics/we-acted-bravely-prof-abdool-karim-reflects-on-sas-covid-19-milestones-and-challenges-ed57e93d-794c-4bda-9b93-28b5aa5945e7.

29. **Nicole McCain**, Professor Salim Abdool Karim announces end of term as co-chair of Covid-19 advisory committee, *News24*. 25 March 2021. https://www.news24.com/news24/southafrica/news/professor-salim-abdool-karim-announces-end-of-term-as-co-chair-of-covid-19-advisory-committee-20210325.

30. **Kyle Cowan**, First take: Prof Salim Abdool-Karim: A complex legacy, but we owe him our gratitude, *News24*. 25 March 2021. https://www.news24.com/news24/analysis/first-take-prof-salim-abdool-karim-a-complex-legacy-but-we-owe-him-our-gratitude-20210325.

31. **Pumza Fihlani**, Ivermectin: South African medics using unproven worm drug to treat Covid-19, *BBC*. 27 March 2021. https://www.bbc.com/news/world-africa-56526632.

32. **Carl Zimmer**, Scientists warn US lawmakers about the continued threat of coronavirus variants, *The New York Times*. 13 May 2021. https://foster.house.gov/media/in-the-news/scientists-warn-us-lawmakers-about-the-continued-threat-of-coronavirus-variants.

33. **Sam Bradpiece**, South Africa's third COVID wave could be the worst yet, *Al Jazeera*. 29 June 2021. https://www.aljazeera.com/news/2021/6/29/south-africas-third-wave-set-to-be-the-worst-yet.

34. **Estelle Ellis**, Should anti-vaxxers working in key sectors submit to mandatory weekly Covid-19 tests? *Daily Maverick*. 25 August 2021. https://www.dailymaverick.co.za/article/2021-08-25-should-anti-vaxxers-working-in-key-sectors-submit-to-mandatory-weekly-covid-19-tests/.

35. **Kelly-Jane Turner**, Inevitable Covid-19 fourth wave predicted for early December – Professor Salim Abdool Karim, *IOL*. 18 August 2021. https://www.iol.co.za/news/covid19/inevitable-covid-19-fourth-wave-predicted-for-early-december-professor-salim-abdool-karim-f34f16fa-440c-4906-af58-18ccfc31144f

36. **Mark Heywood**, Human rights in the response to Covid-19: Are we getting it right? *Daily Maverick*. 24 August 2021. https://www.youtube.com/watch?v=-bmbDhFxagw&t=6s.

37. **Edwin Naidu**, Covid-19: Human rights go hand-in-hand with saving lives, *IOL*. 19 September 2021. https://www.iol.co.za/sundayindependent/news/covid-19-human-rights-go-hand-in-hand-with-saving-lives-09b43d5b-c782-4d83-9b22-9db072a9ad50.

38. **Zainul Dawood**, Epidemiologist Professor Salim Abdool Karim to receive Rhodes honour, *IOL*. 25 October 2021. https://www.iol.co.za/dailynews/news/kwazulu-natal/epidemiologist-professor-salim-abdool-karim-to-receive-rhodes-honour-38593170-3957-4eaa-a4fb-e6c6f961bd99.

39. **Catherine Namirembe**, We need coordinated approach to fight Covid-19 – Prof. Karim, Saturday Vision – Uganda. 13 November 2021. https://www.caprisa.org/DBFile/Files/18ceaace-486b-46ef-a384-9943e3b4e968/Saturday%20Visions%2013%20Nov%202021%20We%20need%20coordinated%20approach%20to%20fight%20covid-19.jpg.

40. **Salim Abdool Karim and Safura Abdool Karim**, Punishing South Africa will harm global pandemic response, *The Times*. 30 November 2021. https://www.thetimes.co.uk/article/punishing-south-africa-will-harm-global-pandemic-response-lvrjk8mkp.

41. **Unathi Nkanjeni**, Prof Abdool Karim says future Covid-19 variants are likely to be 'much weaker' than Omicron, *Times Live*. 13 January 2022. https://www.timeslive.co.za/news/south-africa/2022-01-13-prof-abdool-karim-says-future-covid-19-variants-are-likely-to-be-much-weaker-than-omicron/.

42. **Special Report by Nature journal**, African scientists race to test COVID drugs but face major hurdles, *The Guardian*. 3 February 2022. https://guardian.ng/features/science/african-scientists-race-to-test-covid-drugs-but-face-major-hurdles/?fbclid=IwAR0hbxLxSZtdSpnVg5Rf2GKIFuXg31YMuY0VIKwk7eYHy2Zsge3Qysmq6Gg.

43. **BusinessTech Staff Writer**, When the fifth Covid-19 wave is expected to hit South Africa: Expert, *BusinessTech*. 15 February 2022. https://businesstech.co.za/news/trending/558410/when-the-fifth-covid-19-wave-is-expected-to-hit-south-africa-expert/.

44. **Suthentira Govender**, We did more things right than wrong: Prof Salim Abdool Karim, *Sunday Times*. 3 March 2022. https://www.timeslive.co.za/sunday-times-daily/news/2022-03-03-we-did-more-things-right-than-wrong-prof-salim-abdool-karim/.

45. **Jonisayi Maromo**, Rhodes honours leading epidemiologist, Prof Quarraisha Abdool Karim and her husband Prof Salim Abdool Karim, *IOL*. 8 April 2022. https://www.iol.co.za/education/rhodes-honours-leading-epidemiologist-prof-quarraisha-abdool-karim-and-her-husband-prof-salim-abdool-karim-73d62132-c899-419f-9f88-92c825623da6?fbclid=IwAR2bGHQxYCsw5XtDOrN6Kg8fVmpgjcHSGqJ31ixpRrcDXtrl_kQqpHh3sP8.

46. **Linda Nordling and Gilbert Nakweya**, Standout voices in African public health, *Harvard Public Health*. 12 May 2022. https://harvardpublichealth.org/global-health/25-names-to-know-in-african-public-health/.

47. **Katherine J. Wu**, You are going to get COVID again … and again … and again, *The Atlantic*. 27 May 2022. https://www.theatlantic.com/health/archive/2022/05/covid-reinfection-research-immunity/639436/.

48. **Lebogang Mashego**, Leading HIV expert in South Africa, Prof Karim explains why there's no HIV vaccine yet, *Briefly*. 24 June 2022. https://briefly.co.za/editorial/

explainer/129976-explained-leading-hiv-expert-in-south-africa-prof-karim-explains-why-we-are-not-getting-hiv-vaccine-yet/?utm_source=facebook&utm_medium=ps&-fbclid=IwAR0PWIKiplycDEsxBsgSgAlsOxlkyXc0P1c0Ync9sBvpJrvITJg9vOxQ mhk.

49. **Alicia James**, Who were the expert voices during the COVID-19 pandemic? *University World News*. 30 June 2022. https://www.universityworldnews.com/post. php?story=20220627205743444.

50. **Suthentira Govender**, Japan to honour SA's spouse scientists for HIV and Covid-19 work, *TimesLive*. 3 August 2022. https://www.timeslive.co.za/news/south-africa/2022-08-03-japan-to-honour-sas-spouse-scientists-for-hiv-and-covid-19-work/?utm_term=Autofeed&utm_medium=Social&utm_source=Twitter#Echo box=1659520457.

51. **Tamar Kahn**, Top scientist warns doctors still prescribing ineffective Covid-19 treatments, *Business Day*. 17 August 2022. https://www.businesslive.co.za/bd/national/health/2022-08-17-top-scientist-warns-doctors-still-prescribing-ineffec-tive-covid-19-treatments/?utm_medium=Social&utm_source=Facebook&fbcli d=IwAR1gk2MeY96tKLTxcVxbZjhnloJmToge2VTEK4I-nWEXzE5TqYTE WCO_xVo#Echobox=1660770964.

52. **Ben Farmer**, 'The pandemic is far from over – but this is how it ends', *The Telegraph*. 4 October 2022. https://www.telegraph.co.uk/global-health/science-and-disease/south-africas-top-covid-expert-reveals-how-pandemic-might-end/?fbclid=IwAR1YVxZVjg1SB4 sPGMDAhiAK3RGIQv-bqcgw39lw3JU7-SiiQnOfTxxjZbg.

53. **Jeffrey V Lazarus, et al.**, A multinational Delphi consensus to end the COVID-19 public health threat, *Nature*. 3 November 2022. https://www.nature.com/articles/s41586-022-05398-2.

54. **Katherine J. Wu**, Will we get Omicron'd again? *The Atlantic*. 10 November 2022. https://www.theatlantic.com/health/archive/2022/11/covid-new-variant-winter-wave-omicron-mutation/672075/.

55. **Meredith Wadman**, Small victories, *Science*. 22 November 2022. https://www.science. org/content/article/small-victories-south-africa-struggling-improve-kids-health-decades-apartheids-demise.

56. **Salim Abdool Karim and Quarraisha Abdool Karim**, Ending AIDS for the next generation, *CNBC Africa*. 1 December 2022.https://www.cnbcafrica.com/2022/ending-aids-for-the-next-generation/.

57. **Sameer Naik, Karishma Dipa and Norman Cloete**, Health experts call for calm amid new 'vicious' Covid-19 strain, *IOL*. 3 December 2022.https://www.iol.co.za/saturday-star/news/health-experts-call-for-calm-amid-new-vicious-covid-19-strain-12f47bb6-9646-4e28-bff1-51afcf808d9e.

58. **Salim Abdool Karim and Quarraisha Abdool Karim**, Rising to the challenges of Aids, *IOL*. 4 December 2022. https://www.iol.co.za/news/politics/opinion/

rising-to-the-challenges-of-aids-d92ee578-d023-44ea-873e-f6b90424e168.

59. **Katherine J. Wu**, China's Covid wave is coming, *The Atlantic*. 6 December 2022. https://www.theatlantic.com/health/archive/2022/12/china-zero-covid-wave-immunity-vaccines/672375/.

60. **Estelle Ellis**, Should we stress about Covid-19 this holiday season? Relax, but not too much – experts, *Daily Maverick*. 8 December 2022. https://www.dailymaverick.co.za/article/2022-12-08-should-we-stress-about-covid-19-this-holiday-season-relax-but-not-too-much-experts/.

61. **Wang Xiang**, The surge of Beijing 120 emergency calls is mild or asymptomatic, *Epoch Times*. 10 December 2022. https://www.epochtimes.com/b5/22/12/10/n13882340.htm.

62. **Estelle Ellis**, Sahpra mulls over application to register anti-Covid drug from Pfizer, *Daily Maverick*. 12 December 2022. https://www.dailymaverick.co.za/article/2022-12-12-sah-pra-mulls-over-application-to-register-anti-covid-drug-from-pfizer/.

63. **Nike Adebowale-Tambe**, CPHIA 2022: African leaders, experts meet in Rwanda to appraise public health, *Times Live*. 13 December 2022. https://www.premiumtimesng.com/news/top-news/570325-cphia-2022-african-leaders-experts-meet-in-rwanda-to-appraise-public-health.html.

64. WHO, WIPO, WTO call for innovation and cooperation to support timely access to pandemic products, *Reliefweb*. 19 December 2022. https://reliefweb.int/report/world/who-wipo-wto-call-innovation-and-cooperation-support-timely-access-pandemic-products.

Broadcasting – TV and Radio

1. **Stephen Grootes**, Will the lockdown help flatten the spread of the virus? *Newzroom Afrika*. 9 April 2020. https://www.youtube.com/watch?v=8whEiUHw1Sc.

2. Ministerial Advisory Committee chairperson, Professor Salim Abdool Karim, full presentation on Coronavirus in South Africa, *eNCA*. 14 April 2020. https://www.youtube.com/watch?v=OQ8qb7eGS8c.

3. **Andrew Harding**, Coronavirus: Why South Africa is coming out of lockdown, *BBC*. 1 May 2020. https://www.youtube.com/watch?v=wYHbpaCq8EA.

4. South African epidemiologist Salim Abdool Karim speaks to DW, *DW*. 19 June 2020. https://www.dw.com/en/south-african-epidemiologist-salim-abdool-karim-speaks-to-dw/av-53877315.

5. Listen to the experts, Who gets the vaccine first? Prof Salim Abdool Karim answers, *SA Coronavirus*. 22 December 2020. https://www.youtube.com/watch?v=R2wPeJDESOQ.

6. **Sally Burdett**, Update on SA infections: Prof Karim talks on COVID-19 tests in SA, *eNCA*. 7 August 2020. https://youtu.be/8s-ZAujV5xI.

7. **Andrew Meldrum**, AP interview: South Africa to know true virus toll in weeks, *ABC News*. 18 September 2020. https://abcnews.go.com/Health/wireStory/ap-interview-south-africa-true-virus-toll-weeks-73090239.

8. **Gugulethu Mfuphi**, Top 100 companies in South Africa for 2020, *Sunday Times*. 16 November 2020. https://www.youtube.com/watch?v=Inq_AJw1qoo.

9. **Karima Brown**, Second wave of COVID-19 infections, *eNCA*. 13 December 2020. https://www.facebook.com/watch/?v=163930512145732.

10. **Esau Williams**, South African epidemiologist awarded for 'standing up for science', *BBC*. 16 December 2020. https://www.bbc.co.uk/programmes/p091ms1n.

11. **Michelle Roberts**, New variant South African Covid spreading 'far faster', *BBC*. 12 January 2021. https://www.bbc.com/news/av/world-africa-55633274.

12. COVID-19: What we do know, *Carte Blanche*. 18 January 2021. https://www.youtube.com/watch?v=xhTVvNWh5OE.

13. **Alisyn Camerota**, Prof Salim Abdool Karim clears the air over Covid-19 SA variant, *CNN*. 5 February 2021. https://twitter.com/tomselliott/status/1356932445556375553?ref_src=twsrc%5Etfw%7Ctwcamp%5Etweetembed%7Ctwterm%5E1356932445556375553%7Ctwgr%5E%7Ctwcon%5Es1_&ref_url=https%3A%2F%2Fbriefly.co.za%2F94578-prof-salim-abdool-karim-clears-air-covid-19-sa-variant.html.

14. **John Perlman**, Covid-19 in South Africa: One year later, *Radio 702*, *The John Perlman Show*. 4 March 2021. https://omny.fm/shows/afternoon-drive-702/covid-19-in-south-africa-one-year-later#description.

15. **Faith Mangope**, Professor Salim Abdool Karim has completed his term as co-chair of the Ministerial Advisory Committee, *eNCA*. 25 March 2021. https://www.youtube.com/watch?v=zd5VsfBBNaM.

16. **Melanie Rice**, Prof Salim Abdool Karim steps down, *eTV*. 25 March 2021. https://www.etv.co.za/news/prof-salim-abdool-karim-steps-down.

17. **Nurith Aizenman**, Can vaccines stop variants? Here's what we know so far, *National Public Radio*. 9 April 2021. https://www.npr.org/sections/ goatsandsoda/2021/04/09/985745837/can-vaccines-stop-variants-heres-what-we-know-so-far.

18. **Roxana Rustomjee**, South Africa's response to COVID-19, *Sabin Vaccine Institute*. 20 April 2021. http://ow.ly/ZLHY50EtsCX.

19. **Mark Heywood**, Ending Covid means ending Aids, and ending both means ending inequality, *Daily Maverick*. 14 June 2021. https://www.dailymaverick.co.za/article/2021-06-14-ending-covid-means-ending-aids-and-ending-both-means-ending-inequality/.

20. **Nurith Aizenman**, Protecting the immuno-compromised against COVID could be key to ending the pandemic, *National Public Radio*. 28 June 2021. https://www.npr.org/sections/goatsandsoda/2021/06/28/1011043650/the-key-to-ending-the-pandemic-may-be-protecting-immunocompromised-people.

21. **Arnold Kwizera**, How to build robust healthcare systems in Africa, *CNBC Africa*. 8 September 2021. https://www.youtube.com/watch?v=gZSmGQe4rjs.

22. **Eyder Peralta**, Research shows this drug shouldn't be used for COVID-19, but in South Africa many do, *National Public Radio*. 13 September 2021. https://www.npr.

org/2021/09/13/1036533173/despite-warnings-south-africans-re-using-an-animal-medication-to-treat-covid-19.

23. **Francis Heard**, SA's readiness for COVID-19 4th wave with Prof. Salim Abdool Karim, *SABC News*. 20 October 2021. https://youtu.be/0zzb1zyXf7w.

24. **Becky Anderson**, Why epidemiologist says he's 'quite worried' about new variant? *CNN*. 26 November 2021. https://www.youtube.com/watch?v=sbc8jPAVksM.

25. **Vishnu Som**, African Covid panel member on Omicron, *NDTV*. 1 December 2021. https://www.ndtv.com/video/news/left-right-centre/omicron-covid-variant-african-covid-panel-member-on-omicron-611382.

26. **National Department of Health Media Briefing**, What we know about Omicron Variant, *SABC News*. 29 November 2021. https://youtu.be/bljc6nop0jQ.

27. **Kenichi Serino**, 'Outrageous and an overreaction,' South Africa's top epidemiologist on omicron travel ban, *PBS News Hour*. 3 December 2021. https://youtu.be/gqdDEhfHvZQ.

28. **Jonathan Chang and Meghna Chakrabarti**, What we know about the Omicron variant and the pandemic in South Africa, *National Public Radio*. 7 December 2021. https://www.wbur.org/onpoint/2021/12/07/what-we-know-about-the-omicron-variant-and-the-state-of-the-pandemic-in-south-africa.

29. **Scott Tong**, South African doctors gain insight into 2-week-old omicron variant, *National Public Radio*. 7 December 2021. https://www.wbur.org/hereandnow/2021/12/07/omicron-variant-south-africa.

30. **Stephen Grootes**, Covid-19 in SA and globally, *SA FM Sunrise show*. 12 January 2022. https://www.youtube.com/watch?v=x-msCsMiQrU.

31. **Bongani Bingwa**, Professor Salim Abdool Karim gives more insight on the new detected variant, *Radio 702 Breakfast show*. 12 January 2022. https://www.youtube.com/watch?v=OnR9REp9UaI.

32. **Thabiso Tema**, Prof Salim Abdool Karim gives Covid-19 update, *Power FM Breakfast show*. 15 February 2022. https://youtu.be/sf7NOE_ti3s.

33. **Martin Bester**, Listen: Prof Salim Abdool Karim gives COVID-19 update, *Jacaranda FM News*. 15 February 2022. https://www.jacarandafm.com/breakfast-martin-bester/listen-prof-salim-abdool-karim-gives-covid-19-update/.

34. **O'Neil Nair**, Prof Karim update – Covid-19 fifth wave, *Lotus FM*. 2 March 2022. https://omny.fm/shows/the-breakfast-xpress/prof-karim-update-covid19-fifth-wave.

35. **Michelle Constant**, Catching up with Professor Slim, *SAFM*. 5 March 2022. https://youtu.be/dZ_5k5zvdYI.

36. **Xoli Mngambi**, Two years since SA recorded its first Covid-19 case, *Newzroom Afrika*. 7 March 2022. https://youtu.be/JT-v0NyB0To.

37. **Francis Heard**, Calls for face masks and other COVID restrictions to be dropped: Prof. Salim Abdool Karim, *SABC News*. 7 March 2022. https://youtu.be/UZlLGdj0VFc.

38. **Refilwe Moloto**, Expect 5th wave of Covid-19 by early May – Professor Salim Abdool

Karim, *Cape Talk*. 16 March 2022. https://www.capetalk.co.za/articles/441023/expect-5th-wave-of-covid-19-by-early-may-professor-salim-abdool-karim.

39. **O'Neil Nair**, A fifth wave of Covid-19 is anticipated to hit our shores within the next few weeks, *Lotus FM*. 29 March 2022. https://youtu.be/ydtWjmhUU_E.

40. **Ayanda Nyathi**, International Science Council calling on the UN to establish an advisory board for future pandemics, *Newzroom Afrika*. 18 May 2022. https://www.youtube.com/watch?v=VVHH5jQ9Guk.

41. **Stephen Grootes**, A discussion on the disease outlook for this winter, *SAFM*. 2 June 2022. https://www.youtube.com/watch?v=CDcuto_gh-g.

42. **Sally Burdett**, Japan honours Profs Salim and Quarraisha Abdool Karim for HIV and Covid-19 work, *eNCA*. 4 August 2022. https://youtu.be/GDONkaqBsNc.

43. **Discovery**, The distribution of vaccines: The great injustice, *CBC Radio Canada*. November 2022. https://ici.tou.tv/decouverte/S35E07.

44. **Sally Burdett**, World AIDS Day progress in HIV treatment, *eNCA*. 1 December 2022. https://www.youtube.com/watch?v=t3UFQWVDOOE.

45. **Stephen Grootes**, World AIDS Day, *SAFM*. 1 December 2022. https://youtu.be/7VWknhNlF_s.

46. **Minosh Pillay**, CAPRISA scientists research antibodies that are broadly able to neutralise HIV strains, *SABC News*. 1 December 2022. https://youtu.be/jtP3Z_hVhPs.

47. **Aldrin Sampear**, World Science Forum: CAB-LA is a new anti-HIV jab that eliminates one's chances of contracting HIV, *SAFM*. 6 December 2022. https://omny.fm/shows/beyond-the-headline/sahpra-has-registered-cab-la-a-new-anti-hiv- jab-wh?fbclid=IwAR2yqCQNDAuKje2oRCW7RQqP-ghS8uYVpIQt9t- FWOoZcX0inPNNm5FTgOsg.

48. **Henner Frankenfeld**, South Africa's pandemic hero, *DW*, 22 December 2022. https://www.dw.com/de/s%C3%BCdafrika-ein-held-der-coronapandemie/av-64187541.

Podcasts

1. **Rubin EJ, Baden LR, Abdool Karim SS, Morrissey S**. Audio interview: The Omicron variant of SARS-CoV-2. *New England Journal of Medicine*, 2 December 2021, 385: e96. doi: 10.1056/NEJMe2118839. https://www.nejm.org/doi/10.1056/NEJMe2118839.

2. **Rubin EJ, Baden LR, Abdool Karim SS, Morrissey S**. Audio Interview: Covid-19 in South Africa and a new SARS-CoV-2 variant. *New England Journal of Medicine*, 14 January 2021, 384(2): e14. Doi: 10.1056/NEJMe2100736. https://www.nejm.org/doi/10.1056/NEJMe2100736.

3. **Abdool Karim SS**. Variants and vaccines in South Africa, and comparing the 1918 flu pandemic. *The Lancet Voice*, 11 February 2021, Season 2 Episode 3. https://podcasts.google.com/feed/aHR0cHM6Ly9mZWVkcy5idXp6c3Byb3V0LmNvbS84NjE4NjgucnNz/episode/QnV6enNwcm91dC03ODA5MTgx.

4. **Abdool Karim SS**. Discovering the Omicron variant: The story from South Africa. *The Lancet Voice*, 30 November 2021, Season 2 Episode 25. https://

podcasts.apple.com/gb/podcast/discovering-the-omicron-variant-the-story-from/id1499803146?i=1000543499367.

5. **Gounder C**. South Africa's B.1.351 Variant – Immunity-Evading/ – Abdool Karim SS, Lessells R, Bhiman J, Greaney A. Season 1 Episode 62. https://www.justhumanproductions.org/podcasts/e62.

6. **Abdool Karim SS**. Africa CDC clinical trials for Covid-19 in Africa, 30 July 2021. https://soundcloud.com/user-474037739/building-clinical-trial-capacity-for-covid-19-and-other-vaccines?utm_source=clipboard&utm_medium=text&utm_campaign=social_sharing.

7. **Mia Malan**. Prof Abdool Karim: When will Covid end? *News24*, 5 March 2022. https://www.news24.com/life/wellness/body/condition-centres/infectious-diseases/coronavirus/podcast-prof-abdool-karim-when-will-covid-end-20220305-2.

8. **Claudia Hammond**. The Evidence: How pandemics end, *BBC*. 3 October 2022. https://player.fm/series/series-2685931/the-evidence-how-pandemics-end?fbclid=IwAR0bvwazibzu0a4HWAA3DMUIHzSGP-cdpUXRxP6UxbMysXUBYUnCTqX2s5o.

9. **Holly Sommers**. Science in times of crisis episode 2 – the current clash: Science and the national interest, International Science Council (ISC), 8 December 2022. https://council.science/current/podcasts/science-in-times-of-crisis-episode-2-the-current-clash-science-and-the-national-interest/?fbclid=IwAR0Ng_-4BL7USRadKKWu2P-LTDK3TH-VBLUKDzvJIdt8QGSIrnsTFTpbxVs0.

Notes

Part A: A new pandemic arrives: The first 100 days

Chapter 1 Alert!
1 ProMED
   https://promedmail.org/
2 A new coronavirus associated with human respiratory disease in China
   https://www.nature.com/articles/s41586-020-2008-3
3 Genome Detective Coronavirus Typing Tool for rapid identification and characterization
   of novel coronavirus genomes
   https://doi.org/10.1093/bioinformatics/btaa145

Chapter 2 The reality of the pandemic dawns
1 Characteristics of and important lessons from the coronavirus disease 2019 (COVID-19)
   outbreak in China
   https://jamanetwork.com/journals/jama/fullarticle/2762130
2 Clinical features of patients infected with 2019 novel coronavirus in Wuhan, China
   https://doi.org/10.1016/S0140-6736(20)30183-5
3 A novel coronavirus outbreak of global health concern
   https://doi.org/10.1016/S0140-6736(20)30185-9
4 WHO Director-General's opening remarks at the media briefing on COVID-19 –
   11 March 2020
   https://www.who.int/director-general/speeches/detail/who-director-general-s-
   openingremarks-at-the-media-briefing-on-covid-19---11-march-2020

Chapter 3 The pandemic response – science advice needed
1 Report of the WHO-China Joint Mission on Coronavirus Disease 2019 (COVID-19)
   https://www.who.int/docs/default-source/coronaviruse/who-china-joint-mission-on-
   covid-19-final-report.pdf

Chapter 4 Building while sailing
1 The South African response to the pandemic
   https://www.nejm.org/doi/10.1056/NEJMc2014960
2 South Africa is failing on Covid-19 because its leaders want to emulate the First World
   https://www.bizcommunity.com/Article/196/858/206326.html#

Chapter 5 More than an infection

1 We need a coronavirus vaccine – I just wish we could afford it
https://thehill.com/opinion/healthcare/488646-we-need-a-coronavirus-vaccine-ijust-wish-we-could-afford-it/

2 Report into a nosocomial outbreak of coronavirus disease 2019 (COVID⊠19) at Netcare St. Augustine's Hospital
https://www.krisp.org.za/manuscripts/StAugustinesHospitalOutbreakInvestigation_FinalReport_15may2020_comp.pdf

3 Report into a nosocomial outbreak of coronavirus disease 2019 (COVID⊠19) at Netcare St. Augustine's Hospital
https://www.krisp.org.za/manuscripts/StAugustinesHospitalOutbreakInvestigation_FinalReport_15may2020_comp.pdf

Chapter 6 Not just a disease – an upheaval

1 Ebola co-discoverer Peter Piot on how to respond to the coronavirus
https://www.ft.com/content/de0a7c9e-56ff-11ea-a528-dd0f971febbc

2 Obituary: Gita Ramjee (8 April 1956–31 March 2020)
https://www.tandfonline.com/doi/full/10.1080/0035919X.2020.1773106

Chapter 7 Making a plan

1 Dr Zweli Mkhize recommends the widespread use of cloth masks
https://sacoronavirus.co.za/2020/04/10/dr-zweli-mkhize-recommends-the-widespreaduse-of-cloth-masks/

2 Chapter 5 – John Snow, cholera, the Broad Street Pump; waterborne diseases then and now
https://doi.org/10.1016/B978-0-12-804571-8.00017-2

3 A cluster randomised trial of cloth masks compared with medical masks in healthcare workers
https://bmjopen.bmj.com/content/5/4/e006577

4 Respiratory virus shedding in exhaled breath and efficacy of face masks
https://doi.org/10.1038/s41591-020-0843-2

5 Mask wearing in community settings reduces SARS-CoV-2 transmission
https://doi.org/10.1073/pnas.2119266119

6 The South African response to the pandemic
https://www.nejm.org/doi/10.1056/NEJMc2014960

Chapter 8 'Next slide!'

1 Zweli Mkhize holds engagement on COVID-19 response
https://youtu.be/HLTQeMCtcfo

Chapter 9 Knowledge is power

1 From top scientist to science media star during COVID-19 – South Africa's Salim Abdool Karim
https://sajs.co.za/article/view/8450

2 Peter Bruce: Here's to the health of the nation – and the business it needs
https://www.businesslive.co.za/bd/opinion/columnists/2020-04-15-peter-bruce-heres-tothe-health-of-the-nation-and-the-business-it-needs/

Part B: From reluctant medical student to pandemic science adviser

Chapter 10 Formative early years in science
1 Hepatitis B virus in a culicine mosquito species in the RSA
https://pubmed.ncbi.nlm.nih.gov/3750129/
2 The prevalence and transmission of hepatitis B virus infection in urban, rural and institutionalized black children of Natal/KwaZulu, South Africa
https://doi.org/10.1093/ije/17.1.168

Chapter 11 Lessons from AIDS
1 Seroprevalence of HIV infection in rural South Africa
https://pubmed.ncbi.nlm.nih.gov/1492937/
2 Transmission networks and risk of HIV infection in KwaZulu-Natal, South Africa: A community-wide phylogenetic study
https://www.thelancet.com/journals/lanhiv/article/PIIS2352-3018(16)30186-2/fulltext
3 Get on the fast-track, the life-cycle approach to HIV
https://www.unaids.org/sites/default/files/media_asset/Get-on-the-Fast-Track_en.pdf
4 Phase 1 trial of nonoxynol-9 film among sex workers in South Africa
https://journals.lww.com/aidsonline/Fulltext/1999/08200/Phase_1_trial_of_nonoxynol_9_film_among_sex.11.aspx
5 HIV trial doomed by design, say critics
https://doi.org/10.1038/448110a

Chapter 12 From AIDS to Covid-19
1 These married scientists are leading the way on HIV
https://www.gatesnotes.com/Heroes-in-the-field-Drs-Quarraisha-and-Salim-Abdool-Karim
2 The Huanan Seafood Wholesale Market in Wuhan was the early epicenter of the COVID-19 pandemic
https://www.science.org/doi/10.1126/science.abp8715
3 The strongest evidence yet that an animal started the pandemic
https://www.theatlantic.com/science/archive/2023/03/covid-origins-research-raccoon-dogs-wuhan-market-lab-leak/673390/
4 WHO Emergencies Coronavirus Press Conference COVID19
https://www.who.int/docs/default-source/coronaviruse/transcripts/who-audio_emergencies_coronavirus_press_conference_covid19_origins_mission_30mar2021_(1)_clean.pdf?sfvrsn=8fa8d42e_1&download=true

Chapter 13 A perfect storm
1 78% of South Africans will sacrifice select human rights to fight Covid – survey
https://www.capetalk.co.za/articles/412206/78-of-south-africans-will-sacrifice-selecthuman-rights-to-fight-covid-survey
2 Pope Francis: A crisis reveals what is in our hearts
https://www.nytimes.com/2020/11/26/opinion/pope-francis-covid.html

Chapter 14 Covid-19 scientific contributions

1 South Africa sees Covid-19 fourth wave starting in early December
https://www.bloomberg.com/news/articles/2021-08-17/s-africa-sees-covid-19-fourthwave-starting-in-early-december

2 The South African response to the pandemic
https://www.nejm.org/doi/10.1056/NEJMc2014960

3 COVID-19 affects HIV and tuberculosis care
https://www.science.org/doi/10.1126/science.abd1072

4 New SARS-CoV-2 variants – clinical, public health, and vaccine implications
https://www.nejm.org/doi/full/10.1056/nejmc2100362

5 Future scenarios for the COVID-19 pandemic
https://www.thelancet.com/journals/lancet/article/PIIS0140-6736(21)00424-4/fulltext

6 SARS-CoV-2 variants and ending the COVID-19 pandemic
https://www.thelancet.com/journals/lancet/article/PIIS0140-6736(21)00370-6/fulltext

7 Vaccines and SARS-CoV-2 variants: The urgent need for a correlate of protection
https://www.thelancet.com/journals/lancet/article/PIIS0140-6736(21)00468-2/fulltext

8 Omicron extensively but incompletely escapes Pfizer BNT162b2 neutralization
https://www.nature.com/articles/s41586-021-04387-1

9 OmicronBA.4/BA.5 escape neutralizing immunity elicited by BA.1 infection
https://www.nature.com/articles/s41467-022-32396-9.pdf

10 Clinical severity of COVID-19 in patients admitted to hospital during the Omicron wave in South Africa: A retrospective observational study
https://doi.org/10.1016/S2214-109X(22)00114-0

11 Public understanding of science: Communicating in the midst of a pandemic
https://doi.org/10.1177/09636625221089391

12 Omicron SARS-CoV-2 variant: A new chapter in the COVID-19 pandemic
https://www.thelancet.com/journals/lancet/article/PIIS0140-6736(21)02758-6/fulltext

13 COVID-19 vaccine wastage in the midst of vaccine inequity: Causes, types and practical steps
http://dx.doi.org/10.1136/bmjgh-2022-009010

14 Efficacy and safety of ivermectin for treatment and prophylaxis of COVID-19 pandemic
https://doi.org/10.21203/rs.3.rs-100956/v3

15 Time to stop using ineffective Covid-19 drugs
https://www.nejm.org/doi/full/10.1056/NEJMe2209017

Chapter 15 Global pandemic collaboration

1 Maddox Prize 2020
https://senseaboutscience.org/activities/maddox-prize-2020/

2 Genomic characterisation and epidemiology of 2019 novel coronavirus: Implications for virus origins and receptor binding
https://doi.org/10.1016/S0140-6736(20)30251-8

Chapter 16 Science in the spotlight

1 EFF expresses delight at resignation of SA's top coronavirus advisor
https://www.georgeherald.com/News/Article/National/eff-expresses-delight-at-resignation-of-sa-s-top-coronavirus-advisor-202103250142

2 In the footsteps of Einstein, Sagan and Barnard: Identifying South Africa's most visible scientists
https://sajs.co.za/article/view/3873

Chapter 17 Building trust in science

1 In the footsteps of Einstein, Sagan and Barnard: Identifying South Africa's most visible scientists
https://sajs.co.za/article/view/3873
2 Professor Karim dismisses R944m Bill and Melinda Gates Foundation funding claims as fake news
https://izwi98fm.co.za/professor-karim-dismisses-r944m-bill-and-melinda-gates-foundation-funding-claims-as-fake-news/
3 Forbes Quotes: Thoughts on the business of life
https://www.forbes.com/quotes/1214/

Part C: Challenges at the advice-to-policy interface

Chapter 18 Leading the MAC – attaining sufficient consensus

1 The Convention for a Democratic South Africa – CODESA 1 and CODESA 2 (1991–1992)
https://www.concourttrust.org.za/uploads/files/Background_to_CODESA_1.pdf

Chapter 22 Alcohol and tobacco bans

1 Clinical characteristics of coronavirus disease 2019 in China
https://www.ncbi.nlm.nih.gov/pmc/articles/PMC7092819/
2 Lockdown sensation 'When People Zol' featuring Nkosazana Dlamini-Zuma will lift your mood
https://www.timeslive.co.za/news/south-africa/2020-05-07-watch--lockdown-sensation-when-people-zol-featuring-nkosazana-dlamini-zuma-will-lift-your-mood/

Chapter 23 Getting Covid-19 twice?

1 Coronavirus Disease 2019 (COVID-19) re-infection by a phylogenetically distinct Severe Acute Respiratory Syndrome Coronavirus 2 strain confirmed by whole genome sequencing
https://academic.oup.com/cid/advance-article/doi/10.1093/cid/ciaa1275/5897019
2 Genomic evidence for reinfection with SARS-CoV-2: A case study
https://www.thelancet.com/journals/laninf/article/PIIS1473-3099(20)30764-7/fulltext
3 COVID-19 re-infection is a reality in SA – Dr Yuvan Maharaj talks to us about how his patient tested positive for coronavirus twice in 5 months
https://www.facebook.com/watch/?v=204069474317659
4 South Korea's COVID-19 infection status: From the perspective of re-positive test results after viral clearance evidenced by negative test results
https://www.cambridge.org/core/journals/disaster-medicine-and-public-health-preparedness/article/south-koreas-covid19-infection-status-from-the-perspective-of-repositive-afterviral-clearance-by-negative-testing/9F852F03BCF6CA1D91D30AD32495051B

5   The untold story of Moderna's race for a COVID-19 vaccine
    https://www.bostonmagazine.com/health/2020/06/04/moderna-coronavirus-vaccine/

Chapter 24   A new variant – Beta on the rise

1   New SARS-CoV-2 variants – clinical, public health, and vaccine implications
    https://www.nejm.org/doi/full/10.1056/nejmc2100362
2   Persistence and evolution of SARS-CoV-2 in an immunocompromised host
    https://www.nejm.org/doi/full/10.1056/NEJMc2031364
3   N501Y and K417N mutations in the spike protein of SARS-CoV-2 alter the interactions
    with both hACE2 and human-derived antibody: A free energy of perturbation
    retrospective study
    https://pubs.acs.org/doi/10.1021/acs.jcim.1c01242
4   Deep mutational scanning of SARS-CoV-2 receptor binding domain reveals constraints
    on folding and ACE2 binding
    https://www.cell.com/cell/fulltext/S0092-8674(20)31003-5
5   New SARS-CoV-2 variants – clinical, public health, and vaccine implications
    https://www.nejm.org/doi/full/10.1056/nejmc2100362
6   Appropriate names for COVID-19 variants
    https://science.sciencemag.org/content/371/6535/1215/tab-article-info

Chapter 25   Vaccine rollout fallout

1   Vaccine diplomacy boosts Russia's and China's global standing
    https://www.economist.com/graphic-detail/2021/04/29/vaccine-diplomacy-
    boostsrussias-and-chinas-global-standing
2   With acknowledgements to Dr Tedros Adhanom Ghebreyesus, who I think used this
    term first.
3   Salim Abdool Karim: 'None of us are safe from Covid if one of us is not. We have
    mutual interdependence'
    https://www.theguardian.com/world/2021/jan/10/salim-abdool-karim-none-of-us-
    aresafe-from-covid-if-one-of-us-is-not-we-have-mutual-interdependence
4   Vaccines for South Africa. Now
    https://www.dailymaverick.co.za/article/2021-01-02-vaccines-for-south-africa-now/
5   Silver bullet
    https://en.wikipedia.org/wiki/Silver_bullet
6   Institutional and behaviour-change interventions to support COVID-19 public health
    measures: A review by the Lancet Commission Task Force on public health measures to
    suppress the pandemic
    https://academic.oup.com/inthealth/article/13/5/399/6273788

Chapter 26   Variants versus vaccines

1   Minister Zweli Mkhize gives an important update on Covid-19 vaccines
    https://www.youtube.com/watch?v=LUHlxFt34ZI
2   Dial down the rhetoric over COVID-19 vaccines
    https://journals.co.za/doi/10.7196/SAMJ.2021.v111i6.15740
3   Vaccines and SARS-CoV-2 variants: The urgent need for a correlate of protection
    https://www.thelancet.com/journals/lancet/article/PIIS0140-6736(21)00468-2/fulltext

4 The Lancet Covid-19 Commission Task Force on Public Health Measures to Suppress the Pandemic, SARS-CoV-2 variants: The need for urgent public health action beyond vaccines https://static1.squarespace.com/static/5ef3652ab722df11fcb2ba5d/t/60a3d54f8b42b505 d0d0de4f/1621349714141/NPIs+TF+Policy+Brief+March+2021.pdf

5 New SARS-CoV-2 Variants – clinical, public health, and vaccine implications https://www.nejm.org/doi/full/10.1056/nejmc2100362

6 Coronavirus (COVID-19) vaccinations https://ourworldindata.org/covid-vaccinations?country=USA

7 U.S. ranks 43rd worldwide in sequencing to check for coronavirus variants like the one found in the U.K. https://www.washingtonpost.com/world/2020/12/23/us-leads-world-coronavirus-cases-ranks-43rd-sequencing-check-variants/

8 With most adults vaccinated and case numbers low, Israel removes many restrictions https://www.nytimes.com/2021/06/01/world/middleeast/israel-covid-restrictions.html

9 Coronavirus (COVID-19) vaccinations https://ourworldindata.org/covid-vaccinations

10 WHO calls for moratorium on booster vaccine shots through September, citing global disparity https://www.washingtonpost.com/nation/2021/08/04/coronavirus-covid-live-updates-us/

11 Covax misses its 2021 delivery target – what's gone wrong in the fight against vaccine nationalism? https://theconversation.com/covax-misses-its-2021-delivery-target-whats-gone-wrong-inthe-fight-against-vaccine-nationalism-167753

Chapter 27 Another new variant – Omicron

1 Fact check: Did South African epidemiologist accurately predict nation's COVID surge? https://www.newsweek.com/fact-check-did-south-african-epidemiologist-accuratelypredict-nations-covid-surge-1655486

2 South Africa sees Covid-19 fourth wave starting in early December https://www.bloomberg.com/news/articles/2021-08-17/s-africa-sees-covid-19-fourthwave-starting-in-early-december

3 How the Omicron strain in SA was traced by a missing gene https://www.timeslive.co.za/news/world/2021-11-30-how-the-omicron-strain-in-sa-wastraced-by-a-missing-gene/

4 Pan-sarbecovirus neutralizing antibodies in BNT162b2-immunized SARS-CoV-1 survivors https://www.nejm.org/doi/full/10.1056/NEJMoa2108453

Chapter 28 Miracle treatments

1 Hydroxychloroquine and azithromycin as a treatment of COVID-19: Results of an open-label non-randomized clinical trial https://doi.org/10.1016/j.ijantimicag.2020.105949

2 Official statement from International Society of Antimicrobial Chemotherapy (ISAC) https://www.isac.world/news-and-publications/official-isac-statement

3 Note: the equivalent regulatory body to the FDA in South Africa is the South African Health Products Regulatory Authority (SAHPRA)

4 FDA issues emergency use authorization for convalescent plasma as potential promising COVID–19 treatment, another achievement in administration's fight against pandemic
https://www.fda.gov/news-events/press-announcements/fda-issues-emergency-useauthorization-convalescent-plasma-potential-promising-covid-19-treatment

5 The Covid-19 plasma boom is over. What did we learn from it?
https://www.nytimes.com/2021/04/17/health/covid-convalescent-plasma.html?smtyp=cur&smid=fb-nytimes&fbclid=IwAR07XAuR-hNm7JQYnjpTHnDmFz7qTkie5cmrssYQlZOdC6_HkNJrMHy7bNw

6 The coronavirus 'vaccine' Ekurhuleni wants to import doesn't exist
https://www.news24.com/news24/the-coronavirus-vaccine-ekurhuleni-wants-to-import-doesnt-exist-20200327

7 Pharmacologist investigated for alleged bogus anti-Covid-19 treatment
https://www.iol.co.za/sunday-tribune/news/pharmacologist-investigated-forallegedbogus-anti-covid-19-treatment-c1830deb-9a6f-413a-9d3a-6d8d7d739081

8 Pharmacologist investigated for alleged bogus anti-Covid-19 treatment
https://www.iol.co.za/sunday-tribune/news/pharmacologist-investigated-for-allegedbogus-anti-covid-19-treatment-c1830deb-9a6f-413a-9d3a-6d8d7d739081

9 Apology
https://www.scribd.com/article/496025605/Apology

10 Systematic review and meta-analysis of ivermectin for treatment of COVID-19: Evidence beyond the hype
https://bmcinfectdis.biomedcentral.com/counter/pdf/10.1186/s12879-022-07589-8.pdf

Chapter 29 The disinformation bandwagon

1 Coronavirus misinformation: Quantifying sources and themes in the COVID-19 'infodemic'
https://int.nyt.com/data/documenttools/evanega-et-al-coronavirus-misinformationsubmitted-07-23-20-1/080839ac0c22bca8/full.pdf

2 SA researchers say lockdown 'nearly 30 times more deadly' than disease
https://www.thesouthafrican.com/news/is-lockdown-working-south-africadeadly-disease/

3 Pandemics data and analytics vs Daily Maverick
https://presscouncil.org.za/Ruling/View/pandemics-data-and-analytics-vsdaily-maverick-4548

4 Kung-Flu Panda: Dodgy analytics or pandemic propaganda?
https://www.dailymaverick.co.za/article/2021-02-28-kung-flu-panda-dodgy-analyticsor-pandemic-propaganda/

5 COVID-19 vaccine hesitancy in South Africa: How can we maximize uptake of COVID-19 vaccines?
https://doi.org/10.1080/14760584.2021.1949291

Chapter 30 The Good, the Bad and the Complicated

1 Conspiracy theorists burn 5G towers claiming link to virus
https://apnews.com/article/health-ap-top-news-wireless-technology-international-news-virus-outbreak-4ac3679b6f39e8bd2561c1c8eeafd855

2 KZN cellphone towers torched as 5G conspiracy theories ignite
https://www.dailymaverick.co.za/article/2021-01-08-kzn-cellphone-towers-torched-as-5g-conspiracy-theories-ignite/

3 Are South Africans becoming immune to COVID-19?
   https://ewn.co.za/2020/09/14/
   south-africans-covid-19-immunity-caused-by-exposure-to-previous-coronaviruses
4 Brazilian Amazon city of Manaus may have reached Covid-19 'herd immunity', study says
   https://www.france24.com/en/20200924-brazilian-amazon-city-of-manaus-may-
   havereached-covid-19-herd-immunity-study-says
5 Delhi approaches herd immunity, vaccine shortages, China deploys anal swab tests:
   COVID-19 global update
   https://www.medscape.co.uk/viewarticle/delhi-approaches-herd-immunity-vaccine-
   shortages-china- 2021a1001qy1
6 Resurgence of COVID-19 in Manaus, Brazil, despite high seroprevalence
   https://www.thelancet.com/journals/lancet/article/PIIS0140-6736(21)00183-5/fulltext
7 One virus, two countries: How the misuse of science compounded South Africa's
   COVID crisis
   https://theconversation.com/one-virus-two-countries-how-the-misuse-of-
   sciencecompounded-south-africas-covid-crisis-173079
8 https://www.caprisa.org/Covid-19-Weekly-Updates/

Part D: Lessons for the future

Chapter 31 Contemplating the paths forward

1 Oral nirmatrelvir for high-risk, nonhospitalized adults with Covid-19
   https://www.nejm.org/doi/full/10.1056/nejmoa2118542
2 Paxlovid significantly reduces COVID-19 hospitalizations and deaths
   https://www.epicresearch.org/articles/paxlovid-significantly-reduces-covid-19-
   hospitalizations-and-deaths
3 Pfizer and the Medicines Patent Pool (MPP) sign licensing agreement for COVID-19
   oral antiviral treatment candidate to expand access in low- and middle-income countries
   https://www.pfizer.com/news/press-release/press-release-detail/pfizer-and-
   medicinespatent-pool-mpp-sign-licensing

Chapter 32 Learning from the past to prepare better for the next pandemic

1 As head of the Anti-MERS MERS Headquarters, I will address even the smallest
   problems
   http://english.seoul.go.kr/will-take-care-even-small-details-head-anti-mers-
   mersheadquarters/?cat=928
2 S Korea cuts interest rates to record low amid Mers concerns
   https://www.bbc.com/news/business-33089930
3 During MERS, Park's approval rating plummeted … Corona 19 Yen Wen's approval
   rating rather rises
   https://www.hankyung.com/politics/article/2020030620737
4 South Korea's implementation of a COVID-19 national testing strategy
   https://www.healthaffairs.org/do/10.1377/hblog20210521.255232/full
5 There's still time to beat Covid without lockdowns
   https://www.bloomberg.com/features/2020-south-korea-covid-strategy/
6 Trump's faulty testing claims
   https://www.factcheck.org/2020/03/trumps-faulty-testing-claims/

7 Air, surface environmental, and personal protective equipment contamination by Severe Acute Respiratory Syndrome Coronavirus 2 (SARS-CoV-2) from a symptomatic patient
https://jamanetwork.com/journals/jama/fullarticle/2762692
8 Ranking the effectiveness of worldwide COVID-19 government interventions
https://www.nature.com/articles/s41562-020-01009-0

Chapter 33 Science – the universal language of fellowship
1 COVID-19: Collaboration is the engine of global science – especially for developing countries
https://www.weforum.org/agenda/2020/05/global-science-collaboration-opensource-covid-19/
2 WHO Director-General's remarks at the press conference with President of the European Council to discuss the proposal for an international pandemic treaty
https://www.who.int/director-general/speeches/detail/who-director-general-s-remarks-atthe-press-conference-with-president-of-the-european-council-to-discuss-the-proposal-foran-international-pandemic-treaty

Index